Power Yoga Warrior Stren

Power Yoga is moving, breathing, flowing gets your heart pumping and your muscles m series is a great way to start or end your day with c_____ and strength.

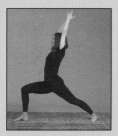

- **Spear thrower.** In spear thrower, imagine lining up your target with your forward hand and foot, then reaching back with your back hand to throw the spear.

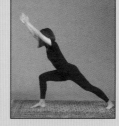

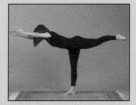

- **Swordsman.** In swordsman, the entire body faces the lunging leg with both arms raised overhead as if grasping a sword in readiness for battle.

- **Extended warrior.** For extended warrior, move into swordsman with hands apart, then angle the body over the front leg to create a straight line from the back heel up through the fingertips.

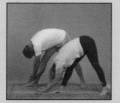

- **Bent knee forward bend in warrior.** Bent knee forward bend is the counterpose to extended warrior, bringing the body down rather than up. The arms can be held behind the back, with hands on hips, or extended over the head toward the floor.

- **T-balance.** In T-balance, the body forms the shape of the letter "T." This challenging balance pose is the culmination of the warrior series.

alpha
books

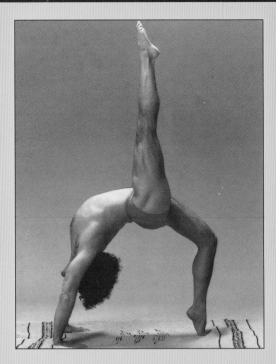

Geo's Thirteen Steps
for More Natural Living

1. Recognize how you can improve your life.
2. Live simply.
3. Follow the yoga abstentions: not harming others, not lying, not stealing, not lusting, and not being greedy.
4. Follow the yoga observances: be pure, be content, be disciplined, be studious, and be devoted.
5. Move your body.
6. Learn to breathe correctly.
7. Observe yourself.
8. Practice concentration and meditation.
9. Know that we are all one.
10. Eat well.
11. Get up with the sunrise each morning.
12. Go to bed by 10:00 P.M. each night.
13. Cultivate a positive attitude.

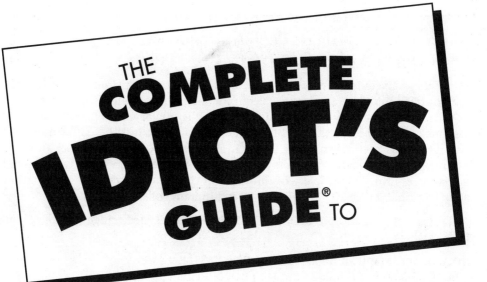

Power Yoga

by Geo Takoma and Eve Adamson

alpha books

Macmillan USA, Inc.
201 West 103rd Street
Indianapolis, IN 46290

A Pearson Education Company

International Standard Book Number: 0-02-863188-9
Library of Congress Catalog Card Number: 99-65048

01   00   99   8   7   6   5   4   3   2   1

Interpretation of the printing code: the rightmost number of the first series of numbers is the year of the book's printing; the rightmost number of the second series of numbers is the number of the book's printing. For example, a printing code of 99-1 shows that the first printing occurred in 1999.

Printed in the United States of America

Note: This publication contains information based on the research and experience of its authors and is designed to provide useful advice with regard to the subject matter covered. The authors and publisher are not engaged in rendering medical or other professional services in this publication. Circumstances vary for practitioners of the activities covered herein, and this publication should not be used without prior consultation from a competent medical professional.

The authors, book producer, and publisher expressly disclaim any responsibility for any liability, loss, injury, or risk, personal or otherwise, which is incurred as a consequence, directly or indirectly, of the use and application of any of the contents of this book.

Alpha Development Team

Publisher
Kathy Nebenhaus

Editorial Director
Gary M. Krebs

Managing Editor
Bob Shuman

Marketing Brand Manager
Felice Primeau

Acquisitions Editors
Jessica Faust
Michelle Reed

Development Editors
Phil Kitchel
Amy Zavatto

Assistant Editor
Georgette Blau

Production Team

Book Producer
Lee Ann Chearney/Amaranth

Development Editor
Lynn Northrup

Production Editor
Christy Wagner

Copy Editor
Abby Lyon Herriman

Cover Designer
Mike Freeland

Illustrator
Wendy Frost

Cartoonist
Jody P. Schaeffer

Photographer
Richard Chang

Photographer's Models
Katresha Moskios, Catherine Grace,
Barbra Kawamura, Kristin Hickson,
Sharon Larimer, Trisha Hoyt Purpura,
Nicole Gruver, William Tappé

Book Designers
Scott Cook and Amy Adams of DesignLab

Indexer
Riofrancos and Company Indexes

Layout/Proofreading
Darin Crone, John Etchison

Contents at a Glance

Contents

Appendixes

Foreword

When I first met Geo Takoma in 1996, I was visiting the Ashram in California, where he is a group leader and a Power Yoga instructor. I thought he was one of the most amazing people I had ever laid eyes on.

During the first of my many rigorous hikes at the Ashram, my group approached the peak of a very steep and seemingly treacherous mountain. I suddenly encountered what I thought was a vision sent from above. As I neared this image, I saw a man with crazy, curly hair and a gleaming smile bursting with vitality. Though I felt as if I were going to drop from exhaustion, I still found the strength to grab a small portion of a protein bar from this strange apparition that appeared before me. All at once he spoke: "Here honey, take this—you'll make it, don't worry." Then he smiled and said, "I'm Geo." I was awed at the energy that exuded from this man. Though it may not seem like much now, Geo's small donation and words of encouragement were more than enough to help me make it through to the end of the hike.

As the week went on, Geo instructed my group in Power Yoga in the mornings before our hikes and again in the evenings. Trust me when I say Power Yoga was an absolute necessity to get us through the rest of the day's activities. Not only did I learn how to successfully use Power Yoga and integrate it into my life, I also discovered a new friend in the man I found on the mountain.

Before I met Geo, I had heard of Power Yoga, but never really understood the meaning of the words until I tried the workout. Once I felt comfortable with the program, I discovered that Power Yoga enabled me to discover a whole new physical existence that I wasn't capable of before. I found that my body was more relaxed and flexible and that I was able to deal with daily stress more easily. Another benefit of Power Yoga is what it did for my appearance. My muscles became more toned and resilient, and my energy level increased as I continued the training. Lastly, I found that Power Yoga ignited the light inside me; it sparked a spiritual glow that others soon recognized too.

Geo's methods are simple. He explains things thoroughly and in easy terms so that anyone—even those who have no experience—can follow instruction almost effortlessly. He is able to make Power Yoga fun, invigorating, relaxing, and effective all at once. I know from my workouts with Geo that his kind words of encouragement have enabled me to push myself to reach higher levels of Power Yoga.

When I heard Geo was doing a book, I wondered if his incredible energy and presence would translate to the page. I wasn't disappointed. This book is fantastic. It takes you through the entire scope of a comprehensive Power Yoga routine, with room to adjust, shorten, lengthen, and challenge yourself in whatever way you need. The pictures make each movement easy to follow, and best of all: Geo's voice, spirit, and passion come through on every page. This is a workout to challenge the most fit, but even a beginner can feel at home with this book.

I hope you enjoy *The Complete Idiot's Guide to Power Yoga* as much as I did. I loved it! It is certainly worth your time and every penny. Geo is my spiritual mentor and a friend that I hold close to my heart. He has helped me to empower myself by using Power Yoga, and he can do the same for you.

I love you, Geo-daddy-o!

Supermodel Amber Valletta

Supermodel Amber Valletta began her modeling career at age 15 when she enrolled in modeling school. After a stint in Milan and her high school graduation, she moved to Paris and graced the covers of the top magazines in the business—*Vogue, Harper's Bazaar, Elle, Allure, W Magazine,* and *Glamour.*

Ms. Valletta has worked with some of the most prestigious companies, photographers, and designers in the world. She has appeared in major advertising campaigns for Versace, Prada, and Chanel, among others. Her international fashion house runway appearances include: Prada, Armani, Versace, Calvin Klein, Chanel, Helmut Lang, Donna Karan, Dior, and Givenchy. She has garnered international fame as the exclusive image for Elizabeth Arden in skincare, makeup, and fragrance.

In addition to being an accomplished model, she is also known as a champion of causes, including Dishes, the Covenant House, St. Jude Children's Hospital, The World Wildlife Federation, Habitat for Humanity, the Special Olympics, the Nina Hyde Foundation, the Tibetan Children's Village Charity, and Nelson Mandela's Children Fund. Ms. Valletta lives in New York City.

Introduction

These days, the news about yoga is everywhere. Celebrities, medical professionals, even your friends and neighbors are raving about the benefits of yoga. But you aren't sure. You have a busy, hectic life, and frankly, you like it that way. You thrive on the move, and although you occasionally wish for a few moments of peace, you think sitting in the lotus position for an hour sounds like a big bore.

Guess what? This isn't the yoga you thought you knew. This yoga moves, breathes, bends, arches, swings, sways, flows, and dances. This yoga speaks to you in a language you understand. In a world that moves as fast as this one does, where information is transmitted from continent to continent in a few seconds, where people eat on the run, work on the run, and then go running, few people feel they have the time to spend in a class that forces them to be still. We don't remember how to be still!

Power Yoga allows us to move, work our muscles, and really get somewhere. Power Yoga builds strength and endurance fast, giving you the results you want quickly, but it also works another kind of magic on the hurried, frayed, overworked bodies and minds of those who practice it. Gradually, subtly, it teaches you how to slow down when you need to slow down. It gives you control over the body you thought had taken the reins of your life. It calms, clears, and brightens the mind so that you can work smart and live in a healthy way. It clarifies.

Welcome to the new yoga, the yoga for the twenty-first century: Power Yoga. You'll be glad you found us.

How to Use This Book

The Complete Idiot's Guide to Power Yoga is divided into six parts that introduce you to Power Yoga and then gradually build your strength, flexibility, and confidence until you are doing movements and positions you never thought possible. Each part of this book has a different purpose, and each part is important to the development of your Power Yoga practice. This book is designed to be read in order, but once you've got the basics, you can skip around to find your favorite routines and make them your own.

Part 1, "Feel the Power," introduces you to Geo and the story of how Power Yoga evolved in his life. In it, you'll learn how movement is natural to the human body, and how the movements of Power Yoga, in particular, are innate to each of us. Power Yoga is particularly suited to the impossibly busy and spiritually hungry character of the world in the twenty-first century. Learn how your own fitness level fits into a Power Yoga plan, whether your attitude is holding you back or not, how to start slow and gain strength fast, and all about the life force energy that is in you and around you.

Part 2, "First Moves: Developmental Poses for Building Strength," shows you how to begin building strength through basic routines of standing poses, bends, warrior poses, tilts, twists, arches, and a prowling tiger series that will help you get in touch with your primal nature. You'll also learn where your seven chakras are located, the color of each chakra, and how to test your own chakras for blockages. Finally, learn how to heal your chakras with color.

Part 3, "Stand Up and Take a Bow," takes standing poses one step further. Salute to the light within is a series based on the traditional yoga sun salutation, but re-designed to match any fitness level. Warrior series taps into your courageous side, honing your confidence as well as the muscles in your legs, arms, and torso. Next, you'll learn some power balances, incredible strengtheners for the entire body and excellent for developing focus and concentration. Angle and triangle poses stretch the sides of your body and help to release and stimulate your internal organs and glands.

Part 4, "Your Animal Nature," introduces you to several routines based on poses that imitate the forms and movements of our fellow creatures in the animal kingdom. From monkeys and pigeons to dogs and alligators, learn how to gain incredible strength and endurance by getting down on all fours. You'll also learn Geo's 13 steps for natural living. Suggestions such as simple living, a positive attitude, eating well, meditating, and going to bed early will help you regain your natural rhythm.

Part 5, "Get Down," brings you to the floor with powerful sitting, stomach-strengthening, side-stretching, and back-building exercises. You'll also find yourself in some incredibly powerful inverted positions: shoulderstands, headstands, and when you are strong enough, the truly impressive feathered peacock, scorpion, and dolphin poses.

Part 6, "Winding Down," begins the process of a well-deserved rest. First, learn to take in more energy and nourish the body by breathing correctly. Most people don't breathe the way their bodies were designed to, but a few adjustments in your technique may be all you require to reap the full benefits of the breath. Learn breathing techniques that rejuvenate the body or calm the mind after just a few minutes. Then, come down into relaxation poses. Last of all, learn to meditate, the final payoff of Power Yoga.

After you've mastered the routines in this book, Appendix A will offer you some "Alternate Power Plays" to vary your routine. In Appendix B, you'll get a comprehensive glossary of all the Power Yoga terms used in this book. In Appendix C, you'll find out more about how to study with Geo in person.

Power Parcels

Throughout this book, you'll see four types of extra information in boxes, to further enlighten you to the power possibilities.

Power Words

These boxes define the terms we use in this book that may not be familiar to you. Whether anatomical or physiological, Sanskrit words, or names for new concepts, these boxes will explain their meanings.

The Right Moves

Not sure you're doing a move right? Looking for some special tips, tricks, and guidance? You'll find that information in these boxes.

The Wrong Moves

Avoid injury and get the most out of each exercise by checking out these boxes, which will warn you, let you know what to watch out for, positions to avoid, and the best ways to solve your power problems.

Geo's Journey

Extend your knowledge with extra information and personal anecdotes from Geo's life experience.

Acknowledgments

Thanks to everyone who made this book possible. To my friend Lloyd Short, who opened the door; to Gary Krebs, for calling me through the door; to Lee Ann Chearney at Amaranth and all the people at Alpha Books. Special thanks to Eve for all her input and work, and to Wendy Frost for her illustrations. Thanks to all my teachers: Indra Devi, Swami Vishnudevananda, and the Venerable Vera Dharmawara. To my mother, my first teacher, and my dad, for my strength. Special thanks to my wife, Katresha, the goddess in my life. She has always believed in me. To my students, who unknowingly taught me more than I taught them; to Richard Chang, the best photographer I've ever seen, and his wife Barbara for her help; to all my beautiful models: Bill, Barbra, Sharon, Katresha, Nicole, Kristin, Trish, and Catherine. To Ann Marie Benstrom for paying me to hike and teach yoga at the Ashram; to Catarina Headburg for giving me time off to work on this book; to Vince McCullough for his friendship, and to Jean Cotner, who first guided me into yoga and built my foundation. Love and light to you all!

—Geo

Special thanks to my mother, who kept the kids at bay; to my father, whose loyal practice of his own form of Power Yoga is an inspiration; to my baby, Emmett, who demonstrates to me each day how innate Power Yoga really is to the human form; to my three-year-old, Angus, whose enthusiasm for yoga is unbridled and who can do a lovely wheel pose; to Lee Ann, who made my wonderful career possible and who always bestows verbal applause when I need it most; to Kathy, for leading me to Lee Ann; to Joan, for all she has taught me about yoga; to Katresha, for launching Geo, unawares, into the information age; and to Geo, whose inner light illuminates every page of this book.

—Eve

Trademarks

All terms mentioned in this book that are known to be or are suspected of being trademarks or service marks have been appropriately capitalized. Alpha Books and Macmillan USA, Inc. cannot attest to the accuracy of this information. Use of a term in this book should not be regarded as affecting the validity of any trademark or service mark.

Part 1

Feel the Power

What is Power Yoga, and how is it different from every other type of yoga you've seen, read about, or tried? Power Yoga is a unique, dynamic system of movement based on the body's innate movements. It is uniquely suited for the twenty-first century because it starts big, it moves fast, it offers a challenge, and it eases you, almost imperceptibly, toward more serene control of your inner and outer being.

In this section, I'll take you through the personal journey that helped result in the development of this system of Power Yoga. I'll help you assess your own fitness level, I'll give you a basic lesson in anatomy and physiology, so you know what body parts are working and how, and I'll tell you all about life-force energy—how it powers you, drives you and fills you with vitality, and how you can get more of it into your body every day.

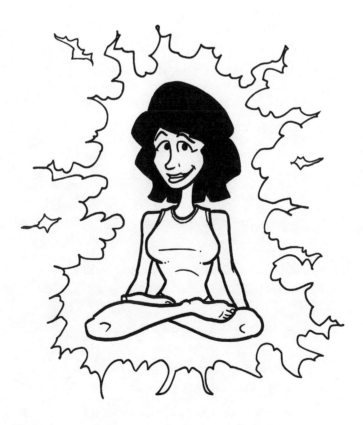

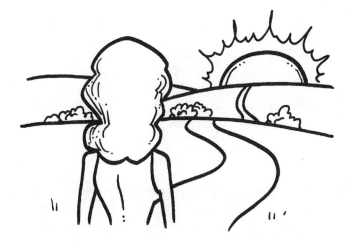

Chapter 1

The Journey Begins

> **In This Chapter**
>
> ➤ Power Yoga is a journey
>
> ➤ Movement is natural
>
> ➤ The power of yoga can be your power
>
> ➤ Geo shares his journey to Power Yoga with you

Yoga is a journey into the magical side of the self. Because every self is different—because I am different from you—my journey will not be the same as yours. Yet, our journeys might take parallel paths, and that is my hope for this book. My journey can become a roadmap for your journey, and then your journey can grow and evolve into what is necessary for you.

The Evolution to Power Yoga

Yoga is also a journey into the magical side of a culture. It is not just "something from India," although it has meant, and continues to mean, much to that culture. It has also become a part of Western culture, through its unique evolution in the West. Yoga is evolving differently here than it has evolved in the East, which is appropriate given its nature. Yoga is flexible, changeable, adapting to different individuals, situations, and societies in unique ways.

Power Words

Yoga is from the Sanskrit word *yuj,* meaning "to yoke." Yoga is just that—a yoking of the different sides and forces of the self, through various techniques. Most yoga practiced today in the West, including Power Yoga, is based on a type of yoga called Hatha Yoga. The root *ha* means "solar" and the root *tha* means "lunar." Hatha Yoga, then, is the balancing or yoking together of the solar and lunar aspects of the self. All forms of movement yoga are based on Hatha Yoga.

Power Words

Power Yoga is a moving, flowing form of yoga that is almost dance-like in its grace. In Power Yoga, we tie traditional (and nontraditional) yoga poses together to affect many different aspects of the body with an entire routine. Traditional Hatha Yoga tended more to work specific areas and hold poses to strengthen certain areas. Power Yoga strings these together to bring out the natural, innate power of movement in the human body.

Yoga has become a mirror for the spiritual consciousness of the culture in which it grows and changes. And right now, here, in the West, yoga is changing, growing, and evolving into something that is indeed magical in the way it changes the body and the mind, refining and smoothing, adding grace and power, strength and vitality. Many like to call this evolving form Power Yoga.

The term *Power Yoga* means different things to different people. Many equate the term with Astanga Yoga, a form of yoga based on an ancient eight-limbed system of yoga and more recently advanced by Pattabhi Jois and popularized by such fitness gurus as Beryl Bender Birch. For some, it means a form of aerobics using yoga poses, and for others it means very difficult yoga poses. I can only relate what it has come to mean to me and to those I have taught. But before I launch into your introduction to Power Yoga techniques, I'd like to introduce myself and give you insight into my own evolution as a practitioner and Power Yoga teacher.

Power Yoga is not something I concocted to give my yoga classes a gimmick. Neither is it something I learned from someone else and am now repeating to you. Instead, it has come about through a long, slow process of personal physical and spiritual experimentation.

Power Yoga is an outgrowth of my tendency to push the limits. When what I am doing, physically, isn't enough to germinate the seeds of spiritual growth—because the body and the spirit are inextricable and what grows or shrinks one will grow or shrink the other—then I will push and test and explore until I find my way to the next level. In other words, if my body isn't working, my spirit isn't working. By pushing my physical limits, I push my spiritual limits as well, and that's good for the whole self.

My guess is that you are something like me when it comes to testing limits and pushing yourself. Many of us living in this fast-paced culture spend much of our time testing our limits—of strength, endurance, and ability to hold up under pressure. Are you going, going, going, all the time? If you are, the idea of a yoga class may seem tedious, too slow, requiring too much patience, flexibility, and inner quiet. You want to move, get things done, accomplish, achieve, and then get on with the next item on your to-do list. I hear you! And believe me, Power Yoga is for you. It helps you test your limits in a context you can relate to. It is the continuing exploration and evolution of you.

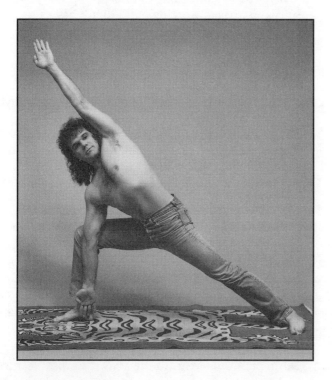

Geo moves into extended angle pose.

My First Steps

I first took a yoga class in the 1970s (like so many others!), but that was not the beginning of my yoga evolution. I feel that I began yoga the moment I was born. Every movement of the infant is an attempt to grow, explore, and evolve, which is the essence of yoga.

I was instinctively meditating at four years old, and as a very young child, I remember having the first experience of leaving my body and going into an owl. I remember looking back at my body and seeing it below. That was a part of my evolution.

When I was seven years old and living in Portland, Maine, I woke up one morning and I heard a strange noise that seemed to surround me. At the time, I didn't know what the sound was; it was indescribable. Yet, even to my young mind, it was clear that everything in the universe was coming together in that one tone. I didn't know

Power Words

Om is a Sanskrit word that yoga practitioners have used for centuries to describe the resonating sound of the universe. Saying "Om" on the exhalation while you're doing Power Yoga can help you focus on your breathing and get in tune with the universe.

until 15 years later that this sound has a name, *Om*. I don't know why I was, for those few moments, able to actually hear the tone. All I know is that I heard it and internalized it, and so it became a part of me.

When I was 10, I became interested in physical pursuits and I began working out. I didn't have a set plan or lessons or a sport, I just started working, making movements that felt natural, exploring the range of motion and the internal prompts that urged my body to move.

At 15, I became interested in athletics and began playing football. In college, I was a gymnast. In between, I joined the Marine Corps, and that experience also had a profound effect on how my physical body learned to move in response to, and sometimes despite, my spiritual body.

Semper Fidelis: *Always Faithful*

In some ways, being a Marine echoed my childhood play. I remember, growing up with my brothers and friends, that we loved to play warrior games. We would shoot bows and arrows, throw spears and lances, and have mock sword fights and fencing matches. We loved to fight. It wasn't fighting out of animosity or violence, of course. It was pure, joyful, natural play, yet it spilled out of us in the form of combat. And in the midst of our combat, I remember having a sense of and understanding that life was perfect, and that everything is a part of it.

The Wrong Moves

Stillness can teach us about balance and strength. But we get restless when we sit, stand, or sleep in one position for too long. Don't try to hold a yoga pose so long that you lose concentration, or your balance! Keep moving. Make it a smooth, graceful dance.

During my three years in the Marine Corps, I learned much about what the body can do well, and what it is not meant to do. I learned about the forms of combat, and much about personal discipline. We were often made to stand at attention. Attention means to stand up perfectly straight and perfectly still. It's a lot like what people call the mountain pose in yoga today.

I remember one Marine drill sergeant telling me one day that you can't make a platoon of men and women stand at attention for very long. So, when they really wanted to make us suffer, they had us stand at attention for a long period of time. Pretty soon, people would start falling over.

Later, I realized that when a body tries to stand perfectly still, straight, and at attention with all the muscles straight, strong, and tight, at some point, no matter how hard the body tries to stay motionless, it will begin to move into a kind of spiral. The bodies of these Marines would start spiraling from the feet up. The spiral would be small at the feet and get bigger and wider as it went up the body, and sooner or later, the body would spiral to the point of falling down!

You see, bodies are never still—it's impossible. The only still body is a dead body. As long as breath lives in the body, it affects the natural flows and motions of the body, moving it in a natural way, massaging and stretching and toning and traveling through the body. The very process of breathing necessitates movement. We are never still, and that is an important component of Power Yoga. But more about that later.

Another thing I learned from the Marine Corps is how natural and innate it is to move like a warrior. At some point, when we grow up and no longer play at fighting, and when there are no wars to fight or countries to defend (or we have chosen not to actually engage in violence), all that remains is the beautiful, flowing motions of the warrior. These movements needn't have anything to do with violence. They are movements of the spirit, engaging the body in life.

In Chapter 12, "The Warrior Within," when I introduce you to the Power Yoga series of movements called the warrior series, you may find yourself very attracted to these motions, but you aren't a violent person! Of course not. In fact, yoga advocates nonviolence. The warrior movements are more a matter of empowering the body, strengthening the muscles, and imbuing the mind with confidence. Warrior poses engage both of the feet in a way that suggests stepping out into new territory, courageously and without fear, while remaining rooted in the self at the same time. The warrior in the modern world is the active, engaged, courageous body and spirit.

This can be you. This *is* you, even if you don't feel particularly brave at this moment. Power Yoga can help you move through your fear and stagnation into a state of strength, courage, and grace—not to mention glowing health.

Geo's Journey

I can understand how T'ai Chi evolved from Kung Fu, a martial art form that has become an important part of exercise for the Chinese and for many Westerners as well. Far from being combative, T'ai Chi is a beautiful dance of flowing poses. When combat isn't necessary in life, the movements of combat can still be an integral part of the body's need to move, strengthen, stretch, and grow. Power Yoga is similar to T'ai Chi in that it takes movements that are organic or natural to the body and gives them a structure and flow, a systematic and beautiful path to better health and strength.

Essence of the Warrior

Warrior poses require incredible strength and power in the legs. Too many people are weak in the legs, and the legs have huge power potential. In fact, in Greece, there is a phrase referring to the point when a person is ready to die that can be loosely translated as "He has lost his legs."

The legs are like the second heart. The heart mostly pumps blood down to the extremities, but the legs pump the blood back up. The thighs contain the largest set of muscles in the body, and these muscles do incredible work for the body, especially if you really use them. Moving through the warrior poses and cultivating power in the legs is another important component of Power Yoga.

I like to call this warrior pose the spear thrower. The back arm is ready to throw the spear, while the front arm and the front foot line up the target. This pose is easy for beginners, but it is also an incredible source of power.

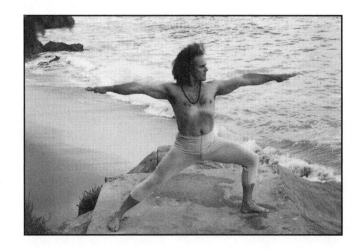

As I looked at the warrior poses from my ex-Marine, warrior point of view, I began to see how one movement was a raising of the sword, one movement a throwing of the spear, one movement a lunging of the sword. That's what they were; that's what they evolved from. I began to understand at that point that yoga has evolved from natural human positions. It works so well and has lasted so long because it's simply natural for human beings. It doesn't work because it's a fad right now, or because it's "cool" to be involved in something "Eastern." It has always worked because it has always been a part of us. It's something we're *meant* to do.

How long has it been since you moved your body in a natural way, just because your body wanted to move? Maybe you danced around your living room when no one was looking. Maybe you started to stretch out your muscles one morning just because they felt they needed it. Or maybe it has been a while since you've done anything that feels "natural." Although you probably don't remember, when you were an infant, your movements were completely natural, coming out of what your body needed. You lifted your head up to look around. You stretched your arms and legs up as you lay on your back. You crawled on all fours. This is where Power Yoga starts.

Just because you grew up doesn't mean you have to lose a sense of what your body wants to do and needs to do to stay strong and healthy.

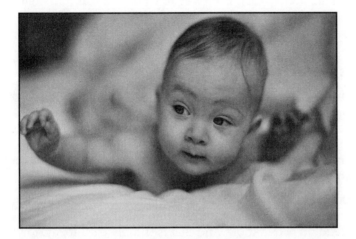

Power Yoga uses the natural poses we performed effortlessly as infants and toddlers.

Going Through the Motions

Finally, in the 1970s, in California, I began to learn yoga. I took classes, and eventually, I began to teach classes, too. My practice grew and grew and became very successful. People knew who I was. And yet, something was missing. I decided to follow my intuition and study with the teacher within me rather than continuing solely as a student of others. I spent more and more time each day at it, holding poses, then resting. Holding poses, then resting. Holding poses for long periods, and longer periods. Getting more and more intense. Holding. Still.

Soon, I was practicing yoga for about eight hours each day. Eight hours, can you imagine? It didn't leave much time for anything else. I wasn't able to spend much time teaching. I wasn't able to spend much time with my wife. I just kept practicing and practicing. I was looking for something, but I had hit a plateau, and all the yoga I had learned wasn't helping me to move beyond it.

I became frustrated with my teaching. I felt I'd been simply relating what I had learned from my teachers, rather than internalizing those teachings and allowing them to resurface into something new, something transformed and representative of true growth. I felt I wasn't doing my students much good, and I knew I wasn't doing myself any good. I hit a wall.

So, I got out my sledgehammer and knocked down the wall. In the late '70s, my wife, Katresha, and I left our successful yoga practice and moved to the mountains of Colorado. We were ready to start again, to allow the transformation we felt was necessary if we were to continue growing.

Making a major life change isn't easy. Anyone who has done this knows what I mean. Whether you looked in the mirror one day and knew you were going to get in shape for real this time, or you knew you had to change jobs or marry the person you loved or do anything else that steered your life in a direction of new growth, you surely remember that change, although rarely easy, is the key to vitality. If your life stops moving, you stop living. If your life doesn't work anymore, you may need to shake things up to see things from a fresh perspective. It's all about movement.

The Evolution of a Body

It took three months for me to completely transform my body. My wife and I spent our days hiking in the mountains and getting stronger. We ate an excellent diet of pure, natural foods and really "cleansed" physically and mentally. For both of us, it was a turning point. Yet, it wasn't really a conscious decision, to make this radical life change toward a more spiritual existence. It was almost as if we didn't have a choice. Everything seemed to push us in that direction. We could hardly do anything else.

I had felt like a broken record, teaching yoga in California. Instinctively, intuitively, I felt I didn't deeply understand what I was doing or talking about. So I went away to Colorado to better understand, to better know. And that is still my path today, toward better understanding and knowing.

In Colorado, I really began to see the world through cleansed eyes. I looked at everything in the nature around me. I spent a lot of time in a large wilderness area in southwest Colorado and was able to watch the animals that lived there. I began to think about how the animals lived naturally.

The Nature of Powerful Movement (and Living!)

I remember once walking up a mountain above Durango, Colorado. I was leading a group of people, and we were all huffing and puffing. We were at about 12,000 feet, and I remember stopping and looking up at the mountain peak, which was another thousand feet away. "It's going to take at least another hour to get up over that guy," I thought. Then, suddenly, out of nowhere, an elk appeared. We spooked him, and he began to run. Up and up he went as we watched him, and in five minutes, he was over the top of the mountain.

The elk and his remarkable flight didn't leave my thoughts for a long time. I had just been contemplating the hour's hike ahead, and then the elk so effortlessly shot to the top. The miracle of that movement was incredible to me.

This led me to wonder why my dogs looked so great right up until the day they died. They always looked strong and healthy, then suddenly, it was their time and they were gone. I thought about all the other animals out there. I realized that I never look at a wild animal and think, "Gee, that looks like an *old* wild animal." Rather, I usually look at them and say, "Wow, look how beautifully they *move,* how graceful and naturally powerful they are."

The more I thought about it, the more I came to see that animals maintain their vitality because they live naturally. It wouldn't occur to them to live any other way! The elk behaves the way an elk should behave. It eats what an elk should eat and drinks what an elk should drink. It lives where an elk should live and exercises in a natural way by going about its life in the hills and on the mountains, the way an elk should.

Yet, isn't "should" such a human word? The elk doesn't feel an obligation to eat healthy foods or get up from the couch, turn off the television, and exercise. That's absurd! An elk simply *is*. He is saturated with *elkness*.

I went back to my house that day with these thoughts lingering in my mind. The next day, I lay down on the ground in my yoga practice for awhile and watched my breath and just meditated on it all. For some time, yoga has been a thing that has been instinctive for me. I don't have a set routine. I often just lie down and my body will start to move in a way it needs to move. And it starts with the breath.

The Right Moves

Go out and take a nature walk today. Compare the instinctive movement of the natural environment to your own daily patterns of movement. How "natural" is your experience of motion? Do you sit in front of a computer all day, or behind the wheel of your car? Power Yoga helps you get back in sync with your body's natural motion. You'll feel refreshed, activated, and engaged with the power of being human.

I began looking at the natural motion of my breath that day. How could I become saturated with humanness, the way the elk was saturated with elkness? What was truly natural movement for me?

You might want to try this right now, especially if the question engages you: What is a truly natural movement for you? One answer lies, quite literally, within you. Breathing is one of the most basic natural movements we have. Lie down on your back on the floor or another relatively firm surface. Now, without controlling your breath in any conscious way, try to become aware of your breathing. What does your body do when you inhale? What moves and what stays still? What happens when you exhale? Concentrate on your breath for a minute or two and really feel it moving in and out of your body. Notice how the movement engages more than your mouth and nose and upper chest.

Now, imagine breathing with your entire body. Your lungs are like two balloons, filling and deflating with each inhale and exhale. What if your entire body was a balloon? Imagine inflating and expanding with each inhale, deflating and collapsing with each exhale. Stay here another minute or two. Now you're moving naturally, even if it doesn't feel like much movement. Sometimes it's good to start small.

Our Human Experience: Born with Power

My experience with the elk and my examination of my own breathing led me to examine what would constitute natural living for humans. And, of course, that prompted me to start looking at babies, for what more natural form of a human exists?

I began to look at the way babies lie on their bellies, then start to get lonely or hungry and lift their heads up to look around. I saw how that beginning motion began the process of building their muscles, shaping their spines, their necks, their arches. I watched how they lie on their backs and bring their legs up, how they move their arms and legs and can do it all day long—with plenty of naps in between, of course! Later, I even developed a pose I call yoga walks, which mirrors what babies do.

The yoga walks pose mirrors the developmental process of babies as they learn and grow.

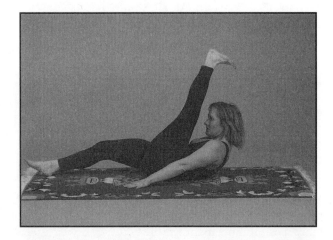

Cobra pose is a natural!

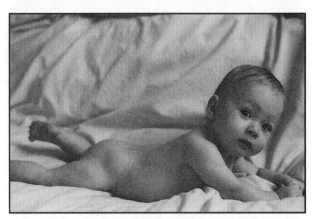

Then I began to think about how babies get into their crawl and squat positions and how and why they move. I really saw and understood that yoga is not something new to us. We've all done yoga; it's innate, part of us. My own yoga teacher once told me that yoga was put into me before I was born. That applies to all of us. We're meant to be able to move in every direction, but as we get older, we begin to lose that capacity. Our bodies become less flexible. One of the most noticeable things about babies is their flexibility. As we mature, we get bigger, stronger, harder muscles that can stretch and flex less and less. They get harder, and older, and eventually they die.

Geo's Journey

Indra Devi was the first woman to study with the renowned Sri Krishnamacharya, the teacher of many of those who have developed the influential yoga systems of today. Born in 1899, Indra Devi started teaching yoga in the 1930s and was among the first yoga teachers in Hollywood (her pupils included Gloria Swanson and many other movie stars). Still teaching and traveling around the world, Indra Devi is now 100 years old. I studied with her in the 1970s.

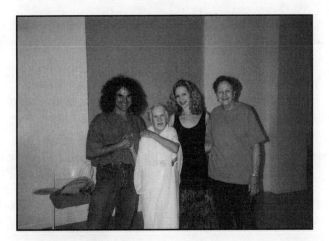

Geo with his teacher Indra Devi, his wife, Katresha, and his mother-in-law, Mavis Gilleland.

As I began to move, there in my house in Colorado, and as my body began to move through its natural arches, the arches became stronger. As I inhaled, my spine lengthened even more, allowing me to breathe more deeply down into my belly. I could feel my lungs opening as I opened my chest at the top of each inhalation. Then, as I exhaled, I began to focus on the collapsing of the breath and the motion of the diaphragm. I began to help the movement along. As I exhaled, I sucked in my belly. As I inhaled, I consciously expanded my body and continued to move with the breath.

Soon, I began to feel great power inside myself. Things were shaking up inside me, moving deep down. My whole body felt activated. The endorphins began pumping and I felt a wonderful, excited sense of pleasure and health. "How many people get to feel this sensation?" I thought. It was so easy to attain, a subtle feeling but wonderful. Anyone could do it, even on their first day of a yoga practice. Anyone could release this energy, if they knew how to do it. You can do it, and I'll show you how.

Moving Toward Power Yoga

Traditionally, yoga has always been taught in a way that poses are held for long periods of time, with rest between each pose to allow the body to adjust to the changes the pose has effected on the body. Holding poses is a valuable way to practice yoga. It builds strength in and applies pressure to particular parts of the body.

For years, I practiced yoga in this traditional way. The advantage to the years of practice was that I became consciously able to notice the effects of each pose. If you lie in a forward bend over your right leg with your left foot up in a half lotus position between your thigh and your hip, after 5 or 10 minutes you will notice that your leg will start to go to sleep because the arterial blood flow that would normally pump down the femoral artery into the foot is dammed up. That damming of the blood activates and puts more pressure on all the lower glands and organs, especially down in the lower abdominal area. These are some of the facts that I grew to understand about many of the yoga poses, what they were doing in my body and how they felt when I was really "in" them.

But at some point, those parts get strong enough and don't need that much time, pressure, or strengthening anymore. When we move into those poses, the body has a memory of them and just goes right back to the memory as we move easily through and out of the pose. If we structure the yoga poses properly, the well-trained body will allow each pose to fold out of or evolve into the next pose.

Still, a yoga practice based more on movement needn't require years of traditional yoga practice first. With the right training and guidance, the body can find the right position even without holding it for long periods of time. Indeed, holding for long periods may be the more difficult method because the body is so dynamic. The body wants to move, and the breath is the impetus.

I knew that if I could create a series of poses and counterposes that would move naturally with the inhaling, arching, expanding, then exhaling, rounding, and contracting flow of the body—in which each pose sets up the next pose and a kind of lovely, life-bestowing, and strengthening dance evolves—I would create a new kind of dynamic, cardiovascular (of the heart and lungs), movement- and breath-based practice: *Power Yoga.*

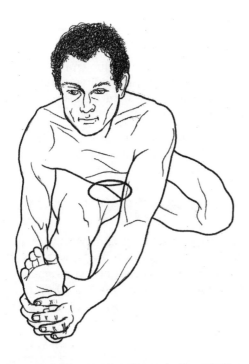

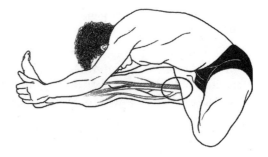

Holding a forward bending pose dams the flow of arterial blood to increase pressure on the lower glands and organs.

The Journey Continues

As you can see, Power Yoga has come out of a lifelong process for me. I am finally to a stage in my physical and spiritual development where I recognize that yoga should consist of natural human movements, lifting the weight of the body, manipulating the weight of the head or the shoulders, stretching the back, stretching the body by using weight, pressing on things, pushing on things, turning things, rotating things— all in healthy, activating ways.

Soon, I found myself naming the positions and movements I had developed from nature, such as prowling tiger. I began to work with releasing the *chakras* (see Chapters 9, "Chakras and the Power of Color," and 10, "Chakra Testing for Power Healing") through movement and teaching that the physical affects the mental, emotional, and spiritual.

All of the realms of the self are directly connected at all times, and directly affecting and being affected by each other at all times. It is difficult to affect the emotional or the mental with some people, and with others, it's difficult to even touch the

Power Words

Chakras are energy centers located along the body's spine that are activated for the benefit of mind-body well-being. The spine is the human nervous system's powerhouse, funneling energy transmission from the brain to the whole body.

spiritual (which is too bad), but we can always start from the physical. You can start there today.

As I mentioned before, I changed my whole body, my whole being, my whole nature in three months. I committed to it and worked on it every day. But doing it *every day* is the reality. It does work. It works in amazing, miraculous ways. But just thinking about it won't do much for you at all. You have to do it.

A few years ago, Dean Ornish came out with his program for reversing heart disease, and it, too, seemed like a miracle, but people found it very difficult to follow because they had to *do* something. They couldn't just take a pill and keep on watching TV. That's the reality with yoga. The results are phenomenal, but you've got to do it. It's a process, and it's up to you to get up off your buns and get started. Take responsibility for your life.

A 20-minute Power Yoga workout every morning, especially when combined with a walk in the fresh air, is enough to keep anybody healthy and fit for life. Most people don't do any physical exercise at all, and the thought of a vigorous fitness program may be intimidating. But 20 minutes of yoga? Anyone can do it. In fact, a 20-minute Power Yoga program is something you can do even when you are 90, or 100, or older. And that's the kind of fitness program that makes sense—something you can do for life.

The scorpion pose isn't as difficult as it appears, once you've acquired the proper strength and balance.

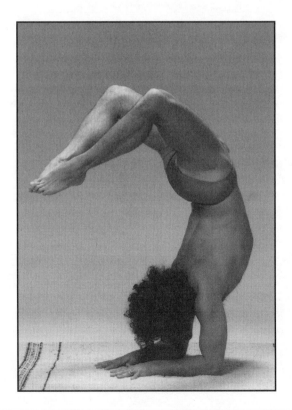

Power Yoga is a natural way of manipulating and moving the body to strengthen, to stretch, to tone, to keep the body healthy, to awaken the brain, to enliven the glands and organs, to juice the joints, to move the natural hormones and endorphins through the body so the body is healthy and happy in whatever path it chooses, whatever work it has to do. It's the most natural exercise imaginable, and its power can be your power.

The Least You Need to Know

➤ The ancient practice of yoga has evolved in a way that is relevant, fresh, and exciting for us today.

➤ Power Yoga has many practitioners and interpretations, but one basic commonality: movement.

➤ Power Yoga is a journey of self-exploration that requires you to move with your body.

➤ Using the human body's natural power and movement, through Power Yoga poses that understand the body's physiology, creates incredible results and promotes physical and mental well-being.

➤ Just a 20-minute daily Power Yoga workout is all you need for physical fitness, mental health, and personal well-being!

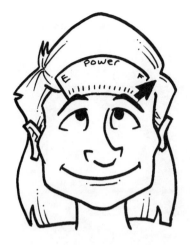

More Power to You!

In this chapter, I'd like to go into a little more detail about what, exactly, Power Yoga *is*—and, while I'm at it, what Power Yoga *is not*. Yoga means different things to different people, of course. But to me, yoga is a journey into the magical side of the self. It helps move the body and the mind into a more balanced and, consequently, happier state. It is about fitness, but not *just* about fitness.

Everyone who writes about or teaches yoga tries to explain what yoga is. However, defining it is as difficult as explaining what love is or what God is. Our limited, rational minds feel a compulsion to explain concepts and put boundaries around them so we can grasp them, but some things our minds may never be able to grasp. And yet, I'll take my turn at an explanation, too.

In yoga, as in everything, we start with a form. The form is the body. This form has its limits, but as we work with the form and test those limits, the form evolves. It will always change, thank God! How terrible to become static.

This concept is the secret to Power Yoga—the resistance to stasis. Power Yoga is about movement. It is the most natural thing in the world for our forms, our bodies, because they are built to move. Bodies aren't built to sit at desks all day, typing on computer keyboards. Bodies aren't meant to sit on couches all evening, staring at the flickering lights of a screen in a box. If your body has forgotten this basic principle, you can "re-mind" yourself by beginning a Power Yoga practice.

Bodies are meant to move, bend, twist, arch, stretch, and strengthen.

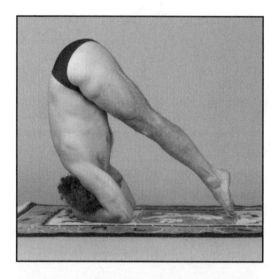

Why remain upright all day long? Our bodies are meant to move through and to hold a much wider variety of positions than most of us practice.

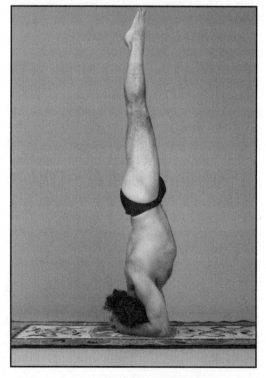

Power Yoga: Yoga, American Style

Many of us may have developed a negative opinion of the word "power" in the 1980s. Power meant to control the people, places, and things around us. Having power meant having the most money, the most influence, the ability to get whatever material possessions you wanted, and the respect you wanted.

In the 1990s, however, even the word "power" has evolved. The kind of power in Power Yoga isn't the kind used to conquer and subdue, or the kind used for personal gain. It isn't stepping on people to reach the top of some proverbial social, financial, or corporate ladder. Instead, it is the power to live fully, to be fully in our bodies, awake to the experience of life, to live as fully flowered human beings.

Geo's Journey

Just as every animal on earth has a natural, innate grace and power, so do we. When someone has this kind of power, it isn't scary or intimidating. It's beautiful. It comes naturally when the spirit is able to freely experience and relish its humanity without the barriers of an unfit body or an excessive attachment to material things. It is a spirit free from pettiness and filled with life.

How do you get this kind of power? For many of us, it requires an altered point of view. Instead of looking from the outside in, wondering what's going on inside our bodies and spirits, we must look from the inside out. We must live in our bodies and in our souls, so familiar with who we are, how we move, how we feel, think, and live that we feel absolutely at home in our bodies and our minds, living and experiencing each moment of existence. We are not gross humans grasping for some higher spiritual existence in the next life, but powerful spirits who have chosen to experience humanity. If we don't experience it, we are missing a wonderful opportunity for spiritual growth! We are missing our calling.

Power Yoga is a way to help move your perception inward so you can experience life in a more loving, energetic, and healthy way for the rest of your life.

The Right Moves

How do you know if Power Yoga is for you? The same way you know whether anything else is good for you: Something is good for your life if it makes you stronger, healthier, more energetic, and happier. Something is bad for your life if it makes you weaker, sicker, less energetic, and less happy. Sounds obvious, but if you examine your life, you may find plenty of activities you keep doing even though they have made a negative impact on your life.

Catch the Power Yoga Train

Most of my students are successful, busy people who have found that they need to spend some time alone. Yet, the pulses of the world are constantly affecting their physical pulses. These people are constantly moving. If I were to say to them, "Be still and know that you are God, the universal" it would be like telling a freight train barreling along the tracks as it carried its load of coal from one coast to the other to stop moving for a moment and consider the nature of the coal it carries.

Everyone knows life is stressful these days, but how often do we recognize the effects of stress on our own internal rhythms? I'm talking about your pulse, your heartbeat, your breath, all the rhythms and movements associated with being alive. Each of us has a very personal, individual rhythm that is right for us, but the frantic rhythm of modern life is often louder and more insistent than our internal rhythm. One way to work toward better health and well-being is to learn how to tune out the incessant rhythms of an obsessed and fast-paced culture, at least for a little while each day, and get back in touch with our own, individual rhythms.

Spend some time each day listening for your internal rhythms.

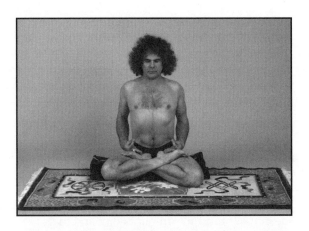

Power Words

Metabolism is the process, occurring in all living things, by which food is broken down in the body and converted to energy.

A train must move to do its duty, and humans, too, must move to fulfill their destinies. In order to reach these folks, to awaken them to the stillness within them, we have to start with movement. It is the language they speak. It is the language of the world in the twenty-first century.

Movement is also the language of Power Yoga. Power Yoga is a moving, flowing yoga that affects every corner of our beings in a natural, non-competitive way. We stimulate, strengthen, stretch, twist, juice, focus, and balance every gland, organ, vessel, muscle, joint, and bone in our bodies.

We also move to create heat. The process of burning our food for energy is called *metabolism*. Metabolism dictates the speed at which we live. It is responsible for fueling all our bodily functions. Therefore, to keep the metabolism "up" is to keep living. Power Yoga keeps the metabolism stoked and ready to burn.

Of course, all yoga, including the ancient forms, consists of flowing movements. Even when you hold a pose, you are continuously moving as your breath and blood move. You move in and out of poses, even if you hold the poses themselves for a long period of time. But in Power Yoga, the movement is greater, bigger, faster, stronger—more like our daily lives.

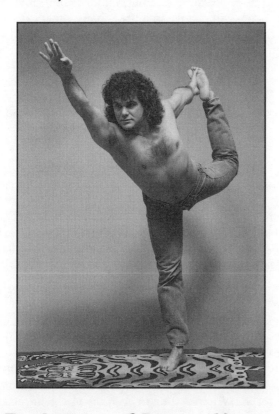

To move is to live, and strong, powerful movements are the best way to begin a dialogue with the body that can result in more strength, greater health, and a heightened sense of personal well-being.

The Evolution of Power Yoga

Power Yoga is part of a process that is, and has always been, happening in the yoga world. Some love it, some hate it, but no matter what this or that yoga teacher or yoga student may think, Power Yoga continues. That's not to say Power Yoga is the only path. It is simply a way many have chosen to follow.

I see Power Yoga evolving in a world that is moving, in the midst of its commercialism and mass production and depersonalization, toward a more natural way of life. To cite a contemporary example, you can now buy veggie burgers and baked potatoes at many fast-food restaurants. People are looking for a more natural way to live and be healthy. They are seeking their true nature and asking the question, "How are humans meant to live?"

Demographically, a large percentage of Americans are reaching their 50s. Yes, I mean the war babies, the baby boomers, that group you may well be a part of or have heard about. This generation (of which I'm a part) has always refused to change with the times, but has instead actively changed the times and redefined the world as it moved through different periods of life.

I've heard it said that every seven years we come to a new and different time. At the age of 49—the end of the seventh "era" of change in a life—many Americans are finding that the second half of their lives is beginning. The first half of life was a movement from spirit to human, and the second half of life is a movement from human back to spirit.

Geo's Journey

Humans are moving quickly into a time when being a centenarian (reaching the age of 100) will be normal, even expected. Scientific advances in health, longevity studies, and a greater focus on natural health and relieving the debilitating effects of stress may all contribute to increased life expectancy. With the help of yoga, humans won't just live longer. They can live better, healthier lives, far into old age.

Most of us in this time of life have raised families, found our professions, bought houses, and are now looking at a new millennium as an opportunity for a major shift in the movement and purpose of our lives. The seeds for this time were planted in the 1960s and 1970s, but the productive movements of this period were mislaid by distractions such as drugs and many other mistakes of youth and being human. Then the responsibilities of life set in. Who has time to keep up a yoga or meditation practice when the rent is due, when the roof leaks, when the baby is hungry?

As a generation, I think we have done a fantastic job. And here we are, in the most prosperous of times. We've accomplished a lot! Yet, many of us have paid for these prosperous times with our health. We aren't in shape. We don't feel energetic. And we may feel spiritually out of shape, too.

It's no surprise, then, that baby boomers, and those generations surrounding the boomers, too, have a renewed interest in yoga. However, the yoga of choice these days isn't always the yoga of the 1960s and 1970s. While yoga has always been a tool for creating better health, Power Yoga is a more contemporary form.

If you are interested in wine, you may know that grapevines taken from the hills of France and planted in California or Australia or Chile soon evolve into different grapes. The grapevine is just one factor in the resulting fruit. The environment—the soil, the water, the sun—all contribute their influences. Yoga has changed in this same way, now that it has "lived" in the West for so many years. Power Yoga has become the new "yoga for Americans."

Geo's Journey

The original book, *Yoga for Americans,* was written by my teacher, Indra Devi, the first woman to be taught yoga by the great Krishnamachara. At 100 years old, she's still doing well, traveling, giving seminars, and living her yoga. Up until Krishnamachara accepted her as a student, it was absolutely taboo to teach a woman yoga. Indra Devi's movement of yoga into Western culture and Hollywood had a significant effect on yoga's popularity and familiarity in the United States. She set the stage for many of us teaching yoga in Hollywood today. Her teacher's training course, one of the first of its time, was largely based on her book, *Yoga for Americans.*

The Great Balancing Act

The word "yoga" comes from the Sanskrit word *yuj,* which means "to yoke." For example, if two oxen are yoked together, they can pull a plow or cart more evenly and with greater strength through a field or down a road.

I like to think of that field or road as our lives. The oxen are the male and female sides of the self—the earthly/heavenly, the right brain/left brain, the inward-looking/outward-experiencing sides. When we live our lives in a balanced way, we radiate health, energy, happiness, and a sense of well-being.

A lot of this balance work is spiritual. We come into this world as a particular spirit with a certain nature or personality. That personality then adjusts to live in a certain environment and with the different personalities around it. In order to find balance, that personality or nature must continuously adjust, change, *move.* Often we'll be moving back toward a center between opposing poles, finding a balance to the extremes that enter our lives and environments. Moving toward a center encourages greater stability and balance.

The Wrong Moves

It's a competitive world, and all that competition is stressful. In Power Yoga, however, competition is irrelevant. Power Yoga is not a contest or a race. You can only win, so leave your competitive mind at the door.

However, if you've spent most of your life hanging out at one end, it isn't easy to move toward the middle, or even to find the middle point at all! Picture this balance as a swing. If you're swinging back and forth, way up high, you can't just suddenly stop so that your swing immediately hangs straight down in the center of the arc. You have to let the swing slow down gradually until you at last come to rest in the center.

Power Yoga, too, starts with big movement and works gradually toward a smoother, more gentle rhythm. It helps you to find your center at a pace that works for you. After a Power Yoga workout, you'll find it is much easier to be still, or at least a little quieter.

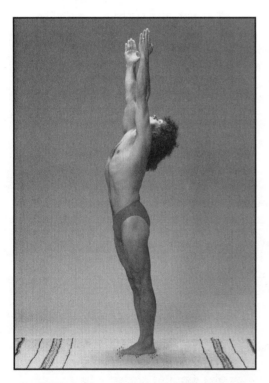
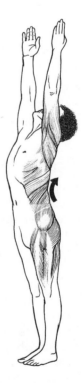

Your Power Yoga routine should be personal, moving to the beat of your own internal rhythms and expressing your physical, mental, and spiritual self.

Power Yoga: The Rhythm of Life

To me, Power Yoga should be a ritual, one that's personal—just between you and your God. A ritual requires rhythm, but it has to be your own rhythm to be performed most appropriately. It must also contain your own beautiful, personal series of movements.

That doesn't mean, of course, that Power Yoga consists only of the poses your body finds easy. If you aren't in shape or aren't used to certain types of movements, your muscles may resist at first. Your mind and even your instinct must be allowed to take over to some extent, so that your body can be directed into the positions it requires.

For example, what I call four-legged poses are the poses that create the most heat in the body because they're the most difficult for us. These poses involve walking on the hands and feet, like a bear. But we're not used to walking on our hands anymore, and at first, it's tough! Maybe our primate progenitors were more accustomed to using hands as tools for locomotion, but in the twenty-first century, arms and hands are usually used for working the computer, writing checks, waving, shaking hands—pretty lightweight stuff.

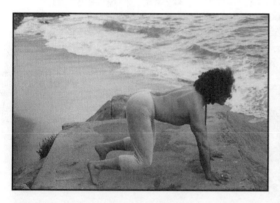 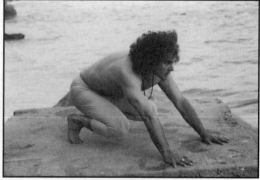

Bear pose looks easy at first, but is actually an incredibly powerful, strengthening pose. Here, Geo performs the pose. Inhale during the left movement and exhale as you move into the position shown in the photo at the right.

Even if we do exercises, a few push-ups each night, lifting weights, or hoisting groceries and kids around, we still aren't used to using our muscles in the way they are used if we walk on all fours. You probably haven't done that since shortly after you learned to walk! So, bear poses aren't easy, but they create a lot of strength, a lot of power, and a lot of heat in the body. We're working very hard when working on our hands. Would you think to include such a movement in your personal power ritual? Perhaps not at first.

The Right Moves

People under a lot of stress find meditation difficult. It may surprise you to learn that the road to meditation is to focus on rhythm, not stillness. Once you find the appropriate rhythm of life for you, meditation follows naturally and easily. You'll be awakened, stimulated, strengthened, and exuding inner energy. You'll be able to sit peacefully and reflect on your inner self as it functions the way it was meant to function.

But an important first step to crafting a Power Yoga ritual is learning a basic repertoire of poses and routines, then practicing them so they become so well memorized that they feel like second nature (see Chapters 6, "Stand for It," 7, "Tilts, Twists, and Arches," and 8, "Prowling Tiger Series," to begin building your repertoire). Just as a dancer needs to have mastered basic techniques, positions, and moves, but can then improvise a dance of beautiful spontaneity and artistry, so you can eventually create your own Power Yoga routines once you've mastered the basics.

Yogis believe there is a little god residing inside each of us, and the process of yoga is, ultimately, about discovering that god and allowing that god in each of our hearts into the world. I believe we have free will, a choice. We can choose to reflect in any way we like. You can be the meanest, nastiest demon of all time, hateful and horrible in every way, sending fear in every direction. Or, you can reflect the most wonderful god that's ever been in this universe, all-powerful, all-loving, all-compassionate, happy wherever he or she goes, bringing and creating goodness in the world.

Geo's Journey

The physical, mental, emotional, and spiritual are connected and always affecting each other. In essence, you have no separate parts, and neither does the universe. You are personally integrated, you are one with your fellow humans, with the natural world, and with the universe itself. No matter what personal beliefs or spiritual theories you subscribe to, you can understand some version of the concept that we are all part of something bigger, like individual cells in the body of God.

Most of us are somewhere in the middle, somewhere along the path between demon and god, closer to creating goodness, but still creating a little badness now and then (intentionally or not). We're all somewhere along that continuum.

Wherever you are, yoga can help you to find the self you want to be. Yoga is a process of enshrining the body-mind and the spirit. We start in the body, with the materials of the body. We start reorganizing, building, creating a strong, balanced, sacred temple, almost like a pyramid, in which we can sit and meditate.

As long as we live, the temple is never fully built. But, far from being frustrating, I find the continual construction, creation, and re-invention of the body incredibly exciting and inspiring. Movement is life. When you are completely still, you are no longer alive.

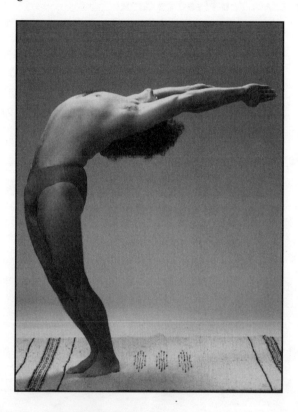

Power Yoga is a process in which you learn the limits of your body, then learn how to expand those limits, a little further each day, until you are evolving and transforming yourself with each new workout.

Living: Just Do It

I've learned an important lesson in my years of experience, from childhood, to Vietnam, where the fear of death was my constant companion, to my ongoing physical and spiritual journey: No matter what the circumstances of your life may be, the only way to live is to continue to move upward and outward, looking for life. Death will come on its own, at some mysterious time. It doesn't warrant your consideration. All you need to do is seek movement, vitality, life. Never stop moving, never stop seeking.

This continuous movement doesn't mean you will be restless or discontent. On the contrary, the search for more life can grant you supreme contentment at any given moment because you know you are spending your time in the way you were meant to spend it. We are meant to move, to learn, to live. So let's embrace the moment!

The Least You Need to Know

➤ Power Yoga and life share a basic principle: To move is to live.

➤ Power Yoga is part of yoga's evolution, a form that works best for our modern world where everyone is always moving, thinking, doing, acting, and rushing around.

➤ The word yoga means "to yoke," and yoga yokes together opposing sides of the self for greater balance and harmony.

➤ Power Yoga teaches you to find a personal, rhythmic ritual.

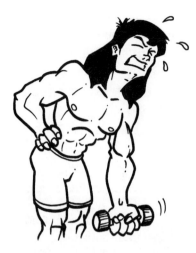

Chapter 3

Assess Your Fitness Power

In This Chapter

➤ The meaning of "in shape"

➤ How do you stand?

➤ What the mirror is telling you

➤ The importance of leg strength

➤ Muscle testing with a friend

➤ Test your attitude

You've probably seen this warning on every kind of fitness program and diet aid: Before attempting this (*fill in the blank*), please consult your physician. Consulting a professional is so often recommended when new exercise or diet regimens are under consideration because we aren't all the same. Big surprise? Of course not—but we are all different in ways more obvious than hair color, height, weight, and personality.

Every body has a different fitness level, and this fitness level may change from day to day, even from hour to hour. Whenever you do something your body isn't used to doing, you take a risk. Keep in mind, however, that risks aren't necessarily bad! Attempting an exercise you've never done before that is too difficult for your current fitness level will risk injury, and that's bad. But attempting something new in a logical progression, as part of a sequence of fitness growth, allowing your muscles, joints, bones, circulation, and even your mind to reach new levels of movement and understanding—well, that's good. That's great!

In this chapter, you'll learn your current fitness level and where your individual fitness profile needs tweaking, adjusting, or reviewing. Where are you strongest? Where should you concentrate your efforts? Those are the questions we'll address in this chapter.

What Kind of Shape Are You In?

The term "in shape" is a little strange. In the shape of what? A human? What shape is that?

As you know, humans come in many shapes and sizes, heights and weights, and girths. Many of these shapes are perfectly healthy. Some of the shapes you might see more often on TV or on the pages of fashion magazines might not be the healthiest or strongest shapes they could be. Some of the shapes you see in a gym might not be the most flexible or aerobically conditioned shapes. Some shapes that would, by some standards, be considered less than beautiful are both strong and flexible. Any shape, no matter how perfect or imperfect by current standards, could belong to someone who is happy or someone who is unhappy. And every shape, no matter how "in shape," houses a beautiful spirit.

The Right Moves

Even a disabled body can find its strengths and develop these to the fullest for a personal level of health that works for the individual. Whether you have a sensory or a mobility impairment, or just a bum knee or a bad back or asthma, Power Yoga can become a part of your life. Just find the movements that work for you, or adapt movements (check with your physician, physical therapist, or experienced teacher) to bring more power to the resources you have.

But a spirit in a healthy, flexible, strong body will be better able to express itself, so the spirit in a healthy, flexible, strong body will probably have a better shot at maintaining a level of happiness. I'm not talking about looks here. I'm talking about health, and the glow and joy it imparts to the person who has it. I'm talking about a body that works in concert with the mind, a mind/body that can move and bend and stretch and run as it needs to, as the soul dictates, or as life's circumstances require.

Before you begin a Power Yoga routine, you should assess your own fitness level. Visiting your health care practitioner for an overall health assessment is always a good idea. Knowing that your blood chemistry is where it should be or that it needs some adjustment, that your weight is in a healthy range or could go up or down a bit, or that your internal organs and structures all seem to be functioning as they should when subjected to stress tests, sugar tests, reflex tests, and so on, are all things your physician can assess. But there is more to your health than what a battery of medical tests will tell you.

You can also form your own picture of your fitness level and individual health profile, to "color in" the results of a physical. Your own assessment may be just as valuable, if not more valuable, in determining the level at which you can begin a fitness program and how fast you can move through the program toward greater health.

Are you healthy? The answer to this question is a matter of degree, and differs greatly from individual to individual. You can begin to answer this question for yourself with a few simple tests.

Up Against the Wall!

The first way to assess the basic state of your body's health is to stand against a wall in what yoga traditionally calls the mountain pose, but what I like to call the Marine pose, because this is the pose in which we always had to stand in the Marine Corps.

The Wrong Moves

Power Yoga can be challenging, and trying poses and sequences of poses that are beyond your fitness level can result in an injury that will keep you sidelined. Listen to your body and don't make any movements that are too difficult for you. A slow progression will get you to those challenging poses soon enough. You have your whole life to do yoga.

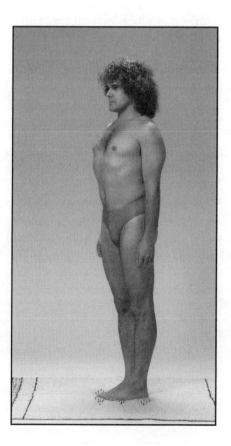

In Marine pose, the body is held straight and upright, at "attention." It forms a base for correct posture and is a starting point for many Power Yoga movements.

Find a space along a wall with no molding at the base (a closed door may work well). Put your heels up against the wall, and stand with your calves, buttocks, shoulders and upper back, and the back of your head touching the wall. Try to center your weight on your feet so you aren't forward on the balls of your feet or backward on the heels. Turn your arms so that your palms face front, opening your chest. Imagine a string attached to the crown of your head suspends you, and adjust your posture accordingly.

How does it feel? Natural? Unnatural? Strained? Easy? Like you're about to fall forward? Write your first, general impression here:

_____

_____

_____

Head, Shoulders, Knees, and Toes

Now let's get specific. We will begin with your head. Does your neck feel craned back? If you can do this exercise looking in a mirror, even better—make sure your head is touching the wall in a way that will allow you to look straight forward, not up or down. Do you feel like you would tip over backward if the wall weren't there, or do you fall forward unless you move your feet away from the wall slightly? Does your spine feel as if it is in a brand new position? Balanced? Unbalanced? Does your neck or back hurt? Describe how your head, neck, and spine feel in this position:

_____

_____

_____

_____

The Right Moves

When performing the wall test, depending on your body shape, you may need to stand with your heels about an inch or so in front of the wall to keep from pitching forward when pressing your head, shoulders, and buttocks against the wall. When your body gets into better condition, you should be able to stand against the wall and feel balanced.

Press your shoulders firmly against the wall. Do you feel as if you are sticking out your chest unnaturally? Does this position hurt your upper back? Are you able to pull your shoulders back far enough to touch the wall, or does your body resist this position? Would you feel silly walking around in this position, or does this feel like your normal stance? Does anything feel like it is going numb or tingling? Do you feel more energized? Describe how your shoulders and back feel in this position:

_____

_____

_____

Now focus on your hips. Are your buttocks keeping you from getting close enough to the wall? Are your hips bent unnaturally to stay against the wall? The hip/belly area is the center of your body. Do you feel centered here, or somewhere else (or nowhere)? Describe how your hips feel in this position:

_____

_____

_____

What about your legs? Are they shaking, keeping you in this position, or do they feel strong and solid beneath you? Are your knees locked or slightly bent? Are your feet solid on the ground, and is your weight centered over them, or are you forward or backward on your feet? Describe how your legs and feet feel in this position:

_____

_____

_____

Geo's Journey

Your backbone or spine is the bony protection for your spinal cord, which conducts messages from your brain to your body, and vice versa. When your body receives sense impressions, these messages go to the brain, which responds with messages about what to do in response to those sense impressions. A spinal cord injury can cut off communication between body and brain, but many structures are in place to prevent injury. The vertebral bones, fluid-filled spinal disks, and spinal muscles cushion shock to the spinal cord. Keeping the spine and surrounding muscles strong and flexible and keeping your weight in a comfortable range are strong protection from spinal cord injury.

The Shape of Your Spine

Now that you have a pretty clear picture of how this pose feels against the wall, I'd like you to notice a few other things. No writing this time, just awareness.

As you stand against the wall, bring your awareness back to your spine. Try to feel its shape. Does your spine feel filled with energy, or is it strained and uncomfortable? A healthy, strong spine will support the body effortlessly and be shaped like a very gentle, stretched-out S. The first bend in the S is approximately the place where your upper back touches the wall, and the S ends in your tailbone where your lower back touches the wall. Is your lower back unnaturally arched? Does your spine feel weak or uncomfortable in this position? Does your lower back lack energy? Check the boxes to indicate which areas you feel need additional strength:

SPINE: ❏   LOWER BACK: ❏

Shoulder Stories

Now pay attention to what your shoulders are doing. Are they trying to cave inward toward your heart, protecting this vulnerable area, or are they thrown back naturally to let your solar plexus meet the world? Do they feel strong and filled with energy, or are they ready to collapse, pulling your spine into a more exaggerated shape, as soon as you step away from the wall? Does your upper back feel strong enough to give your shoulders the support they need? Check the areas that feel weak or lacking in energy:

SHOULDERS: ❏   UPPER BACK: ❏

Foot Notes

Now, bring your awareness to your legs and feet. Are your legs supporting you with strength and energy, or do you feel wobbly? Do your knees feel comfortable? Is your weight centered over your feet? Does anything hurt? Are your feet having trouble supporting you with strength and energy? Are you rolled over onto the sides or in towards the arches? Check any areas that feel weak or lacking in energy:

LEGS: ❏   KNEES: ❏   FEET: ❏

At last, you may step away from the wall, but do so with awareness. Does your entire body collapse with relief, or do you step away and remain in about the same position? If standing against the wall was a real effort, you could probably use some all-over strengthening.

Keep in mind the areas you checked, so you know where to start working once you begin a Power Yoga routine.

The You in the Mirror

But wait! Your self-assessment isn't over yet. The state of your physical being is reflected in more ways than your posture. You can tell a lot from just looking in the mirror.

Find a mirror that allows you a well lit, full view of yourself, and take a good look. Pretend you are looking at someone else, so you can be more objective. First of all, what is your general impression of the health of your reflection? Do you look sallow? Slumped? Dull? Or vibrant, rosy, full of life? Write your general impressions here:

_____

_____

_____

_____

The Right Moves

One important key to success in Power Yoga is to start working in the areas where you aren't as strong. Remember, balance is the key. If you concentrate on the areas where you are already strong, you'll just become further out of balance. Strengthen the weak areas to bring your whole body into a more unified state.

Your Soul Windows

Now look at your eyes. I used to study *iridology,* which is the study of the iris, or colored part of the eye, for clues to overall health. According to iridology, the state of health of every system of the body, even down to the individual organs, is reflected in the colors and fibers of the eye's iris, and knowing how to read the iris is a way to detect which areas of the body are healthy and which are more subject to developing certain health problems.

Look closely at the iris of your eyes. Although I won't get into the details of an iridology analysis here, some basics to look for are:

➤ **Clarity.** Look for clear whites and clear colors. As you become healthier, you'll notice your eyes become clearer. Murky eyes are a sign of ill health.

➤ **Dense fibers.** Look at the iris of your eye as a wagon wheel with spokes. In someone with a strong constitution, the "spokes" will be close together. A body with a constitution more delicate or vulnerable will sport eyes with "spokes" farther apart. Such a person can still be perfectly healthy, but may not be able to get away with careless health habits.

Power Words

Iridology is the study of the *iris,* or colored part, of the eye. The root *iri* comes from the word "Iris," which was the Greek name for the goddess of the rainbow. The root *ology* means "study of."

➤ **White space.** Everyone has spaces in their eyes that look like little holes. These holes show us the areas of our bodies that need a little more strengthening. An iridologist can analyze what holes in different areas mean, and some even claim they can see tumors in the eyes! The blacker the holes, the more the corresponding area needs strengthening and balancing. As health increases, the black spots will turn gray and eventually white. White spots in the eyes reveal that the body has generated enough energy to start some serious healing. You may experience a healing crisis—a three-day cold, for example, as your body purges toxins—shortly after you notice white areas in your eyes.

➤ **The inner circle.** The inner circle of the eye, just around the pupil, corresponds to the colon and intestines. If the area around your pupil is very dark, you probably need to purify your digestive system. Try eating better, fresher foods and drinking lots of water.

➤ **The outer edge.** The perimeter of the iris represents the circulatory system. When someone suffers from poor circulation, the outer edge of the eye will become light and chalky looking.

The Skin-ny

Next, look at your skin. Everyone has a different natural skin tone, so yours may tend to be darker, lighter, more olive, more rosy, or whatever your genetics bestowed upon you. But beyond your natural skin tone, the condition of your skin can reveal your general state of health.

According to some health theories, the skin is the first organ to reveal an internal imbalance, like an early warning system. If you are often victim to rashes and break-outs, your body may be trying to tell you something. Very dry skin can reveal that you aren't well hydrated and should up your intake of clean water and add more healthy fats, such as olive oil, to your diet. Acne can reveal a hormonal imbalance, and many skin conditions, from hives to blisters, can be evidence of an allergic condition, which is an inappropriate response by your immune system to a harmless substance such as pollen, milk, or wheat.

Although many of these conditions can't be cleared up through improved diet and a good exercise plan, they may be significantly improved by an overall improved state of health. When your body is working at its healthiest, it will be best able to take on its own internal problems.

Take a good look at your skin, on your face, your neck, your chest, your arms, your legs, your torso. What do you see?

_____

_____

_____

Hair Raising

Now let's look at your hair. Long or short, black or blonde, straight or curly, your hair is also an indicator of general health. Is it shiny, strong, and flexible? Or is it dull and does it break easily? As much as hair product companies would like you to believe a shampoo, conditioner, or other product can turn dull weak hair into Rapunzel's locks, the truth is, hair condition is largely related to your hormonal state and your health. Vibrant health, vibrant hair. What do you see when you look at your hair?

_____

_____

_____

Weighty Issues

Now we come to the issue many health and fitness books put right up front: your weight. Weight is another indicator of health, but I hope you aren't looking for a chart that will tell you exactly what you "should" weigh. Not in this book! Weight is a highly individual matter. For one person, 150 pounds might be the perfect weight to maintain ultimate health, strength, and vitality. For another person, 150 pounds might be too heavy, and for still another, it might not be enough. Height alone is not an indication of what your weight should be. Weight charts might give you a general idea of a sensible range, and being too far out of that range is probably unhealthy, but again, much depends on your individual structure, your musculature, your build, your activity level, your diet, and even simply who you are.

But you can detect signs that you are over or under the best weight for you. You'll need a full-length mirror for this one. Stand up straight, and look at yourself from the front, the sides, the back. You don't need to strip down, but clothing that allows you to see your body shape will make this analysis easier.

The Wrong Moves

Weight is a sensitive issue for many people. Before analyzing your body condition in the mirror, try to cultivate an attitude of self-love. If you are overweight or underweight, it doesn't diminish in any way the beauty of your spirit. In analyzing your weight you're determining how to best maximize your physical side so the beautiful you can be most effectively expressed. That's all. Your weight is just one small factor in the complex picture that is you.

When standing up straight with your feet touching, examine the shape and tone of your stomach, your hips, your buttocks, your thighs, your upper arms, and your calves. Does your body hang down where it should stand up, or cave in where it should stand out? Are your bones obvious, or completely hidden? Are the shapes of your muscles visible, or are they indistinguishable? Look at your overall body profile.

Does it need some trimming or some fleshing out? Write your general impression here:

_____

_____

_____

Power Parts

You've got two areas of your body where strength is of the utmost importance. Without strength in these two areas, you will find it difficult to be strong anywhere else. I'm talking about your legs and your heart.

Geo's Journey

Muscles mean movement. Muscles are responsible for almost all movement of the body, internal and external. Muscles help you breathe, move, digest, excrete, and keep your skeleton from tumbling to the ground. Muscles make up approximately 50 percent of your total weight and use most of the energy from food and oxygen you take in. You have over 600 muscles in your body. Keep them strong, flexible, and in motion, and your body will be powerful!

Leg Strength

Power Yoga builds strength in the legs first. The buttock muscles, or *gluteus maximus*, are the largest muscles in your body. These muscles help to move and rotate the thigh muscles outward, and give your movements tremendous power. The thigh muscles, or four *quadriceps* muscles, are the largest muscle group in the body. These muscles help you to extend your knee and help to power movements from squatting to standing. These areas must be strong to form a solid base for the body, providing a foundation of strength for all other movements. This is why we concentrate on standing routines and lunges before we work on smaller areas like the back and arms.

These are the muscles that move you! Concentrate your efforts here first and everything else you do will take less effort. A magnificent statue will fall over if it doesn't have a strong, solid base.

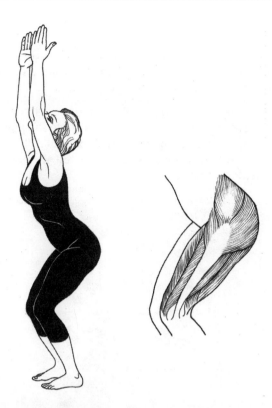

The muscles of the hips and the thighs provide a strong foundation of strength.

Heart Strength

Your heart is a complex, four-chambered, fist-sized muscle in your chest. Without it, your body can't function. The heart pumps blood through the body's arteries, veins, and capillaries, nourishing the internal organs and facilitating all the processes of the body.

Heart strength and leg strength are closely related. The large muscles in your legs work to pump blood back up to the heart, which mostly sends blood downward. The heart supplies the legs with the blood and nutrients they require, and the legs return the favor. Think of your legs as the heart of your lower half.

When these two parts work together, you're talking about real power. Nutrients, oxygen, and glucose can freely circulate to every part of your body, from your scalp to your toenails! Muscles will be nourished, and better able to flex, contract, and strengthen.

Power Words

The **gluteus maximus** is the buttock muscle, the largest muscle in the body. It extends from the lower back to the top of the thigh and is responsible for extending and rotating the thigh and supporting and extending the knee. The **quadriceps** muscles are the largest muscle group, which include the rectus femoris, the vastus lateralis, the vastus intermedius, and the vastus medialis. These four thigh muscles extend the leg at the knee.

Muscle Testing and Mind Power

You can do a lot to keep your body in shape, physically. But did you know that your mind alone can undo much of that hard work? It's true. Your mind has a strong affect on your body and its ability to move, be strong, and stay healthy.

I've seen the effects of mind power on the body myself. I've mentioned before that I used to perform muscle tests in front of my yoga classes, to demonstrate the power of the mind on muscle strength. For me, muscle testing was a teaching tool. When I spoke in a positive manner to the person I was testing, his muscles would test stronger. When I spoke in a negative manner, his muscles would test weaker.

Muscle testing is a simple process that you can try at home. All you need is a partner and a little imagination.

Try muscle testing with a partner.

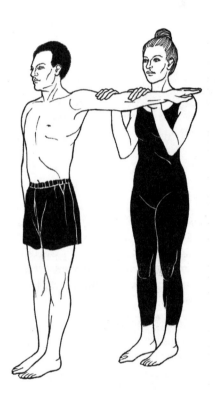

How to Muscle-Test Yourself

At home, you can try the same experiment we performed at the Ashram. Here's how it works:

> ➤ One partner stands up straight and lifts one arm out to the side, palm down, so the arm is parallel with the floor. The other partner places his or her hand on

the arm and gently pushes it down. Both partners should notice how much work it takes to push the arm down.

➤ Now, have the testee think negative thoughts. These can be anything, from imagining the taste of some unpleasant food to a confrontation with an unpleasant person. Test again. In most cases, the arm will be easier to press down.

➤ Now, try the test one more time, after the testee thinks positive thoughts. The most effective are to think about a loved one. The muscle will usually test stronger, the arm becoming more difficult to push down.

You can try variations on this test as well. Have the tester say negative and positive things, or simply think negative and positive thoughts without telling the testee what the thoughts are.

Indra Devi and the Power of the Word

My teacher, Indra Devi, used to perform a similar demonstration with muscle tests. The last time I saw her do this was at a yoga conference in Marietta, California, in the early 1990s.

Indra Devi is a small woman, and she would usually choose a rather large volunteer. She would ask him to hold his arm straight out to the side, and she would try to push the arm down. Not only could she not push the arm down, she could even swing on the arm!

Then, she would ask the volunteer to leave the room for a few minutes. Then, she would have the entire class think negative thoughts. When the volunteer returned, he had no idea what went on in the room when he was gone, but when Indra Devi tested him again, guess what? She could push his arm down easily. Somehow, the negative energy in the room had weakened the man's muscles, even though consciously, he didn't know the negative energy was there! His muscles knew. His body could sense it. That's how powerful our thoughts can be. They can work for or against our health.

To return the volunteer to a state of strength, Indra Devi would have him leave the room again. She then instructed the class to fill the room with our positive thoughts. And when the volunteer returned, he was strong. She could swing on his arm, once again!

You can use this power to your benefit, or to your detriment. Positive thoughts and a positive attitude can enhance your fitness efforts, and a negative attitude can foil your most dedicated attempts toward health. Isn't it worth trying to cultivate a positive attitude and fill the universe with thoughts of goodness?

Geo's Journey

The notion that the mind and the body are connected isn't just a matter of mystical speculation. In fact, a new field called psychoneuroimmunology studies how the body's immune system is partially regulated by the nervous system, which regulates the brain. In other words, the brain is linked to the immune system. This field of study finally makes clear, in "scientific" ways, that what we think and feel, and what happens to us, can all impact the state of our health.

Attitude Adjustment: Do You Need One?

Indra Devi's telling demonstration brings me to the last aspect of our self-analysis, which has to do with what's going on in your mind. What were you thinking as you surveyed your physical body and its current state? Where you berating yourself for being in such lousy shape, or where you getting fired up about improving your health? Are you a "glass-is-half-full" or "glass-is-half-empty" type?

How you perceive yourself and your experiences can make a huge difference in how effective any efforts toward improving your health will be. Constant negativity can undermine the most rigorous fitness program, while a positive outlook can make the most out of even small movements and steps toward better health.

Do you need an attitude adjustment? Take this quiz and find out.

Attitude Quiz

Choose the answer that sounds the most like you:

1. You've got your whole day mapped out: go to the gym, grab breakfast, go to the office, lunch with friends, a brisk walk after work, then a trip to the market on the way home. You get up early, put on your workout clothes, and get into the car. It won't start. What do you do?

    A. The whole day is ruined. Now you'll have to sit around and wait for someone to come fix the car; you won't get to the gym; you'll be late for work; your coworkers will be annoyed; you won't be in the mood for a social lunch; and you'll be in no state to go to the market because you certainly won't want to cook. Just your luck!

B. Run back inside, call someone to jump-start your car, and, as long as you've got your workout clothes on already, take a brisk run around the neighborhood. After the car is started, take a quick shower and head off to work feeling great. Maybe a nice stir-fry for dinner tonight...

2. You've got a great new plan for how to improve things at work, but your boss isn't impressed. What do you do?

A. Your boss may not have given your presentation her full attention—she does have a lot going on right now. But why not look your ideas over to see if you can make them even better? Then you can present a fresh approach, because you really have confidence your ideas are great!

B. How typical, to have your great ideas ignored again. Your boss must have it in for you. She's a rotten boss, anyway, and doesn't know quality when she sees it. Well, you might as well just forget the whole thing. If they don't want to use your ideas, it's their loss.

3. You've gained five pounds without realizing it, and your clothes feel a little tight and uncomfortable. What do you do?

A. Come to think of it, you haven't been spending much time moving around lately. Too much sitting! You decide to take a long walk in the fresh air and have a light dinner. You go to bed feeling great.

B. Oh, that's just wonderful. Now, on top of all your other stress, you're getting fat. Well, you're probably destined to gain weight as you get old, so you might as well accept that your prime is past and order that big, gooey dessert.

4. You're having a bad day. Everything seems to be going wrong. Everything takes more time than you planned, a huge unexpected expense arises, and a friend snaps at you. You go home exhausted. What do you do?

A. Arrange for some serious personal time. Take a long, hot bath, listen to relaxing music, take a leisurely walk in the park, call a trusted friend to talk over your feelings, meditate. Remind yourself that tomorrow will be better and life is full of challenges.

B. Snap back at everyone you meet, go home and fume, then stay up late staring at the television because you aren't in the mood to deal with anything or anybody.

5. You began your new exercise class with high hopes. You would become strong, fit, and healthy. But after a few minutes, you are huffing and puffing. This is harder than you thought! What do you do?

    A. Forget this. This is too hard. Everyone else is better at this than you are! You watch the clock and make plans to quit and try something easier.

    B. A challenge! You slow the pace and try to adapt the movements to your own fitness level. You watch the teacher and the other students for inspiration. Someday soon you'll be able to move like that!

Now, tally your answers as follows:

1.:	A: 0 points	B: 1 point
2.:	A: 1 point	B: 0 points
3.:	A: 1 point	B: 0 points
4.:	A: 1 point	B: 0 points
5.:	A: 0 points	B: 1 point

Your score: _____

If you scored between zero points and two points: You need an attitude adjustment, all right. Small challenges throw you off, and big challenges destroy your day. You tend to see the negative in events and in yourself before you see the positive. I could just say, "change!" but I know it isn't that easy. Everyone has certain tendencies, and you are who you are. In some cases, pessimism can even be beneficial. You are probably cautious, prudent, even street-smart.

On the other hand, extreme pessimism can make a good day seem miserable and can quickly sap a life full of potential. You can begin making small changes in your life to help you see the brighter side. Remember, you are the one who attaches "good" and "bad" to your life experiences. Even when something is, in your mind, clearly "bad," fume for awhile, then sit down and consciously try to see what good could come of your situation. Make a real list if you have to, then act on it. A positive attitude is, to a large extent, a matter of retraining. It just takes a little effort. You may always tend to be a pessimist, but that doesn't mean you can't take control of your mindset and make it more productive.

If you scored a three: You are straddling the fence between optimism and pessimism. When you are in the mood for it, you can see the bright side and rally your internal forces to make the best of any situation. When you aren't in the mood, however, watch out. You can be as irritable and self-doubting as can be. You have an advantage over a full-time pessimist, however. You know what it feels like to take the up-side. Conscious effort to be positive even when you don't feel like it will make any situation better, less damaging to your psyche, and more productive for your life. Keep working on those optimism skills!

If you scored between four and five: You are an optimist who doesn't have too much of a problem seeing the bright side of any situation. Sure, sometimes you feel down, but most of the time, you take the positive route. You probably consider yourself a happy person, in general, and as you work toward better health and a higher level of physical and spiritual fitness, you'll find that your natural aptitude for optimism makes the road a lot sunnier. You can maximize your body's potential! But I don't have to tell you that. You already know you can do it.

Powering Your Practice

Working with a combination of a positive attitude, dedication, and an awareness of your current fitness level is the key to powering your Power Yoga practice. Listen to your body, progress at a pace that makes sense for you and lessens the likelihood of injury, and fill your mind and the room around you with positive thoughts. Concentrate on your weak areas, build a base of leg strength and cardiovascular fitness, keep one eye on the mirror to assess your progress, and keep working. Power Yoga is a lifelong commitment, and the fun is in the process. You'll just keep getting stronger, healthier, and more alive. What a way to live!

The Least You Need to Know

➤ Assess your current fitness level so you know where to start, how fast to progress, and what areas need the most work.

➤ Your posture, spine shape, eyes, skin, hair, and weight all reveal your current fitness level and state of health.

➤ Build leg strength first to provide a strong base for all other physical activity.

➤ A positive attitude can increase muscle strength and eventually overall health. A negative attitude can decrease muscle strength and eventually overall health.

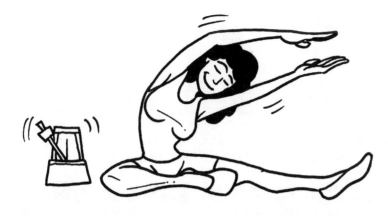

Chapter 4

Power Pacing

In This Chapter

➤ The importance of starting slow

➤ Where are you strong, where are you weak?

➤ A body lesson

➤ Locating your gastrocnemius (and your other muscles, too)

In addition to an understanding of your personal fitness level, you need two things to help you most effectively proceed on your journey toward better health: smart pacing and body knowledge. This chapter is about pacing and also about the body.

Pacing is a crucial part of any fitness program, including Power Yoga. If you do too much too fast, you're going to get hurt. If you don't know your body, you're going to get hurt. And if you get hurt, you'll probably end up sitting on the sidelines with a bag of ice or a heating pad on whatever body part you've injured, wishing you were back in the game and wondering why your body broke down. Getting injured is no fun, and it certainly isn't an indication that you are "giving it your all" or a sign of your dedication to your sport or fitness program. It is only a sign that you weren't listening to your body.

Body knowledge is equally crucial. The more you know about the human body, including the locations and movements of the various muscles, bones, and joints, the better you'll understand how your own body moves and what your individual potential is. We'll wind up this chapter with a mini anatomy lesson. Don't worry, I'm not talking about a boring lesson irrelevant to your life. Anatomy is about you, your body, your muscles, your bones, your ability to move, grow, and be alive!

Fly Like an Eagle

First let's get back to the concept of pacing. I used to love a yoga pose often called the eagle pose. It involves standing on one leg and wrapping the other leg around the standing leg, then coiling both arms around each other. Then one day I was having my class do this pose, and a student popped her knee out. I rushed over and popped her knee back into place. I still remember the sound. After that experience, I wasn't quite as fond of the eagle pose as I had been.

I have since modified the pose to be done in a prone position in conjunction with a sit-up exercise, a movement I call eagle crunchers. However, I'm not saying the eagle pose is a bad pose; it is simply an advanced pose, and isn't for someone just starting out.

Eagle crunchers are a modified version of sit-ups in which the arms and legs are twisted around each other. This pose is safer for the beginner than a standing eagle pose.

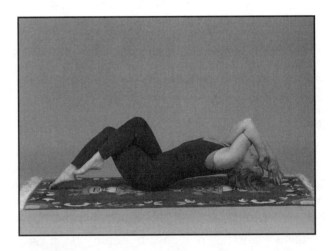

Why Start Slow?

I've already warned you about the possibility of injury when you push your body into movements it isn't ready for, but that isn't the only reason to start slow. Everyone has certain strengths and certain weaknesses—even the fitness gurus you see on television. You might not yet know where your weaknesses are, so a careful progression can uncover what areas need more attention before those areas are given more than they can handle.

Also, because yoga is by nature non-competitive, a slower pace will help you keep from competing with your fellow power yogis, or even with yourself. Move with an attitude of harmlessness. Yoga isn't a game to "win" or "lose." It is organic fitness, movement as it was meant to be, as the body requires to stay healthy.

The mind benefits from a careful pace as well. Attempting movements beyond your current fitness level can engender frustration—a negative emotion that won't help your practice or your stress level. You'll be more likely to view your yoga experience as unpleasant, and you'll probably give up. When your mind is telling you to slow down, listen! Keep it feeling great—challenging, but great.

Where to Begin

How do you know what level is right for you? We've labeled all our Power Yoga series and poses with difficulty levels from I to V, but are you a I, a II, a IV? How can you tell?

A little experiment is in order. Start with the very first poses, the poses in level I. Don't just assume they'll be easy. Really work on them seriously for a while, until you feel very confident that you have mastered the basics. Then move up to the IIs. Master those. And so on.

When you get to a level where you can't actually perform the series as pictured in the book, try some of the modifications I suggest to make the poses more basic. If you still find them too difficult, step back a level. You've found your limit.

Work at this level. Keep up the basic work on these poses, but continue to cultivate the poses that are slightly above your ability. Keep practicing. Like anything else, the more you practice, the better you'll get. When at last you've mastered poses you couldn't perform at first, you'll feel a great sense of accomplishment, and your reward will be moving to the next level.

Your Power Practice

Once you've determined your fitness level and the level of poses and pose series you are able to perform safely, you can begin to develop your own power practice. Remember, the key to yoga is to work on your weaker areas, to bring your whole system into balance.

The Wrong Moves

Never apply heat to an injury that is swelling, such as a sprained ankle. Heat increases swelling. Reserve heat for areas that need to relax, such as cramped muscles, and put an ice pack on areas that are swelling. Better yet, avoid injury by moving within your limits!

The Right Moves

Some athletes swear that visualizing themselves successfully performing an activity before the actual performance—whether the execution of a Power Yoga routine or a game of basketball—greatly increases the body's ability to perform. Before you begin your workout, spend a few minutes relaxing, eyes closed, and picturing yourself moving through your activity of choice with strength, power, and skill. You might be surprised at the results!

In the previous chapter, you already pinpointed some of the areas you think need a little more work. Here are a few more pointers to help you determine which body parts and which chakras (see Chapter 9, "Chakras and the Power of Color," for more about chakras) need to become more of a focus during your workout.

What Do You Protect?

One way to tell if an area is weaker is that your body will protect it. People with heart disease tend to roll their shoulders inward, protecting their hearts. When you injure something, your body tends to protect the area, bending over it, rubbing it, covering it.

The Wrong Moves

Some of the exercises in this book are very challenging. I've labeled these as level V poses. Please don't attempt these poses before you are ready. Work up to them so they are only a small step away from the poses you've mastered, rather than a giant leap.

If you stand in front of a mirror and consciously survey your posture, as you did in the last chapter, it may not be immediately apparent what your body subconsciously protects because you will be aware that you are looking at yourself, and you'll be standing up straight. A better way to "catch" yourself in protective mode is to glance at yourself in a mirror, or even a storefront window, as you are walking along naturally attending to your business.

You might be surprised how different you look when you catch a glimpse of yourself. Any time you look in the mirror, you probably prepare yourself first, even if you don't realize it. Your face and your body get ready to be seen. Catching yourself unaware is a whole different story, however. Don't be surprised if you see a surprising slump, a poochy stomach, swayed-back hips, a lopsided stance, hunched-up shoulders, even a strangely blank expression. Yikes! Is that you?

On the other hand, you might be pleased with what you see. Just be sure you catch yourself when you aren't getting ready to be seen.

A crooked, swayed, slumped posture is very telling. Where do you slump? Over your stomach, your abdomen, your heart? Each of these areas contains a chakra, or energy center, that emits certain aspects of our personality. The seven primary chakras are located in the lower abdomen, the navel area, at the solar plexus, near the heart, in the throat, in the forehead, and at the crown of the head. Protecting one could mean you have a physical problem in this area. Each chakra is associated with certain gland and organ systems. Each chakra is also associated with certain emotions, feelings, urges, and other less physical aspects of our being.

Geo's Journey

I once took a seminar from Dean Ornish, the renowned physician who has studied the many ways to reverse heart disease. He has seen heart patients who protect their hearts by hunching their shoulders forward, as if their bodies instinctively knew their own weakness. If you've ever watched a boxing match, you know the "boxing stance." Boxers also protect their hearts, their emotional centers, from physical blows by rolling their shoulders inward and placing their arms in front of their bodies.

For example, if you tend to slump your shoulders forward to protect your heart, you could have some emotional issues you aren't allowing to come forward—a "broken heart," or a fear of vulnerability, for instance. Protecting the abdomen could reflect a repression of your more basic, primal instincts. Perhaps you have issues about sex, self-control, or rage. Protecting your stomach could reflect more than digestive difficulties. It could mean you have problems letting things go.

Of course, a slump could just be the result of years of bad posture habits. Only you can determine if your emotional life is reflected in your posture. Check out Chapters 9, "Chakras and the Power of Color," and 10, "Chakra Testing for Power Healing," for more information on what the various chakras mean. For now, just become aware of what areas you are protecting, and use your intuition to determine what your protection instincts say about the bigger picture of you.

Strong Parts

Although bringing balance to your system is the order of the day, it won't hurt to notice, and even feel proud of, your strengths. Don't just focus on what is lacking in your self-analysis. Where are you strong?

Do you throw your shoulders back proudly and lead with your solar plexus, ready to meet the world and all its challenges with gusto? Is your stomach a seat of strength for your body? Are your legs powerful and strong? Do your hair and eyes reflect glowing health? Do you stand up tall? Don't be afraid to relish your strengths as you work to balance your whole self. Feeling good about yourself will make you a more positive person, and confidence is an important part of any plan to attain better health.

Geo's Journey

In her influential book *Don't Shoot the Dog* (Bantam, 1985), behaviorist and animal trainer Karen Pryor describes the benefits of positive reinforcement for training anything, including yourself. She tells the story of a friend who decided to use positive reinforcement to improve his racquetball game. Instead of cursing himself every time he made a mistake, he praised himself every time he did something right—even patting himself on the back when no one was looking. Soon his game was so improved that he was beating opponents who, not long before, were playing far above his ability. Why not try the technique on yourself? The next time you do something well, let yourself know: "That was a beautiful wheel pose! Look how flexible I've become! Congratulations, me!"

See It, Strengthen It

The next step to bringing your system into balance is to know how to gain strength in the areas you have identified as weak. Knowing your shoulders roll forward is one thing. Knowing your latissimus dorsi muscle in your back or your deltoid muscle in your shoulder needs more work is quite another.

If you can visualize a specific muscle, joint, or organ, knowing what it looks like, where it is, and exactly what it does, you'll find that physical activity takes on a whole new dimension. You'll be able to target your mental efforts more specifically to the area you are working. Visualizing a particular muscle becoming stronger as you work it can really make a difference in your rate of progress and the way you feel about your body.

With that premise in mind, I'd like to introduce you to your body on a whole new level.

A Body Lesson

A lot of people like to compare a body to a machine. I'm not so sure I like the comparison, because a machine doesn't have consciousness, and our physical natures are so interwoven with our consciousness that they can never be completely distinguished from one another. Yet, to some extent, bodies are like machines—self-aware machines, perhaps, which makes them even more complex and awe-inspiring than a computer.

Your body is, on a basic level, a skeleton filled with and surrounded by organs that regulate the entire system, connected by a vast network of connective tissue, nerves, and blood vessels of all sizes, then covered with skin and hair. No part of your body exists on its own. Each organ has its jobs to do. While the circulatory system nourishes the whole, the nervous system is hard-wired to let us think, act, feel, and move according to cues from the external world.

Any system this complex is bound to have a few glitches here and there—we all have them. No body is flawless, although you might think some look that way. Occasionally, bodies fall prey to infections and viruses. Tendons and ligaments can become strained, sprained, or torn. Bones can break. Muscles can become strained. The kidney, the liver, the pancreas, the heart, the lungs can all malfunction. The skin can become injured and bleed. The circulation can become blocked and areas of our bodies can become nutrient-starved, for a short while or permanently. We can feel pain and not know why.

When you are down with a sprain or the flu or something worse, you may feel like bodies don't work very well at all. But think what your body is still able to do! Look how it is fighting to heal you!

In general, the whole system is pretty miraculous. Let's take a closer look.

Anatomy 101

Many of you probably took an anatomy class sometime during the course of your education, but you might not remember exactly what anatomy is all about. *Anatomy* is the study of the structure of the body and each of its parts.

To be a more effective practitioner of Power Yoga, you don't need detailed knowledge of anatomy, but some basics sure help when you are moving those parts in ways you've never moved them before. So, here are the basics:

Power Words

Anatomy is the study of the structure of bodies, including humans, other animals, and plants.

➤ On a very basic level, you are a collection of cells. These cells perform chemical reactions that take nutrients—food—and turn them into energy, then get rid of whatever is left over that the body doesn't need. This process is called metabolism.

➤ The next level is tissue. Cells form all the tissues of the body, which include skin, connective tissue, and membranes, which hold everything in and bind everything together; cartilage and bone; muscle tissue; nerve tissue; and the liquids of the body, such as blood and lymph. Tissues are the nuts and bolts of the body, or the "ingredients" of the body's physical structure.

➤ Made of tissue, but each with its own function, the body contains organs—including the brain, heart, lungs, kidneys, liver, pancreas, eyes, stomach, sex organs, glands, and skin.

➤ Organs also work together, forming organ systems: the skeletal system, the muscular system, the circulatory system, the nervous system, the endocrine system, the digestive system, the respiratory system, the excretory system, and the reproductive system.

➤ The next level is the external aspect of the body. Human bodies have a head with a skull that holds the brain and is fronted by the face. A spine extends down from the head, and along the spine are the thorax or chest area, the abdomen, and the pelvic girdle, or hips. Bodies also have extremities: arms, wrists, hands, legs, ankles, feet.

Whenever you move, all aspects of your anatomy are involved. Your skin moves to accommodate you. Your skeleton is moved by your muscles, which move according to cues from your brain. Your organs are along for the ride, of course, and every body part may become pushed, pressed, expanded, contracted, flexed, strengthened, or stimulated, depending on what kind of movements you make.

Even though your whole body is involved when you do Power Yoga, certain parts are certainly more involved, and more instrumental in helping you to become stronger and more vital. Your muscles are probably the tissues most intensely affected by Power Yoga, and the circulatory system is the most directly affected organ system, although other systems, such as your immune system and your skin, will enjoy a host of positive effects as well.

Geo's Journey

Visualization is a powerful skill. Your brain can affect your body processes, helping them along or hindering them. Biofeedback is a perfect example. You learn to "feel" certain internal processes, such as your heart rate or blood pressure, and can then affect them with your consciousness. Several studies in which surgical patients were taught how to visualize specific healing actions revealed that these patients recovered more quickly from surgery. Why not use this power to increase the benefits of Power Yoga?

As we get into the series of poses themselves, I'll be clueing you in to which aspects of your anatomy are involved in which poses. One pose might strengthen your quadriceps muscles. If you can visualize your thigh muscles becoming stronger as you perform the movement, with the knowledge of how these muscles look and move, you can help your body strengthen this area. If you can feel the oxygen-rich blood flooding your brain during a headstand and visualize it as it happens, your brain may benefit to an even greater degree.

Physiology: To Live Is to Move

When you are thinking about anatomy, don't forget about *physiology.* Anatomy studies the actual structures of the body, but physiology looks at how those structures move, interact, and function. Muscle anatomy is knowing where the muscles are and what they are called. Muscle physiology is understanding how the muscles move.

In the next section, we'll give you a brief description of both: muscle names and locations and muscle movements. First, however, a little movement vocabulary will help you:

➤ **Extension.** Increasing an angle at a joint. For example, coming out of the chair pose increases the angle of the knee from bent to straight.

Power Words

Physiology is the study of the processes and mechanisms of life in humans, other animals, and plants.

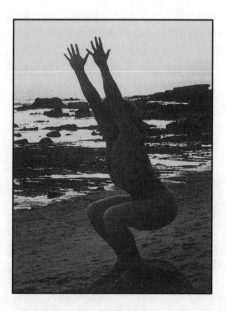

In chair pose, the legs are bent at the knee. Coming out of chair pose to a standing position involves extension of the knee joint.

➤ **Flexion.** Decreasing an angle at a joint, such as the angle between your thigh and lower leg, by drawing the lower leg up toward the thigh. Moving into the spear thrower position decreases the angle at the knee as you lunge forward.

In spear thrower pose, the leg bends at the knee joint as the body lunges over the front leg, causing flexion in the knee joint. The arms move away from the midline of the body, an example of abduction; and when coming out of the pose, the arms move back toward the body, an example of adduction.

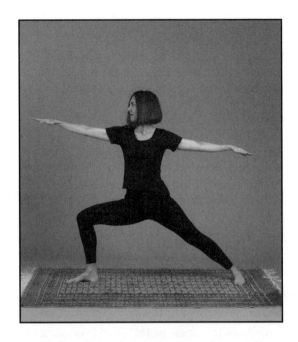

➤ **Rotation.** Revolving a body part on an axis, such as rotating your head to look to the right or left. Some rotation is called external or internal, depending on whether the motion moves the body part away from or toward a midline. An example of a midline is a line between your two feet. Turning your feet outward is external rotation; turning your feet inward, toward the midline, is internal rotation. Rotating your head at the neck to look up in angle pose is an example of rotation.

In angle pose, the head rotates on the neck to look up toward the extended arm.

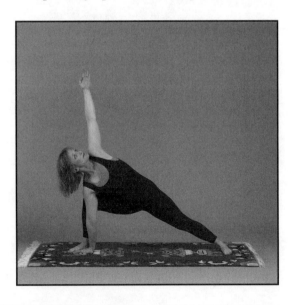

➤ **Abduction.** To move a body part away from the midline. For example, imagine a line through the center of your body. Lifting your arms out to the side away from this line, as you would for the spear thrower movement (see preceding photo), would be abduction.

➤ **Adduction.** To move a body part toward the midline. Returning the arms to the sides as you move out of the spear thrower movement (see photo on previous page) would be adduction.

➤ **Pronation.** To move a body part downward, toward the floor. For example, turning your torso toward the floor in the bent knee forward bend.

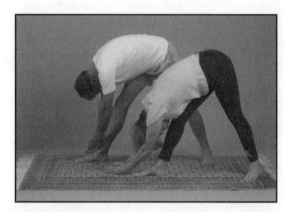

In bent knee forward bend, the torso moves toward the floor, an example of pronation.

➤ **Supination.** To move a body part upward, toward the sky. For example, turning your torso upward, as in revolving triangle.

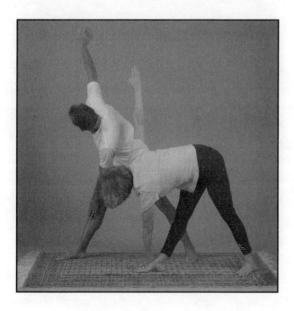

In revolving triangle, the torso turns upward, an example of supination.

➤ **Protraction.** To move a body part forward, such as opening the chest in exalted warrior.

In exalted warrior, the chest moves forward, an example of protraction.

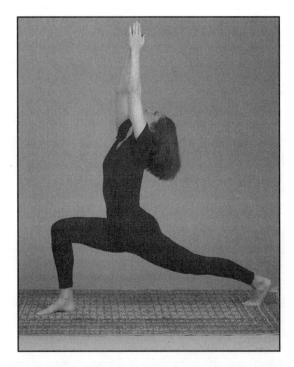

➤ **Retraction.** To move a body part backward, such as caving in the chest with cat pose.

In cat pose, the chest caves in, an example of retraction.

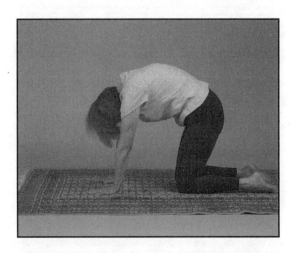

Learning the Perfect Body

No body is the same as any other body, of course, but at some level, we are all perfect, unique, and special. Of course, we all have certain individual physical strengths and areas that need to build strength. To best know your physical body, follow a general model of the muscles of the body. The major muscles, the ones I'll mention frequently when describing how to move in and out of Power Yoga movements, are labeled in the following list. Study them and refer back to the following illustrations often. When performing a Power Yoga movement series in which these muscles are used, remember these illustrations and visualize how the muscles are moving in your own body.

Following the illustrations is a description of each of the major muscles and what they do. We'll move from front to back as we work our way down, showing you the muscles that balance each other.

> **The Wrong Moves**
>
> Muscle strains, the most common muscle injury, occur when muscles are torn or pulled. Strains can range from a few over-stretched muscle fibers and a little pain to actual muscle tears that you can feel on the outside of the skin, loss of muscle function, and severe pain. Avoid muscle strains by warming up with slow, controlled movements before attempting larger, faster movements.

➤ *Sternocleidomastoid* is the neck muscle that runs along the front of your neck from your ear to your chest. It helps you to flex your neck and rotate your head.

➤ *Splenius capitis* is one of the larger neck muscles responsible for rotating the head and drawing it back.

➤ *Trapezius* is a large muscle that attaches along your spine and stretches all the way over your shoulder to your collarbone. This large muscle helps move your shoulder blades, and also your head.

➤ *Deltoid* is the large, rounded muscle that covers the top of your shoulder. This muscle is largely responsible for the movements of your shoulders and arms.

➤ *Biceps* is the large muscle in your upper arm that you think of when you imagine people "showing some muscle." This muscle flexes and supinates (turns upward) the forearm.

➤ *Triceps* is the smaller muscle on the back of the arm that balances the biceps. The triceps muscle helps to extend the forearm.

➤ *Pectoralis major* is the primary chest muscle, extending from the center of your ribcage to your underarm. This muscle is also influential in moving the arm, primarily in forward and downward motions.

➤ *Rhomboids* are on the other side, helping to power the upper back. These muscles help to move the shoulder blade toward the spine.

➤ *Latissimus dorsi* wraps around the torso from front to back, moving the arm backward and downward and rotating the arm inward.

➤ *Rectus abdominis* are the stomach muscles that run vertically, from the pubic bone to the ribs. This muscle helps to flex your torso and tense your abdomen. These muscles are also used in certain yoga breathing exercises (see Chapter 24, "Breath of Life").

➤ *Transverse abdominis* is the abdominal muscle that runs horizontally, tensing the abdomen from the pubic area up through the lower ribs.

➤ *Internal* and *external obliques* are the muscles along the sides of the torso that flex the upper torso and spinal column.

➤ *Gluteus maximus* is the "buns" muscle, and the largest muscle in the body. It abducts, rotates, and extends the thigh.

➤ *Gluteus medius* runs along the side of the hip and abducts and rotates the thigh.

➤ *Quadriceps* are the four muscles of the thigh, and the largest muscle group in the body. These muscles extend the knee joint.

➤ *Biceps femoris, semitendinosus,* and *semimembranosus* are the three muscles that make up what is commonly called the "hamstrings." These muscles flex the knee and extend the hip.

➤ *Gastrocnemius* is the muscle of the calf. This muscle helps to flex the knee and the foot.

➤ *Achilles tendon,* while not a muscle, is nonetheless instrumental to movement and an important area to keep limber and flexible. This tendon attaches the gastrocnemius or calf muscle to the heel bone.

As you read about each muscle, find its location on your own body. Feel it. Move it. Flex and contract it. Get to know your muscle, and they'll respond. Give them what they need to become strong and flexible—challenging movement appropriate for your fitness level, good nutrition, and your attention—and they will transform your body.

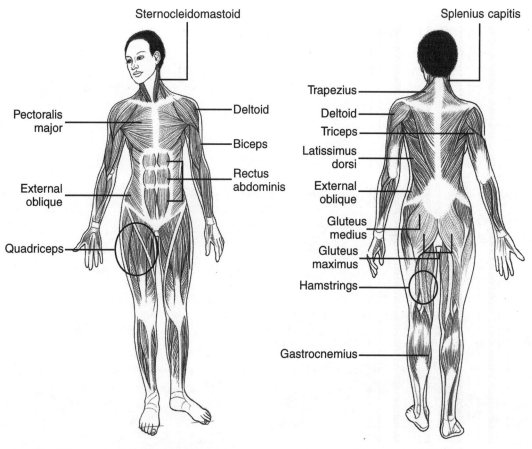

The major muscles, front and back.

The Least You Need to Know

➤ Moving beyond what is appropriate for your fitness level risks injury and frustration.

➤ Analyze the weak spots and strengths of your physical body for a smarter and more enlightened approach to your Power Yoga workout.

➤ A basic familiarity with anatomy and physiology will make your workout more effective. Learn where your muscles are and what they do.

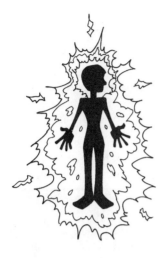

Chapter 5

A Word About Energy

> ### In This Chapter
>
> ➤ What is energy?
>
> ➤ Prana, chi, and the life force
>
> ➤ Cultivating your force for life

A book about yoga wouldn't be complete if it didn't discuss energy. Energy means different things to different people, but to yogis all over the world, energy is something very specific, powerful, universal—the power behind yoga, the power behind human life, even the power fueling the universe.

What is this mysterious force? Does it have something to do with your "get up and go" (or lack thereof) each morning? Sure. Does it have something to do with your will to stay alive and thrive even under adverse conditions? You bet it does. Does it have anything to do with the proliferation of life on this planet? That, too. But I'm getting ahead of myself. Let's talk first about what we Westerners generally think of when we hear the term "energy."

Energy Potential

Energy is a hot commodity these days. You hear about it all the time. Save energy, get more energy, eat this for energy, don't eat this or you'll lose energy, spend energy to get energy. But what is energy? You can't touch it. You can't point to it and say, "Look! There it goes!" It doesn't have a color or a shape.

Power Words

Metabolism is the process in living things by which food is broken down to release energy.

Is it *metabolism?* Metabolism has to do with energy. It is the rate at which your body burns nutrients to make energy. But energy is more than calories burned.

Is it heat? Exercise teachers are always telling you to "warm up" before you exercise. Heat is one form of energy, but you can be quite warm and not feel very energetic, so that's not very helpful.

Is it an attitude? Attitude can help your energy, but if your energy level is truly depressed, you'll be disappointed if you think you can just "think yourself out of it."

Is it something that comes from exercise? Exercise can certainly boost energy, as well as mood. Studies show it can help alleviate the effects of depression and many regular exercisers claim they wouldn't have the energy to get through the day without their daily workout. You've probably noticed that the less you exercise, the less energy you have.

But exercise isn't the only factor, either. All these factors—metabolism, heat, attitude, movement—affect the ebb and flow of energy in your body. But what is the energy itself?

Geo's Journey

One of my favorite exercises, besides Power Yoga, is hiking. I love to hike in the mountains, and I often take groups of people from the Ashram on long hikes. Hiking is a great exercise because it not only gives the body a great workout, but it allows your body to take in fresh, pure, clean air (rather than stale, indoor "gym" air, as you might breathe at a health club). It also allows you to exercise surrounded by breathtaking natural beauty, which is great exercise for the soul. If you don't live near the mountains, a walk outside in a park, by a river, in the country, or even around your neighborhood can also be soul-inspiring and great for your energy level.

Energy = Living

Energy is a nebulous term. Even the dictionary's definition is somewhat of an enigma. My dictionary calls it "force of expression," with a second definition, "inherent power; capacity for action." I like "inherent power," but even that doesn't quite say it all.

Energy is waiting inside us to be released and used. It is also all around us. Just ask a physicist. Potential energy surrounds a ball at the top of a slope, an unlit match, a rocket. Potential energy surrounds us and waits within us, too.

But how do we activate it? How do we push the ball, light the match, launch the rocket? It may help to learn a little about the nature of energy.

In the short term, energy is like a resource that you use until it is gone. You run until you are tired, lift weights until your muscles are exhausted, stay awake until you can't stay awake any longer. In the long term, however, energy behaves quite differently. The more you use it, the more you have. Using energy actually prompts your body to generate more.

And if you don't use energy? If you stop taking in energy, and stop expending it? Eventually, you die. In other words, energy equals living. Not life, the noun, but living, the verb. Energy is vitality.

Many cultures have observed this phenomenon and have attempted to harness energy's amazing quality of proliferation. Many names have been bestowed upon energy. These words sometimes also refer to a person's inner spirit, or the spark that indicates life.

The yoga word for energy is *prana* (pronounced *PRAH-nah*). Other cultures have different names for it. For example, the Chinese call it *chi* (pronounced *chee*). Although you'll probably find varying definitions for both prana and chi depending on where you look, I see them as different words and interpretations of the same thing: the life force energy that fills us, surrounds us, and flows through the universe.

Force for Living

One way this force manifests itself is in the force to live. We all have the instinct to live, the survival instinct. All organisms, from tiny, one-celled organisms to giant blue whales have it—and we are no exception.

You may have heard lots of stories about people doing incredible things either to stay alive or to save someone else's life—the mother lifting the car off her child, the cancer patient overcoming unbeatable odds. Whether they knew it or not, these people were

The Wrong Moves

Your posture can have a dramatic affect on your energy level, so make a conscious effort not to slouch! A slumped posture blocks energy from moving freely through your body. Sit or stand straight and tall, as if you are hanging from the ceiling by a thread attached to the crown of your head, and feel your energy rev up immediately.

Power Words

Prana is the Sanskrit word for energy, while **chi** is the Chinese term. Both refer to energy that flows through the body and also exists outside the body in everything around us.

using prana's potential. Their force to live overpowered other forces working against them.

I used to have a dog named Teko. He was a wonderful, beautiful, big Samoyed, with a glorious, snowy white coat. About six months after I got him, he started having trouble walking. His back legs would cross as he walked. He was clearly in pain, crying all the time.

The vet advised me to put him to sleep. He said he had been born with the worst hips he'd ever seen. Some dogs have a genetic hip condition that gets worse with age and is very painful, and vets often recommend putting these dogs down. They say it is to spare them the pain and the suffering, that they won't have "quality of life."

But I loved this dog. "What is 'quality of life,'" I wondered, "and how can I know whether Teko has it or not?" I wasn't ready to give up on him. I wasn't sure, so I waited, and tried sending him energy. I massaged his hips and touched him constantly, trying to direct my energy into him.

The Right Moves

Try this simple energy-enhancing exercise. Sit comfortably on the floor or in a straight-backed chair, and inhale slowly to a count of five. Then, exhale even more slowly and completely to a count of 10, making a "sss" sound, as if you are a tire leaking air. Continue for five minutes.

Teko didn't seem to be getting better, and I was really struggling with what to do. One day I decided to go hiking and give the matter some serious thought. This was a couple days after the visit with the vet, and his advice was hanging over my head like a cloud. I headed toward a very steep hill. The hill was so steep that it presented a real challenge to me, even though I was in pretty good shape. I actually had to use my hands to climb it, pulling on plants to pull myself up. I thought, "I'll just climb to the top of this hill, really wear myself out, and then maybe I'll be able to think more clearly. Maybe the answer will present itself to me once I've reached the top."

And when I got to the top of the hill, the answer did present itself to me. Teko was there. He'd followed me all the way up that hill, pulling himself up with his front legs. When I got to the top, miraculously, he was there, too, right there with me, and I realized I could not put him to sleep. The dog had a force to live like nothing I've ever seen.

I began to take him on hikes as much as possible, all over the high country. In six to seven months, his body was able to rebuild itself, developing muscles and tissues in places where he didn't have bone. Soon, Teko was running, and for the rest of his long life, he was able to run through the mountains, chase things, and live, live, live. He was an amazing animal because the force for living in him was so powerful.

Maybe you know someone—a person or an animal—in which the force for living is similarly strong. And maybe you know some in which it dwindles at an early age, or never seems very apparent. You can see it in someone's eyes, the sparkle, the light shining out of them makes its existence apparent. Some people might call it charisma. That's the force for living that we all need and seek. We're in this world to live, not just to lie around waiting to die.

I said earlier in this chapter that you can't "see" prana, but in reality, you can see it as it reflects from living things. You can see it in palm trees growing up out of the middle of the freeway, reaching for life. You can see it in people who powerfully manifest themselves, living each moment and finding the joy in being alive despite a physical or mental challenge. That is the nature of power that we're seeking when we practice Power Yoga. We're on a quest to release and free something that is a part of us and something that links us with all of life.

The Right Moves

If you suffer from a chronic medical condition or illness, increasing your life force energy or prana can be a powerful therapy. Don't forget to seek competent medical care, however. Prana can enhance your body's healing efforts, but will do so most effectively if your efforts at healing are guided by a licensed health care professional.

Geo's Journey

I work with prana extensively in my Power Yoga classes, and I often hear yoga teachers and students using the words "life force" and "prana" interchangeably, but even more than "life force," I like to think of prana as a **force toward life.** Just semantics? Not really. Life force, to me, implies something inherent. It's just there, no matter what. But force toward life implies action, movement, a journey toward vitality and the ultimate state of existence. I'll be honest: I don't really know where energy originated. God? The big bang? I'm not a philosopher or a physicist. But I do know that a force for life is out there, and I like to call it "prana."

Prana: Not Just for Yogis Anymore

In yoga, the manipulation and concentration of prana in the body is both an art and a science, and one of the most important parts of a successful yoga practice. Breathing exercises and exercises called *bandhas,* or locks, are used to control prana and draw it into the body, to create greater vitality and energy. Although yoga teaches techniques for drawing prana into the body through the breath, prana isn't the breath. It's something that comes with the breath and runs through the body in

Power Words

Bandhas (pronounced *BAHN-das*), the Sanskrit word for "locks," are exercises used in conjunction with breathing exercises to concentrate and intensify prana within the body. Locks involve setting the body in certain positions—most notably at the chin, the stomach, and the rectum—to keep prana inside and redirect its flow. I'll talk more about bandhas in Chapter 24, "Breath of Life."

Power Words

Sattvic (pronounced *SAHT-vick*) is a term used to describe foods (and other things) that are pure, healthful, and bestowing energy. The word *sattva* is a Hindu word that refers to the purest aspect of the self. Sattvic foods are those that promote life energy, clarity of mind, strength, and inner contentment. Traditionally, these foods are those that are fresh, clean, hearty, nutritious, organic, unprocessed, in natural form, and free of sharp, strong, bitter, pungent, or spicy tastes.

specific ways, depending on our health and how we take care of ourselves.

How you see the energy you have or don't have is largely a matter of perspective. After that breakfast of two doughnuts and two cups of coffee, you feel sapped, drained, void of all energy, no matter what you might call it—prana, chi, whatever. Why?

A nutritionist might say that the empty calories, refined sugar, and caffeine caused your blood sugar to spike, then crash. A doctor might explain why too much sugar puts you at risk for obesity and diabetes. A fitness instructor might say too many calories and not enough protein will add extra body fat which, when coupled with a lack of physical activity, will lead to low energy. And a yogi might say that foods like doughnuts and coffee aren't *sattvic,* or pure, and will drain your prana.

It all comes down to the same thing. How you treat yourself can affect your vitality, which is everything. Eating foods that are close to their natural form, close to the ground, rather than those that have been highly processed or picked and shipped across the country, will increase your vitality, or prana (see Chapter 17, "Thirteen Steps to Natural Living," for more tips on power eating). Moving your body in the ways it was meant to move rather than keeping it static and sedentary all day will increase your prana. Allowing yourself to love others and be loved by others will increase your prana.

Without prana, without vitality, you can't live your life, you can't appreciate the beauty of the world, you can't cherish your loved ones, you can't *move,* and to move is to live. Energy is that important. Isn't it worth pursuing with all the … *energy* you have left?

How to Build Your Prana Power

Power Yoga can help you to bring out your best self, release your potential energy, and be as clear, strong, flexible, open, and naturally powerful as you can be. Power Yoga will maximize your force for living so that it shines out of you like a beacon projecting out into the universe, lighting a path before you.

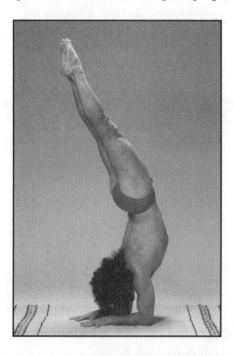

Power Yoga helps you maximize your force for living.

After learning the different movements and the nature of your own body's movements through practice, when you begin to find an internal balance, you'll find that your force for living actually takes over your Power Yoga practice and guides you in which yoga postures you need. At that point, you can create your own routine or flow of movements by following your heart and your energy flow. You'll naturally find the poses that strengthen, stretch, squeeze, turn, or energize the areas most in need of oxygenated blood to keep the life force moving.

But I don't expect you to be at that point just yet. Maximizing your energy is a gradual process. It doesn't happen overnight, and we haven't even started our Power Yoga routines yet! You can begin to maximize your energy by making small changes in your life (see Chapter 17 to read about the 13 steps for natural living). Stand up straight. Cultivate a positive attitude. Eat well. Move. Be open to others, and don't isolate yourself. Don't neglect your spiritual side. Love, and be loved. And it bears repeating: Move!

The Right Moves

Even small changes in your life can increase your energy. Try going one day—just one day—without eating any refined sugar. Studies show that sugar isn't the quick energy boost you may have thought it was. Simple sugars, including table sugar, brown sugar, honey, molasses, and corn syrup, actually promote the production of serotonin in the brain, which has a calming, relaxing effect.

In the next chapter, we get moving. Together, we will start slowly, build a base of strength, and begin to find and release our potential energy, from around us and from inside us. As prana begins to flow more freely in your body and through your life, you'll see how it changes you. You'll feel more alive, more vital, more joyous. Your body will move more easily, and you'll anticipate your workout because of the way it makes you feel.

You'll even find yourself choosing healthier foods and finding the less-pure, more-processed foods you may once have enjoyed less appealing. But again, we'll begin at the beginning. Just turn the page!

The Least You Need to Know

➤ Many cultures have words for energy, but they all refer to the force for living that animates us with vitality.

➤ Prana is the yoga word for energy, and yoga has developed techniques to bring prana into the body and concentrate its power.

➤ A diet of pure, fresh foods and fresh water, regular exercise, a positive attitude, and an open heart will all increase your energy level.

➤ Power Yoga is specifically designed to increase your energy by building a stronger, more flexible body through which energy can flow more freely.

Part 2

First Moves: Developmental Poses for Building Strength

This section starts at the very beginning. You'll move and work, but in ways that won't injure the beginner. These beginning poses, which involve standing, sitting, lying down, twisting, bending, arching, and crawling, will help you build the strength you need for an even more strenuous and challenging workout to come.

We'll also spend time on your chakras. What are they, where are they, and what do they do? I'll tell you. I'll also introduce you to the powerful skill of color healing and show you how to diagnose blockages in your own chakras and begin to open and heal them using a pendulum and a handful of colored stones.

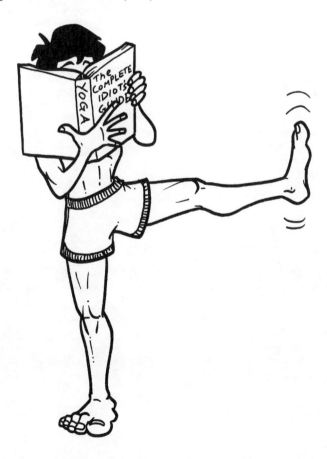

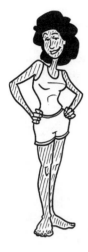

Stand for It

Building a strong, solid base is the most important thing you can do for your Power Yoga routine, and for the strength of your body. Standing in Power Yoga is a truly dynamic experience. You won't be standing casually, jutting out one hip or shifting from foot to foot. The body will remain energized, as you center your weight over your feet and pull upward.

Challenging balance poses may look impressive and a lot more fun than poses labeled "standing poses." If you've flipped through the pictures in this book, you may have spotted a few difficult poses you like. They really are as fun as they look, but don't believe for a moment that I could perform any of them my first time out. Building the strength and balance to achieve these poses took a lot of work, and you know where I started? With standing poses.

Power Stands

As you begin your basic series of poses, keep in mind how your body is constructed, how it moves, and where your center of balance is. The hips are the center of the human body, between the head and the feet. The hips are grounded to the earth, and are the seat of our first chakra, which is our survival center (see Chapters 9, "Chakras and the Power of Color," and 10, "Chakra Testing for Power Healing," for more on chakras). Our appetites come from here, our sex glands are located here, and our most primal emotions come from here. To strengthen this area is to gain control over our survival so that we can live in the best way possible.

Also remember that the area of the heart is the emotional center, where the spirit projects to the world. In the heart, we have the potential to feel good, happy, fearless, and delighted with life. In these basic poses, work on opening the chest by moving the shoulders back rather than hunching them forward. Let your heart open, let your shoulders roll back and away from your chest.

Power Words

Vinyasa (pronounced *vin-YAH-sah*) is the Sanskrit term for a series of yoga poses used in a practice and also for a series of poses performed in a row with flowing movements. The root *vi* means "in a special way," and the root *nyasa* means "to place."

If you are fearless, you will lead with your heart. Your chest will come forward because fear causes the heart to sink in and tighten. The fearful body contracts, as if preparing to be hit. Our hearts sink inward, we roll the shoulders forward, and tighten the muscles in the front of the body. The beautiful arches in the back and the lifting and opening of the heart that draws people to us disappears.

So let's create a routine with these ideas in mind. Once you've mastered the basic stance, which I like to call the Marine pose, you can move on to some basic standing movements. Practice these every day and you'll gain strength and power quickly. Then, you can begin to set up your particular vinyasa, or flow of yoga movements.

The Marine

➤ *Difficulty Level:* I

➤ *Powers:* The posture; also the back, the legs, the neck; frees the breath by allowing more room for the air you inhale.

➤ *Caution:* This pose looks easy, but standing up in the correct form is actually pretty tough for people accustomed to a lifetime of bad posture. Whenever you forget what good posture feels like, go right back to that wall.

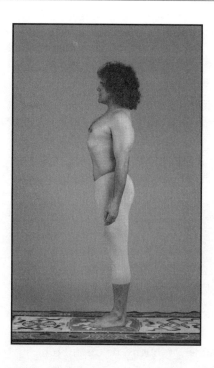

The Marine pose is the core of most yoga standing poses and a good postural model, too.

I always used to say that my mother was my first yoga teacher. She couldn't stand to see us slouch, so she used to make us stand up straight all the time. Little did she know she was moving us into that most basic of yoga poses, the mountain pose.

She'd put us up against the wall and make us feel our back, calves, buns, heels, shoulders, and head against the wall. Remember, I had you do this in Chapter 3, "Assess Your Fitness Power," to help you assess your body's relative strengths and weaknesses. At first it seemed unnatural, didn't it? The more you hold this pose against the wall, the more your body comes to understand how to grow stronger, to become more open, and to find a comfort level that is more natural.

Now that you've tried this pose against a wall, it's time to step forward and try it freestanding. Because the Marine Corps drilled this pose into me after my mother introduced me to it, I like to call it the Marine pose.

The Right Moves

A true mountain pose or Marine pose isn't stiff but naturally straight, like you're hanging from the ceiling by a string attached to the crown of your head. Try to feel the position in which gravity would shape you, rather than the position you must hold with your muscles. I like to ask my students to feel the shape their bodies would take on if they were reaching up toward the heavens, but at the same time, being drawn to the earth by gravity. Pulling one way and being drawn the other way has a powerful opening effect in the body.

Let's start by moving back against that wall or door, heels, calves, and buns against the wall; shoulders, back, and back of the head against the wall. In the Marine Corps they called this the attention pose, so keep that in mind, as well. Pay attention to what your body is doing and how it feels.

➤ Slowly take a step forward, retaining the shape you were in against the wall. Keep pressing out the sway of your lower back, lifting your chest. Memorize this feeling.

➤ This is the most basic, central yoga pose. Every standing pose starts here and ends here, and the feeling of this pose should be present in all your yoga routines. Always move from here.

➤ Hold this pose for five complete breaths, then move into the butterfly pose.

The Butterfly

➤ *Difficulty Level:* I

➤ *Powers:* The quadriceps, the deltoids; adds flexibility and mobility to the shoulder carriage.

➤ *Caution:* If you suffer from shoulder problems, be careful rotating the shoulder joint, and bend your arms slightly at the elbow. If necessary, raise and lower the arms without the shoulder rotation.

Begin butterfly movement with the Marine pose.

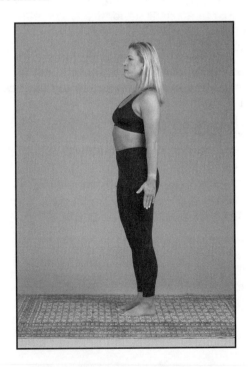

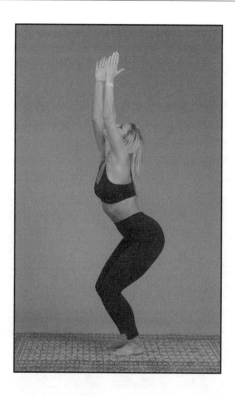

Move the arms overhead and look up to evoke the movement of butterfly wings.

You've just held the Marine pose for five breaths. Now, begin to pay attention to the natural motion of your breath.

➤ As you inhale, slowly begin to bend the knees and squat as if you were sitting in a chair, drawing your hips back and bending at the knees.

➤ Come down just slightly. Don't make a greater than 45-degree angle with your legs. Start small, just coming down a little as if you were just sitting on a barstool, not a chair.

➤ Return to your original position as you exhale.

➤ Continue with this movement until it feels comfortable. With each inhale, draw your hips back, bending the knees just slightly. Let your belly go and feel the chest lift and the whole front of your body puff up.

The Wrong Moves

Don't change the pace of your breathing to match your idea of how fast you should perform the yoga series. Instead, let your movements follow your breath's lead.

➤ As you exhale, stand up straight and strong, pushing your body away from the ground just enough to create a little arch in the tailbone. Feel the stomach pull in, and push away from the ground, squeeze your thighs, and feel your joints beginning to warm up: your knees, hips, and lower back.

➤ Now you're ready to engage the arms. Remember, this movement is called the butterfly. This time, as you come down, gently raise your arms up to either side. Feel the movement softly in the shoulders.

➤ As your arms reach over your head, rotate the shoulder joints so your palms turn toward each other.

➤ As you exhale and stand up straight again, slowly and gracefully bring your arms down, turning your palms away from each other again. Feel your hands moving through the air, the prana, the life force around you, like the wings of a butterfly catching the wind.

➤ Continue with this movement for awhile. Try to imitate the easy, graceful motion of butterfly wings as you move with the natural rhythm of your breath, warming up the shoulder carriage.

➤ After you feel comfortable with the movement, continue for five more breaths, then move into the linebacker.

The Linebacker

➤ *Difficulty Level:* II
➤ *Powers:* The quadriceps, the back; adds strength to the knee joints.
➤ *Caution:* People with knee problems should stick with the butterfly and not tax the knee joints with the deeper bend necessary for the linebacker.

Linebacker pose is inspired by one of the most powerful positions in football.

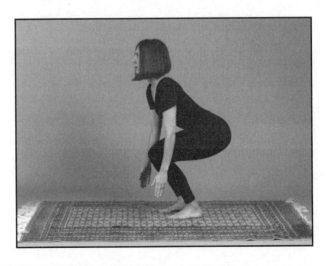

Now your body is warming up, your joints are becoming more mobile, and your muscles are ready to stretch a little further. This next pose, named after a position my body remembers well from my high school football days, is similar to what they call horse pose in T'ai Chi.

Geo's Journey

In high school football, my teammates and I were always told that the defensive halfbacks and the linebackers were the best athletes on the field. The linebacker pose is based on the position they held all the time, all through practice, it seemed. It is a squatting position that builds enormous strength in the legs.

➤ From the butterfly position, open your feet until they are about hip distance apart.

➤ Inhale, drawing your hips back, but sit down more deeply than you did in the butterfly pose. Try to bring your buns and hips down to where they are parallel to the floor (but remember not to bring your knees past a right angle). Pull your breath into your belly.

➤ Instead of raising your arms, keep them at your sides, palms toward your body, fingers together and pointing toward the floor.

➤ Exhale, coming up straight and strong, letting your belly go.

➤ Continue this movement with the natural rhythm of your breath until it feels comfortable. With each inhale, lift your heart, chest, and head, and with each exhale, push down on your feet; stand up absolutely straight and strong, with energy in your arms and hands as they remain at your sides.

Geo's Journey

The basic squat is a natural human position. We were meant to do it. It's a shame that in this country, our bodies are evolving away from being able to do this position comfortably. In many cultures, this position is used to eliminate waste, give birth, cook, garden, work, play—in other countries, you can sometimes see people spending most of their day in this position. Squatting position is vital and good for our bodies.

This movement with breath is a powerful, basic squatting movement that builds strength in the quadriceps, gluteal muscles, hip joints, lower back, upper chest, deltoid muscles, and shoulder joints. As we do it, we move with the natural rhythm of the breath, which also helps strengthen the breathing muscles and smooth the breathing rhythm.

As you grow stronger and are able to sit more deeply in the linebacker position, you'll also get a great massage in the area of your colon, facilitating digestion and elimination, something many people in this country find troublesome. However, if you have knee trouble or have had a knee injury in the past, don't go deeply into this position, at least until your muscles are strong enough to support your weight and protect your knees.

The Wrong Moves

Sitting down on chairs is bad for our bodies, especially when the chairs are comfortable and soft so that we sink down into them. This position destroys the integrity of our spines and blocks the flow of energy in our bodies. I have often noticed that in third-world countries, people's backs tend to be much straighter and stronger. I suspect this is because they don't sit slumped in chairs all day.

Variations: Linebacker with Arms

Once you feel very comfortable with the linebacker movement, you can incorporate your arms into the movement. Lift your arms to the sides as you did with the butterfly, raising your chest even more. Or, rotate your shoulder carriage in a different way by raising your arms in front of you on the inhale with soft palms (relaxed palms) facing forward, and lowering them to your sides on the exhale.

Once you've established a strong Marine pose and feel energetic and powerful doing the butterfly and linebacker movements, you need to balance your strengthening with stretching. You've built up lactic acid in these muscles and they've tired a bit, so let's open them up now and get things moving in the opposite direction.

The Bends

The forward bend is the most basic of stretching poses, and another very natural human movement. Natural though it may be, we need to be careful. Going too deeply into a forward bend before your body is ready can result in a serious back injury. People's backs tend to weaken because of years of crooked posture and sedentary lifestyles. If your back is weak, you can "throw out your back" (anything from a pulled muscle to a slipped disk) just by bending down to pick up something from the floor.

Even if you've been doing forward bends for a long time and you're really good at them—even if you can just lay out over your thighs with no problem—even then, as you warm up your body at the beginning of every workout, you first want to bend the knees gently and stretch over the thighs in a comfortable way so there's no strain in the lower back. And then you have to come back up out of the bend.

As a kid, I used to lift a lot of weights. In high school football, we used to have an exercise called a dead lift. We had to bend forward and pick up a huge barbell. As I recall, it was 440 pounds, and I would pick it up with my back. I'd bend my knees, drop my hips down, lift with my chest and upper back. I'd literally throw the barbell off the floor and then use my legs to push me up. I'm lucky my lower back survived! Not everyone's does.

Although your body probably doesn't weigh 440 pounds, you are doing a similarly hazardous movement when you come up out of a forward bend. Your body weight, no matter what it is, is a lot for your back muscles to lift. When you lie forward from a standing position, half of your weight is lying over your thighs. If you're about 150 pounds, you've probably got 50 to 70 pounds hanging there. Lifting that weight with a rounded spine can really injure any weak spots in your spine, enough to cause a serious injury.

There is a proper way to come out of a forward bend:

1. Bend your knees.
2. Keep your hips down.
3. Lift your head and chest first.

Unfortunately, a lot of yoga teachers and other fitness and even dance instructors will advise you to come out of a forward bend "one vertebrae at a time." This movement can give a nice stretch to a strong spine, but it can also be very dangerous for a weaker spine.

Instead, drop your hips down slightly, raise your chest and head first, then follow your head up out of the forward bend so that your upper back helps support the weight of the head, rather than leaving all the pressure on your spinal column.

The Wrong Moves

The weak back can have problems when it is used improperly. How do you bend down to pick up something? Do you lift the weight of your head, neck, and shoulders with your legs straight and your spine bent? This creates a huge stress on the muscles of the lower back. Instead, whenever picking up anything or coming out of any forward bend, keep your knees bent, drop your hips slightly, and raise your head, following your head up with a flat back.

The Right Moves

When hanging the weight of your torso in a forward bend, make sure your knees remain slightly bent, then increase the bend as you come out of the position. Locking the knees creates a tightness and stress on the knees and calves.

First Forward Bends

➤ *Difficulty Level:* I

➤ *Powers:* The spine and muscles of the back; also floods the brain with blood, nourishing the brain and promoting clear thinking and heightened sensory awareness.

➤ *Caution:* Don't bend farther down than is comfortable for your back and your hamstrings. Some people are naturally more flexible than others. Take it slowly. The more you practice, the more flexible you get. If you try to bend all the way down on your first try, you risk an injury.

In the standing forward bend, the body is folded forward against the thighs.

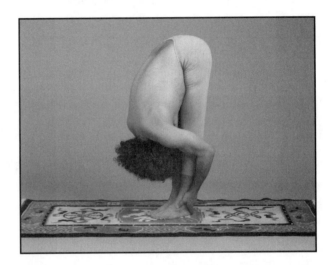

Ready to try it? Begin in the Marine pose, as you did in the first series, with your feet together and your chest lifted.

➤ Reach both arms straight up toward the sky, palms facing each other, and look up. Hold for one breath.

➤ Bending at the waist, bring your hips back slightly and lower your torso, with a straight upper back, toward the ground. Let your arms hang toward the floor, but keep them energized. Eventually, you may be able to hold on to your ankles, or maybe you can do it right now.

➤ Imagine your body folded in half. Let your head hang down and look at your legs. Feel the stretch along your hamstrings and across your upper back. Let the weight of your head gently open the back and stretch your spine.

➤ Hold this position for five breaths.

➤ Shift your hips back, raise your head, and lift your head, neck, arms, and upper back together until you have returned to the beginning position with your arms up in the air.

There is a very good reason for lifting your hands above your head coming out of the forward bend. When you roll forward, you get a lot of blood to the brain. Our bodies have something called basal receptors on the sides of the neck that tell the heart when we're getting too much blood to the head, so the heart will slow down (making forward bends a great way to lower your blood pressure and slow your pulse rate).

The problem is, when you come out of it, all the blood flows back out and gives the heart a jump. That jump can make some people become dizzy and even pass out, especially if they have low blood pressure. The best remedy is to lift your hands above your head when you come out of the forward bend. This movement helps to equalize the blood pressure. You won't get such a buzz, and you won't pass out. We like to stay as conscious as we can in yoga!

The Right Moves

Don't worry if your stomach doesn't come anywhere close to the tops of your thighs, or if your forward bend doesn't look anything like the forward bends you see in this book. Be patient with your body. We all started with that very first reach toward our ankles, and we all thought it looked like a long way down. With patience and persistence, you'll gain flexibility.

The Madonna Pose

➤ *Difficulty Level:* II

➤ *Powers:* The muscles of the upper back, especially the latissimus dorsi; loosens the shoulder carriage, strengthens the neck, adds flexibility to the spine, tightens the gluteal muscles.

➤ *Caution:* If you don't have a firm base in this exercise, you could injure your lower back or your neck. Be sure to squeeze the gluteal muscles and shift the weight of your hips forward as you arch your back, opening your arms and releasing your head back.

In Power Yoga, every motion has a countermotion. This balancing of movements keeps the body balanced and strong in all areas rather than favoring the development of one area over another (which is one of the best ways to injure yourself).

The countermovement to the forward bend is the standing arch, which moves the body in the opposite direction. This movement can flow straight out of the forward bend so that your body moves from one position to the other, back and forth in a continuous motion.

➤ For this series, come out of the forward bend slowly and smoothly by bending the knees, dropping the hips, raising the head first, then coming up following the head and chest with a strong, straight spine and flat back.

➤ Rather than stopping at a straight-up position, continue the arc of movement by arching your back slightly, rolling back into an arch.

➤ When you feel comfortable, gently extend your arms out to the sides, as if preparing to embrace the sun.

The Madonna pose opens the chest and shoulders, adds flexibility to the spine, and strengthens the gluteal muscles.

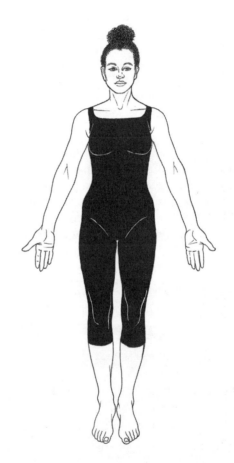

➤ Move very carefully into the Madonna pose, squeezing your gluteal muscles and allowing your body to slowly open. Lay your head back, feeling the muscles in the front of your body carry the weight of the head and get stronger.

➤ Move back and forth between forward bend and Madonna, gently, moving with the rhythm of the breath.

Geo's Journey

Forward bends and arching exercises are always done together. Forward bends close off the heart, so performing an arching exercise afterward is imperative both for physical and emotional balance. Arching exercises are absolute heaven when done properly and if the back is strong enough to do them in the right way. They open up your heart, lungs, even your whole character, nature, and being.

This position opens the heart, the arms, and the shoulders, and works the spine the other way. To really stay strong in this position, engage your gluteal muscles (your buns) to give you a strong center. These large muscles are in the center of your body, and tightening them in this arch will provide both support to the back and a great workout for your stomach muscles, too.

The Right Moves

The Madonna pose looks just like the reed pose (see Chapter 16, "Down on All Fours") but with the arms out to the sides in an open, ready-to-embrace position rather than straight overhead.

The Spear Thrower

➤ *Difficulty Level:* I

➤ *Powers:* The deltoids, biceps, and triceps; the quadriceps; and your personal sense of courage, freedom, and self-confidence.

➤ *Caution:* I recommend coming in and out of this pose with the breath at first, but when doing so, don't let the lunging knee extend past the middle of the foot.

This final developmental standing movement is traditionally called warrior II, but I prefer the more evocative name of spear thrower. I'll go much deeper into the various warrior poses and movements in Chapter 12, "The Warrior Within," but I'd like to introduce you to the basic spear thrower movement here because it is an excellent way to build strength. Perform this movement 20 times every day and you'll feel your power increasing.

Spear thrower evokes the spear thrower's movements by lining up the target with the front arm and foot, and reaching back with the back arm as if to throw a spear.

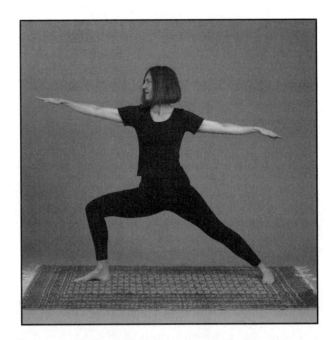

In spear thrower, you are lining up a "target" with your forward arm and drawing back with your back arm as if you were going to throw a spear.

➤ To get into the position, stand in Marine pose, then step out so your feet are three or four feet apart. Turn one foot so that it is perpendicular to the other and you are facing to the side.

➤ Raise your arms, palms down, so that they extend to either side and so that you are looking out over the front arm, and bend your front knee no farther than a right angle.

➤ Keep your body centered, don't lean forward and over-commit or back and create too much arch. Feel your back and hip open, your back leg and gluteal muscles getting stronger, your calves and Achilles tendons filling with power.

➤ Now, move gracefully back into the Marine pose.

➤ Inhale, step out into spear thrower. Exhale, move back into Marine pose. Back and forth, back and forth, in the rhythm of your breath. Feel your muscles working, and feel the strength of the warrior filling you with courage, determination, persistence, and valor.

➤ Repeat on the other side.

These basic positions—Marine, linebacker, butterfly, forward bend, Madonna pose, and spear thrower—are all you need to effect a tremendous change in your body. For the beginner, establish yourself in these first postures. Do them every day without fail until they feel like second nature … because they are! Even though no movement in this chapter is more difficult than a level II, these exercise series are incredibly powerful nonetheless, and will build a foundation of strength, flexibility, and grace in your body.

Later you'll find that as you continue your yoga and get stronger, you'll always start with these poses, no matter how "good" you get. These are the warm-up poses, and a warm-up is imperative. You can't just jump into stretches and poses without warming up the muscles. Like any other form of athletics, you can't challenge your muscles, bones, joints, and tissues with yoga without first getting some blood flowing to these areas, getting the joints juiced and the muscles warm.

Geo's Journey

In all my classes, we use this series of basic movements to create a flow back and forth, over and over. At first, we start very slowly, barely moving into the poses, barely bending the knees. As we get stronger, we can go further into poses, lie deeper into forward bends, straighten legs more, lie back further in the arch, squeeze buns tighter, and create a stronger, deeper arch.

These developmental poses are gradually moving toward a series I call the salute to the light in the heart (sometimes called salute to the sun, this series of poses has a million different variations, but we're going to create our own). See Chapter 11, "Salute to the Light Within," for the salute to the light in the heart series.

The Least You Need to Know

➤ Mastering the basic standing postures will create the strength and flexibility necessary for more advanced movements.

➤ The Marine pose is the basis for all other standing poses.

➤ The butterfly and linebacker poses strengthen the legs, gluteal muscles, and arms, and also work the shoulder and knee joints.

➤ The forward bend and the Madonna pose are counterposes that stretch and strengthen the back and front of the body.

➤ The spear thrower movement strengthens the legs, arms, and character.

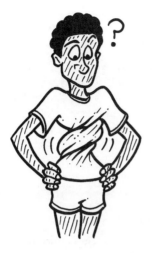

Chapter 7

Tilts, Twists, and Arches

In This Chapter

➤ Tilts, twists, and arches encourage full-body balance

➤ Tilts are more than warm-ups

➤ Arches to balance bends and stretch the body

➤ Twisting your muscles, joints, and internal organs

Back when I was first developing the concepts that led to this organic form of Power Yoga, I spent a lot of time studying what my breath did to the shape and movement of my body. I noticed that each breath would cause my body to move in certain natural arches, and the more I focused on the breathing, the stronger the arches became, even without my necessarily trying to increase or strengthen them. Every inhale lengthened my spine, allowing me to breathe more deeply into my belly. My lungs would open more, my chest would open at the top of the inhale.

With every exhale, I began to focus on the collapsing of the breath and how it moved my body, too. Arches and tilts are natural partners for the breath, which is why we'll talk about them again in the breathing chapter (see Chapter 24, "Breath of Life"). But I'd like you to get the basics down first, so that when you work on advanced breathing exercises, your body will move more naturally, finding and remembering the movements you've learned in this chapter.

Tilts, twists, and arches are all natural body movements that balance their opposites. Something as simple as a small pelvic tilt while lying on the floor may seem like an insignificant movement, but like other developmental poses in this part of the book, even very small, basic movements, performed correctly, build strength and teach your body the right positions so more advanced movements will be easier later.

When people first come to yoga, they often aren't yet very well developed. Pushing a beginner into any extreme pose early on is really a big mistake, although everybody wants to go into extreme poses early on because they look so impressive. I found, however, that it was necessary to first build a base for the power and strength, and that base was a movement called a pelvic tilt.

Pelvic Tilt

- ➤ *Difficulty Level:* I
- ➤ *Powers:* The hips, the lower abdominal muscles, and the lower back.
- ➤ *Caution:* Start very, very small. Even a movement as simple as the pelvic tilt can cause an injury if you do it too quickly, sharply, or move into too extreme of a position. Treat your lower back with care.

For pelvic tilt, gently tilt the tailbone toward the floor with the inhale.

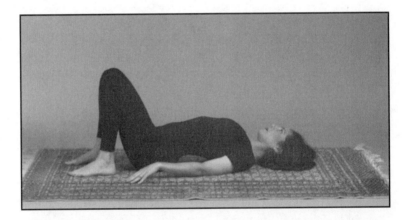

On the exhale, move the hips toward the upper body, pressing the lower back against the floor.

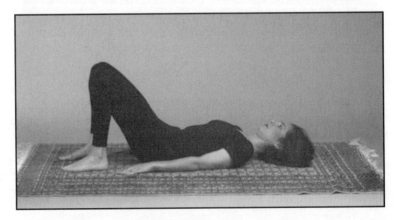

The Madonna pose or standing arch position is just the beginning of a series of tilts, twists, and arches you can do to power your torso and strengthen your center. Your torso muscles, including your *rectus abdominis* and *transverse abdominis,* your *internal* and *external obliques,* and your *rhomboids* and *latissimus dorsi* on the back side will all benefit. In addition, many of your organs and organ systems will be pushed, pressed, and massaged with these movements, activating and stimulating all your internal functions and maximizing your body's efficiency and healing power.

The pelvic tilt is the most basic of these movements, intimately connected with the breath. Pay attention to your breathing throughout this exercise to get the maximum benefit.

➤ Lie down on the ground with your feet apart about hip distance, knees up, hands by your sides with palms facing downward. Feel your spine against the ground and be conscious of flattening it further against the ground.

➤ Slowly but naturally inhale and allow the inhalation to turn your tailbone down and expand your body, elongating the spine. Feel a slight arch developing in your back as you inhale, making space for the breath.

➤ Slowly but naturally exhale and allow the exhalation to tuck your tailbone under, flatten the back on the floor, and very gently tilt the pelvic girdle (your hip bones) up. Don't lift your hips off the floor, just tilt them up, pressing the breath out, rounding the spine, contracting the belly. Make the movement very small.

➤ As you move through the pelvic tilt, feel how this small movement works the muscles on both sides of your torso. Each inhalation stretches and expands the muscles of the back and works to stretch and push out the muscles on the front of the body, too, as if you were a balloon filling up with air. Each exhalation pulls in and tightens the muscles of the abdomen, stomach, and chest while

Power Words

The main torso muscles include the **rectus abdominis** and **transverse abdominis,** which run vertically and horizontally along the stomach and abdominal area; the **internal** and **external obliques,** which wrap around the sides of the torso; and the **rhomboids** and **latissimus dorsi,** which cover much of the back. (See Chapter 4, "Power Pacing," for a more detailed discussion of the muscles of the body.)

The Right Moves

I like to think of the inhale in the pelvic tilt actually expanding the space between the vertebrae of the spine. On the inhale, you should feel no spinal compression at all. Feel, instead, as if you are actually breathing with your back—filling your spine with space.

the back muscles work to tilt the hip girdle forward, pushing out the last of the stale air.

➤ Continue with this movement for 10 breaths, feeling the breath move your body and your body move with the breath.

Power Arches

Don't be in any hurry to move on from the pelvic tilt. It is such a great, basic strengthening exercise that anyone, no matter how fit, can benefit from it.

When you feel very comfortable with it, however, you can move on to more advanced arches. Arches are really just exaggerated tilts. The arch pose I like to teach is called bridge pose, and like many of the poses in this book, it is really more of a movement than a static pose.

Bridge Pose

➤ *Difficulty Level:* II

➤ *Powers:* The spine, the latissimus dorsi muscles in the back, the quadriceps; also gives the neck a great stretch and compresses and stimulates the *medulla oblongata,* which is the mass of nerves that connects the spinal cord to the brain.

➤ *Caution:* As with the pelvic tilt, treat the lower back gently when performing bridge pose, which is really just an exaggerated pelvic tilt. If you feel pain or strain in your lower back, stop what you are doing and counter your movements with a nice, gentle sitting forward bend.

Bridge pose is a strong, energizing, strengthening movement that works the spine, the gluteal muscles, the thighs, and the neck.

The Right Moves

When performing pelvic tilt, you should feel an activation of the back muscles as you inhale, turning the tailbone down. Pelvic tilts are great for strengthening the back muscles, and for people with lower back problems, this is a perfect way to begin—and end!—any kind of exercise program. In fact, your back will benefit if you do nothing other than a pelvic tilt every day for five minutes. Just keep working there, and your back will gain strength.

Power Words

The **medulla oblongata** is the enlarged extension of the spinal cord that connects to the brain. This nerve-rich area is responsible for regulating the heart muscle, constriction of the arteries, and the rate of breathing.

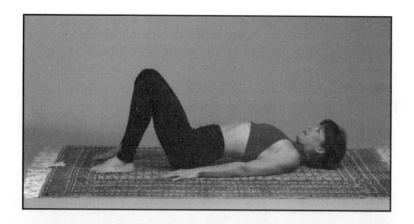

For bridge pose, gently arch the spine with the inhale, as for pelvic tilt.

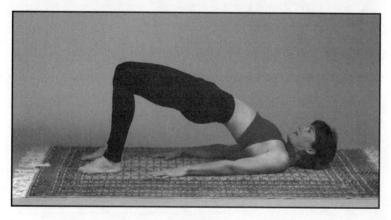

On the exhale, push the hips and spine up, making a bridge with the body.

➤ Begin as you did with the pelvic tilt, lying comfortably on the floor with your feet about shoulder-width apart, knees up, hands to the sides with palms down. Pay attention to your breath and, breathing naturally, begin the pelvic tilt, turning the tailbone toward the floor and slightly arching the back with the inhale, tucking the tailbone under, and pressing the back against the floor with the exhale.

➤ After a few breaths, inhale fully and then exhale and press the hips straight up, pushing down evenly with the heels and pushing up evenly with the hips. Your hands will remain at your sides, but your torso will form a bridge anchored by your shoulders on the ground at one side and your feet on the ground at the other.

➤ Continue raising the bridge on the exhale and lowering the bridge on the inhale. Start with five repetitions and work up to about 20.

Bridge pose is really excellent for the whole back and for the gluteal muscles (your buns), but it also strengthens the thighs, knees, and the back of the neck, something pelvic tilt doesn't do. In addition, because of the weight on the neck, bridge pose massages and stimulates your *thyroid* and *parathyroid* glands, which are located on either side of your trachea and stimulate your metabolism and regulate your blood calcium levels to keep your bones strong.

Bridge pose works the spine, lower back, and quadriceps muscles. It also stimulates the thyroid gland and strengthens neck muscles.

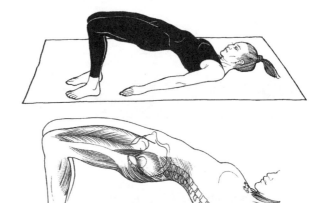

Power Words

The **thyroid** gland is a gland in the throat that produces hormones that stimulate the body's metabolic rate, or the rate at which nutrients are consumed and energy is produced in the body. The **parathyroid** glands are located behind and on each lobe of the thyroid gland. They produce a hormone that regulates the level of calcium in the blood so the bones can absorb it.

Variations: Interlocking Fingers, Closed Knees, and Holds

➤ *Difficulty Level:* II

➤ *Powers:* "Interlocking fingers" adds a stretch to the shoulders and arms. "Closed knees" loosens the hip sockets and strengthens the muscles along the sides of the hips. "Holds" build strength in the legs, shoulders, and neck.

➤ *Caution:* If you have knee problems, be careful with bridge pose with closed knees. Don't close the knees with the feet apart, putting an unnecessary strain on this joint. Instead, perform the pose with both the feet and knees together.

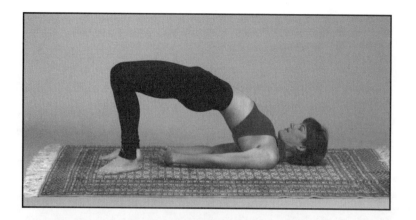

Bridge pose with inter-locking fingers adds a stretch to the shoulders.

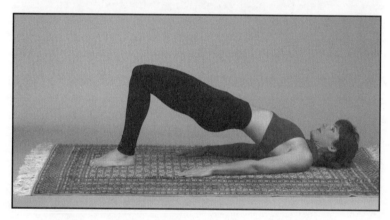

Bridge pose with closed knees strengthens the muscles of the inner thigh and outer hip.

Once you are comfortable in bridge pose, you can try some variations:

➤ **Interlocking fingers.** For an extra shoulder stretch, interlock your fingers underneath your raised torso.

➤ **Closed knees.** To get more strengthening in the inner gluteal muscles and inner thighs, and to get a great stretch in the hip sockets and muscles on the outsides of the hips, keep your feet and knees together as you rise up into bridge pose.

➤ **Holds.** After you feel very comfortable moving in and out of bridge pose, gain additional power by holding the pose for 20 seconds or so at a time, breathing normally.

The Right Moves

Bridge pose is a good warm-up for shoulderstand work (see Chapter 22, "Super-Powered") because it stretches out the neck and shoulders. Don't try shoulderstands until you are very comfortable in bridge pose. Bridge pose puts some of your weight on your shoulders and neck, splitting it with your feet. In a shoulderstand, all your weight is centered over your shoulders and neck, which must be strong and flexible to support it.

The Wrong Moves

In both hug yourself and easy back twist, never force your knee to your chest. Some people are very tight in their hips and bringing their knees to the chest is painful. Let the hips adjust gradually. I put bridge pose in this chapter before hug yourself and easy back twist because it stretches the hips out nicely. After bridge pose, the hips will naturally want to move in the opposite direction, and drawing them to your chest may be easier.

Hug Yourself

➤ *Difficulty Level:* I

➤ *Powers:* Counterbalances arches by stretching the spine in the opposite direction, keeping it loose, flexible, and strong; also a great mood booster.

➤ *Caution:* Don't neglect to counterbalance arches, but don't overdo the counterbalance pose, either. Curl your spine just enough to balance the arch so your body feels centered again.

Every pose has its counterpose, designed to keep the body balanced. After a vigorous series of arches, your body will naturally crave movement in the opposite direction, and the perfect counterpose to bridge pose is a pose I like to call hug yourself because that's exactly what you do.

➤ Lie back down on the floor as if you were about to do another series of pelvic tilts, but instead, draw your knees up toward your chest.

➤ Lift your head to meet your knees.

➤ Wrap your arms around your bent knees, interlocking your fingers.

➤ Hug yourself in this pose, rocking just a little as your spine finds its balance.

➤ If you can't get your knees all the way to your chest or if your head can't reach your knees, that's fine. Just be sure your arms wrap around your knees so your spine can bend in the opposite direction than it was bending in the arches. The more you practice this pose, the easier and more comfortable it becomes.

This pose is also great when you are experiencing stomach distress or even emotional distress. There's nothing like a good hug. Who says you can't give one to yourself?

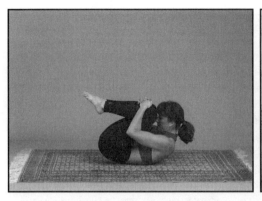 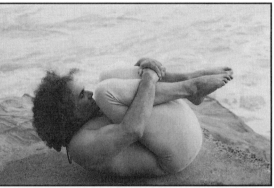

Hug yourself is a cradling counterpose that makes you feel great, physically and emotionally.

Easy Back Twist

➤ *Difficulty Level:* II

➤ *Powers:* The lower back, the neck, the shoulders, and the hips.

➤ *Caution:* Move slowly into this position. Because this position twists your spine, it is a great toner and strengthener for the lower back. Falling carelessly into the position, however, could injure your back. Always perform yoga poses with control and consciousness.

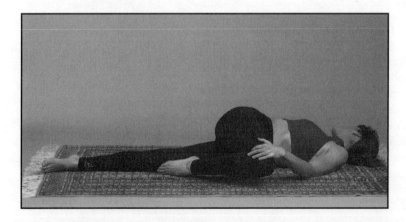

Easy back twist twists and stretches the entire back, loosens the hips, and gently stretches the shoulders.

The last pose in this chapter is more of a true pose and less of a movement. Once you move into the easy back twist, you can relax into it and breathe for a while. This pose gives you a great opportunity to slow the body down even further after the hug yourself pose. If you are just beginning a practice, those bridge repetitions are a lot of work, and you'll need to balance that effort with some stillness.

Yet, of course, your body isn't still when you relax into the easy back twist. It is always moving, and this pose has some phenomenal effects.

The Right Moves

If you've ever been to a chiropractor for lower back pain, you may recognize the easy back twist. This is just the position a chiropractor will put you in to pop your lower back into place. Practice the twist daily, especially if you have lower back problems, to keep your lower back toned, flexible, and aligned.

Power Words

The place where the small and large intestines connect is called the **iliocecal valve**. The **ascending colon** pushes waste matter up the right side of the abdomen. The colon then crosses the abdominal cavity as the **transverse colon** and continues down the left side of the abdomen as the **descending colon**.

One of the body parts most affected and stimulated by twists is the colon, or large intestine, the organ that moves waste matter out of your body. As you draw the knee up, you'll be putting pressure on the base of your *ascending colon,* just at the *iliocecal valve* where the small and large intestines meet. Waste matter then travels up the ascending, across the *transverse,* and down through the *descending* portions of the colon. Your colon is a highly active organ with a great effect on your health. A toned, properly functioning colon moves waste matter through quickly, keeping your body clean and clear. Many people have colon problems, however, ranging from constipation and pain to more serious disorders where areas of the colon lose function. Keeping this area toned and strong will help with all your digestive and eliminative functions.

➤ After hug yourself, lie down on your back, as you did to prepare for the pelvic tilt.

➤ Slowly draw your right knee up toward your chest as far as is comfortable, as if you were doing hug yourself pose, but with only one leg.

➤ Put your left hand on your right knee and bring your right knee across your body toward the floor to your left. Some of you will be able to touch the floor with your knee, others won't. Just go as far as you can without pain, so you are working at the edge of your flexibility.

➤ Once your right knee is to the left, stretch your right arm straight out to the side and turn your head to look down the length of your right arm, so that your entire body is twisted. Turn the palm down to protect the integrity of the rotator cuff and the shoulder.

➤ As you roll over with that twist, you'll feel a nice stretch in the side of your hip and pressure across your ascending colon under your thigh. You'll also be twisting the kidneys, adrenals, lungs, and the organs of the lower abdomen.

➤ Hold the position and breathe deeply for at least one minute, preferably two or three minutes. As you lie in the twist with your right leg rolled to the left, you will be breathing more into your right lung and your liver and gallbladder will be more open, allowing the blood to flow in. Your diaphragm is twisted in this position, too, so breathing will work this large muscle.

➤ Slowly turn your head so you are looking straight up, and with your left hand, lift your right knee back to center. Straighten your leg.

➤ Repeat the entire process for the other side, bringing your left leg up and over to the right, then looking left over your outstretched left arm.

Geo's Journey

Twisting poses are wonderful for anyone with asthma or other respiratory problems. Each side of a twist opens up one lung, allowing you to breathe more freely in that lung. Also, twist poses compress and twist the diaphragm, which is your "breathing muscle," forcing it to work against the compression and gain strength.

When you perform the easy back twist to the right, your left side will open up. Now you'll breathe more into your left lung, and your heart and all its surrounding vessels will open up. Blood flow will increase to this area, nourishing your heart and easing its work for a few minutes.

As you hold the easy back twist on each side, really relax into the pose, allowing gravity to settle your body into this twisting position. Breathe, and with each inhalation, feel your entire body expanding everywhere, putting pressure into all your internal organs and muscles. As you exhale, feel your body releasing and relaxing all over, every organ and organ system releasing and settling.

As you breathe, also be aware of the other pulses of your body. The breath isn't the only internal movement of the body that can direct your conscious movements. The heart beats, the kidneys pulse, the brain pulses; every major organ has its own pulse, and behind all those pulses is the pulse of our spirit.

Even if you can barely get your leg over to one side, just a small twist will still have positive effects. Listen to your body and don't push it beyond its abilities. And remember, if you twist in one direction, always spend as much time twisting in the opposite direction.

The Least You Need to Know

➤ Tilts, twists, and arches balance the body, especially after a session of forward bends.

➤ Tilts serve as a warm-up for arches, but are also strengthening and energizing on their own.

➤ Arches stretch the organs of the torso and work the spine and hips, encouraging flexibility and strength in your body's center.

➤ Twists are a great way to massage, strengthen, and nourish many of the internal organ systems by compressing and then opening each side of the body.

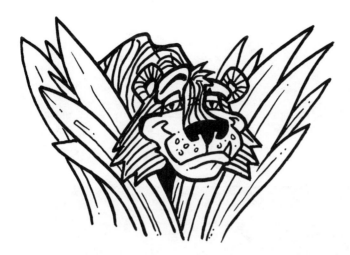

Chapter 8

Prowling Tiger Series

> **In This Chapter**
>
> ➤ Your animal nature
>
> ➤ The strength of sitting
>
> ➤ Suppleness through supplication
>
> ➤ Find the flexibility of a cat
>
> ➤ On the prowl for greater strength and courage

In this chapter, you'll begin the first of many animal poses (see also Chapters 15, "Primates and Pigeons," and 16, "Down on All Fours"). Imitating animals is a great form of yoga. Working your body on all fours is incredibly strengthening—and a lot more difficult than you might imagine! Also, feeling the spirit and movements of our fellow creatures will help you to feel more in harmony with the world around you.

Be a Tiger!

In this chapter, I'll introduce you to the most basic of animal series—the prowling tiger series. This series of movements starts simply but quickly becomes intense. The movements themselves aren't extremely difficult, but the way you perform them can make all the difference. You can do them half-heartedly and get no benefit, or you can do them with commitment, vitality, and spirit. This approach will help you to gain the strength, courage, and spirit of a prowling tiger.

Geo's Journey

Many Power Yoga poses can be held for between one and five breaths, especially after you have gained strength. Many others work best if you move through them, in concert with the breath but without holding. Moving through poses and holding poses each have their own benefits. The ideal workout will combine both approaches.

Prowling Tiger Series

This series starts simply, but quickly moves into the rigorous and primal motions of a prowling tiger. Deceivingly simple, this series will get your heart pumping. Get back to nature by getting down on all fours!

Japanese Sitting Pose

➤ *Difficulty Level:* I

➤ *Powers:* The quadriceps, knees, ankles, and feet.

➤ *Caution:* If your thighs are too thick, especially too muscular, they tend not to be as flexible, and the Japanese sitting pose may cause a separation at the kneecap. Be careful with any kind of squatting movement, where the hips move toward the heel. Start out slowly and gradually stretch out the knees and the thighs, eventually working up to the point where you can sit on your heels. Don't rush it.

Japanese sitting pose is so named because in Japan, this position serves many functions, from eating a meal to praying.

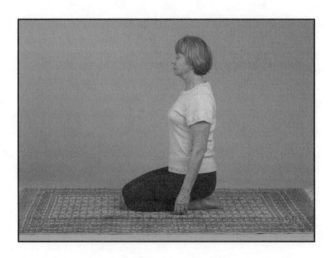

Begin this power series with a simple, centering pose called the Japanese sitting pose. This pose is an easy pose for meditation (see Chapter 26, "Meditation for Your Life") and a great way to work up to a more vigorous workout.

➤ Sit on your heels with your back straight, shoulders back, neck straight, and head in line with the *sacrum* (lower back). Keep your chin parallel to the floor, your shoulders back, and your chest and heart up.

➤ If you find it difficult to sit on your heels, especially if this position hurts your knees, sit on a small pillow or even a small stool or big book placed between your feet.

➤ Hold this position for five breaths, feeling as if you are being lifted upward. Breathe easily and naturally.

Power Words

The **sacrum** is the bony area of the backbone constituting the lower back. It lies between the hipbones. The vertebrae of the spine attach to it extending upward, and the tailbone, or coccyx, extends downward from the sacrum.

Geo's Journey

The Japanese sitting pose is so named because people in Japan use it so often for many activities, from sharing tea and having dinner to prayer and meditation. Try using this pose more often in your daily activities. It is much better for your body than slumping in an easy chair.

Worship to the Supreme

➤ *Difficulty Level:* II

➤ *Powers:* The entire back, chest, neck, arm muscles—a great, gentle, overall upper-body workout; also puts a nice stretch in the quadriceps and inspires a reverence for life.

➤ *Caution:* Keep your gluteal muscles strong and tight when arching back in this pose so your spine is well supported.

Worship to the supreme opens up the front of the body on the inhale.

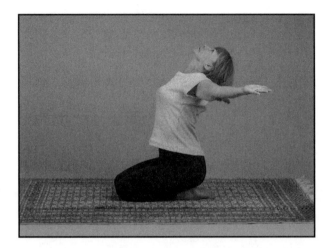

Worship to the supreme opens up the back of the body on the exhale.

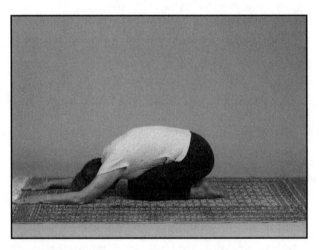

After you feel comfortable in Japanese sitting pose, you are ready to move into worship to the supreme.

This pose is special to me. When I was first developing my personal Power Yoga practice, I spent a lot of time in worship to the supreme, working the basic movement back and forth. Sometimes my entire yoga routine would consist of nothing more than the flow and motion of worship to the supreme, back and forth for 30, 40, and 50 minutes.

Of course, I don't suggest you practice it for that long. Moving in and out of the pose for five breaths is enough and will give you all the benefits of the pose, including a great strengthening of the back and the stimulation of the colon, which is massaged in the forward position of the pose when the abdomen is pressed against the knees.

➤ From Japanese sitting pose, inhale and open your arms out, as if preparing to embrace the sky.

➤ Draw your breath down into your belly, creating an arch in your tailbone by lowering your head back to look up.

➤ Exhale, drop your head, and roll forward over your thighs, reaching your hands over your head into what many yoga teachers call child's pose.

➤ Let the pressure on your abdomen assist your exhalation by pressing the air out.

➤ Repeat this back-and-forth movement several times: Inhale, come up, open the chest, arms, and heart; then exhale, rolling forward.

➤ After you've moved through worship to the supreme a few times, you might want to rest in child's pose for a minute or two. Let your body expand and collapse with the breath in this comfortable meditation position and feel the effects of the movements you've been making.

In worship to the supreme, you are moving the weight of your upper body, most significantly the head (which weighs about 15 pounds), back and forth in two positions that balance each other, a bend and an arch. As you move into the arch, your entire back works to lift that upper body and head weight, and as you move forward into child's pose, your back also works to lower the body's weight with control. Simple as it is, worship to the supreme is a great back strengthener.

It is also a pose that opens your heart and chest when in the arched position. As the back of your body is tightened and contracted to hold the arch, the front of your body is expanding, exploding energy outward, and getting a great stretch, too.

The Wrong Moves

Don't lean back on the inhale farther than you can control. Even a very slight arch in the back while looking up at a 45-degree angle will work for beginners. You don't want to strain your neck or spine.

Geo's Journey

You don't have to be religious to practice worship to the supreme. Although the movement looks like some kind of primitive supplication to a deity, the pose, beyond its physical benefits, can represent an acknowledgment and thankfulness for whatever guiding force you feel is significant to your life: God, nature, the human spirit, love, or anything else meaningful to you.

Cat Pose

> ➤ *Difficulty Level:* I
> ➤ *Powers:* Loosens and flexes the spine, the hips, and the shoulders.
> ➤ *Caution:* When performing the arch with the inhalation, don't sway your back too much or you could strain your lower back. The upward bend on the exhalation is the larger movement.

Cat pose evokes the back-rounding stretch of a cat on the exhale.

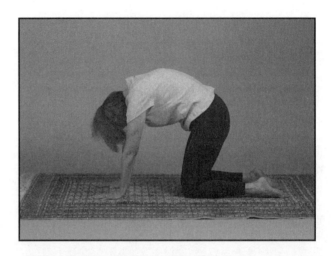

Cat pose bends the spine in both directions for maximum flexibility. The arch on the inhale counters the bend.

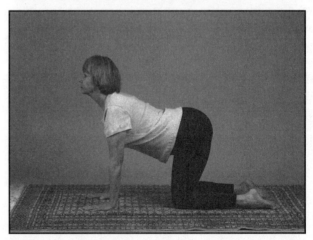

The transition from worship to the supreme into cat pose is simple. You'll be rolling forward onto all fours and moving your spine like a cat. Like in worship to the supreme, where a forward bend balances an arch, cat pose works the spine in both directions, a bend with the exhale, an arch with the inhale.

➤ From child's pose, continue to roll forward and lift yourself up onto your hands and knees. Make sure your hands are centered under your shoulders and your knees are centered under your hips so you have a solid, steady base of strength.

➤ Inhale, and arch your back slightly, raising your head to look in front of you.

➤ Exhale and drop your head down, round your spine, and draw the middle of your body upward like a cat stretching.

➤ Continue to move your body back and forth with the breath, inhaling and raising the head, exhaling and dropping the head while rounding the back.

➤ Repeat for five full breaths.

The Wrong Moves

It's easy to get caught up in the moment and convince yourself you can do a movement or pose that is too challenging, even dangerous, considering your current fitness level. Be cautious with yourself and think instead in terms of your long-range fitness goals.

Prowling Tiger

➤ *Difficulty Level:* II

➤ *Powers:* A great strengthener for the arms, legs, shoulders, hips, gluteal muscles, neuromuscular coordination, and sense of personal power.

➤ *Caution:* Because you will alternate legs in the air on this position, one knee at a time will bear a lot of weight. Perform this movement on a mat or folded blanket to make this movement a lot more comfortable.

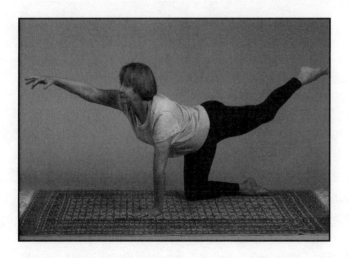

In prowling tiger, the opposing limbs reach outward to evoke the movement of a tiger prowling through the jungle.

With each exhale, prowling tiger moves back into the cat pose position.

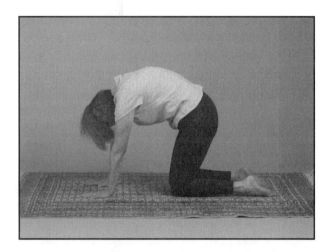

Sharon, my wonderful 68-year-old student who started with me three years ago and is now doing full splits, demonstrates the full range of prowling tiger pose.

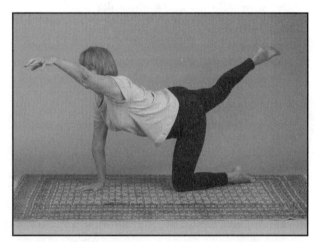

What is a cat's ultimate goal? To become a prowling tiger, of course! The prowling tiger movement comes right out of cat pose and is especially good for people with bad backs because it helps to build and strengthen the back muscles.

It also helps to balance and center the body because it works opposing arms and legs. In fact, anyone who has suffered from a brain injury or who has lost blood to the brain, such as during a stroke, can use this pose to help rebuild neuromuscular function. The cross-crawling technique tunes in to the opposing sides of the brain, helping to coordinate brain function with muscle action.

In my classes, when I have the group perform the prowling tiger, I try to get each person's mind as well as body involved in the spirit of this movement. Imagine being a prowling tiger, moving through the jungle, reaching out with your claws, feeling the sultry air and hearing the sounds of the jungle, feeling the life force energy flowing through you. Pretending isn't just for kids. It can add both power and fun to your workout!

➤ From cat pose, inhale and raise your right arm and left leg. Really stretch that arm forward. You can even make your hand in the shape of a big claw! Imagine your hands are giant tiger paws. Also reach as far back as you can with your opposite leg.

➤ Exhale, and lower your arm and leg, moving forward in a crawl and rounding your back as you did in cat pose.

➤ Inhale again and raise your left arm and right leg. Again, really stretch those limbs outward and feel energy and power flowing through you.

➤ Exhale again and lower your left arm and right leg, rounding your back.

➤ Continue for at least five full breaths. Really feel the power of the prowling tiger. And don't feel self-conscious if a growl escapes you.

You've accomplished something wonderful: You've worked through all the basic developmental poses and now have a great basic repertoire of poses to use in all your future workouts. Keep practicing until you are very strong with these poses, and then you can proceed to the more advanced poses in the rest of the book.

Until then, read up on chakras for an even more complete knowledge of what is happening in your body as you practice Power Yoga, and how you can pinpoint the areas that need work.

The Least You Need to Know

➤ Moving like an animal is empowering for your body and your mind.

➤ The prowling tiger series starts with Japanese sitting pose, moves into worship to the supreme, then into cat pose, then into the crawling movement I call prowling tiger.

➤ Master the developmental poses in this book before moving on to the more advanced poses in later chapters.

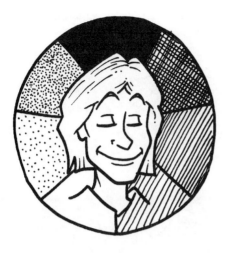

Chakras and the Power of Color

If you've read anything at all about yoga, you may be familiar with the term *chakra*. That doesn't mean you know what chakras are, exactly, and if not, you are not alone. Although chakras are much more familiar to people in this country than ever before, the term still isn't exactly a household word.

But knowing about chakras, and especially being acquainted with the nature of your own chakras, is a powerful physical and spiritual tool. Chakras are energy centers in the body that relate to different aspects of our being. Although the concept of chakras is considered "yogic," chakras exist in everyone, no matter who they are or in what country they live.

Chakra Power

The Native Americans, the Greeks, the Chinese, the Indians all knew about chakras, according to historical evidence. You've probably seen the universal symbol for medicine. It consists of two serpents twining around a staff. Have you ever noticed that the serpents' bodies cross in seven different places? These seven places represent the seven chakras, or energy centers. They are the vortices of the body.

The Caduceus: the universal symbol for medicine.

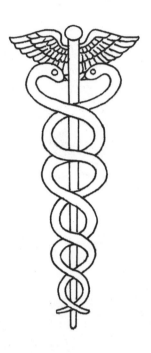

Power Words

Chakras (pronounced *SHAH-krahs*) are energy centers associated with certain glandular and organ systems. Chakras aren't physical structures, but energy vortices that exist along the midline of the body—from the base of the spine to the crown of the head—that store, channel, and release life energy.

My personal understanding of chakras is somewhat different than the traditional Indian system that many teachers understand. I've studied the traditional systems, and my teacher, Indra Devi, taught me the traditional Indian system. If you've taken a yoga class or studied Eastern religions, you may have learned it, too.

But I'm not a Hindu, I don't pretend to be a Hindu, and I don't speak Sanskrit. The system of chakras that I've worked out is my own personal system I've developed by actually working with chakras over the last 25 years. This is a system that relies heavily on color.

One of my first and most influential teachers, the Venerable Vera Dharmawara, was an ancient Buddhist monk and had been so for 60 years or so when I met him. He was 89 and a wonderful, old color healer from New Delhi. When I studied with him, he was the leading color healer in the world. He worked with people like Nehru and Gandhi in India. He was actually Cambodian.

He and I traveled around the country giving seminars on color healing, color meditation, and color awareness. He had amazing auric vision. He could look at somebody and see where he or she had a physical ailment by seeing it in their *aura,* or the energy field surrounding the body like a halo. He would see a gray spot or even dark black when there was a serious problem. This was a method of discerning the location of the ailment in the body.

Power Words

The **aura** is the electromagnetic field surrounding the body. Although some claim that everyone can see auras with practice, some people seem to see them more easily than others. Certain photographic techniques can reveal auras on film.

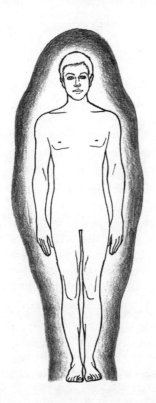

An energy field surrounds the human body, manifesting itself as the aura. The seven chakras—along the midline of the body—center, channel, and release life energy.

I've never achieved that kind of auric vision, but I've never really worked on it that hard. I see auras, but I get a flash of color, and that's about it. So I created this system, to compensate for my lack of vision comparable to that of the Venerable Vera Dharmawara, to read the body and its chakras. This is a system of reading that will work on any part of the body, although we're just going to work on chakras in this chapter. I'll go into more detail about using the system in Chapter 10, "Chakra Testing for Power Healing." But for now, let's first try to understand a little more about chakras.

Geo's Journey

Chakras are not just associated with India. Chakras exist throughout the world, in every culture, in every country. Different cultures, medical systems, and religions have different names for the general areas in which chakras exist, but if you look at the world as a whole, you will see that every culture has, at some level, recognized the existence of chakras.

Chakras 101

Chakras affect and respond to different glands, different organs, and different aspects of our beings. Although an anatomy professor couldn't perform an autopsy and actually point to a physical structure that is a chakra, since chakras exist on an energy level and not on a level of physical matter, chakras are as real as the glands, organs, and other structures and functions they affect. And each chakra has a color.

The Right Moves

If you look at the chakras separately, you'll see that the first chakra (starting at the base of your spine) is red, the second orange, then yellow, green, light blue, indigo, and finally at the crown of your head, violet, just like you would see when light is split by a crystal or by water vapor, creating a rainbow, or the sequence of colors at sunset from the horizon to the night sky.

If you were to look at the aura of a perfectly healthy person, a spiritual being, it would be pure white light. White is the culmination of all colors, and a white aura is the result of all chakras being healthy, strong, and open, radiating their colors. The seven chakras, when viewed individually, display the seven major colors of the rainbow, almost as if the body is a prism separating out each color from the full spectrum light of the spirit.

I like to think of the chakras as the whole human being, not just a particular part. People who know a little about chakras may tend to think, "Oh! The top chakra is the most spiritual, and the color is violet. I'll dress in purple to make myself more spiritual!" The idea of dressing in a particular color to help balance your chakras isn't a bad one. In fact, using colors in your life with the purpose of balancing your chakras is a great idea! However, for one person, purple may not be the right color to wear. For another, it might be just perfect.

In some cultures, red, the color of the first chakra, is the most spiritual color because red is where the light of spirit first reflects from the ground into human beings, when they become human. Wearing the "most spiritual color" doesn't really make much sense anyway. Remember that the truly balanced and perfect spiritual person reflects a white aura. White is the combination of all colors.

For example, if your seventh chakra is already strong, but you are blocked in a lower chakra, you may need to wear more orange or red. Balance is the key, not an overdose of any one color. Finding where you need balance will lead you to the colors you can use to enhance your life.

So, pure awareness is represented by a white aura, which is all the colors. But, as I already mentioned, each chakra has its own individual color. Let's look a little more closely at the colors and the particular energies associated with each chakra. We'll start with the earthly chakras, which are the first three.

The First Chakra: Seeing Red

The first chakra is located very low in the body, around the base of the spine. The first chakra is our grounding, our base, the place where we become human. It's where we feel all those human things—our drives, power, ambition, and anger come from here. It's where we start. To me, the first chakra is the source for our sexual urges, our appetites, our desire to work, fight, and play. It is the passion center, and prompts us to eat, drink, dance, be merry—to be human.

Geo's Journey

In the traditional Indian system of chakras, the sex glands are usually associated with the second chakra. This doesn't make sense to me. For me, the sex glands and sexual urges are based in the first chakra, where our primal human impulses reside.

Red is the color of the first chakra. Red is intense, visceral, and primal. If you are uncontrollably angry, you "see red." Red is also the color often associated with passion. Valentine hearts are red, and many honeymoon suites are decorated in red. Red can also symbolize destruction (it is the color of blood), and all the extremes of human nature, including the survival instinct. It can be uncontrollable, and sometimes intensely pleasurable. People who are strong in this chakra have a great gusto for life and can truly appreciate the sensual aspects of living—the taste of good food, the joy of dancing, passion for another person. Of course, this chakra must also be balanced by the other six chakras, or you could run into trouble! The sex glands are associated with the first chakra, in my system.

Sun pose drives energy right into the base of the spine, the area of the first chakra.

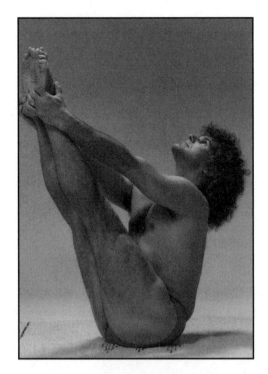

The area of the first chakra.

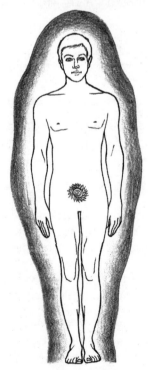

The Second Chakra: Orange

The second chakra sits right under the belly button, just a fraction below the navel. In Power Yoga, we work a lot with this chakra. In *T'ai Chi,* they call this the center for *chi,* or the center for energy. I call this second chakra the furnace. Have you ever looked inside a hot stove, and seen wood or coals pulsing with heat energy? Chances are, they were glowing orange.

We talk a lot in my Power Yoga classes about how imperative it is to keep a strong fire in the furnace. Without a strong fire, disease sets in. To stay healthy, you must be strong in the gut. This is the elimination center and the center for energy in the body. The second chakra helps the body get rid of foods and liquids by burning them off. Even good food can cause disease if you don't have a strong fire in the furnace to burn it off. Conversely, an occasional less-than-good meal probably won't be a problem if your furnace is stoked.

Have you ever noticed how little kids can eat almost anything and it doesn't seem to affect them adversely? Kids are active all the time, because they're fired up in the second chakra. They have energy and life, and their bodies can eliminate anything. They are stoked!

But many adults have lost the intensity of energy in the second chakra that they once had. Many problems arise when this area gets weak. Lower back problems are the result of too much rounding of the spine and crowding in the colon. This second chakra is responsible for getting rid of what we don't need, burning it off. But it needs room to work, and Power Yoga can help give it the room it needs for proper functioning. A tiny, cramped furnace won't be able to heat a whole house!

The second chakra is also associated with letting go, which goes hand in hand with elimination. Letting go is powerful, while holding back is dangerous. The two are conversely related.

These days, it's pretty common to hold back in the area of the second chakra, but when we hold back here, what we are holding back (negative thoughts, pain, etc.) goes right into the back. Have you noticed how many people have lower

Power Words

T'ai Chi is a martial arts system commonly used today in the East and West as a method of moving meditation and exercise. **Chi** is the Chinese word for energy.

The Right Moves

One of the best things you can do for your second chakra, besides practicing Power Yoga, is to drink water to flush out the elimination system. Water keeps things moving and keeps the colon soft. One of the things we really stress at the Ashram where I work is that most people don't drink enough water. A lot of the athletes are the worst—they'll go along without any water at all. We need a lot of water to flush the system, the kidneys and adrenals.

Power Words

The **adrenal glands** are located above the kidneys and produce hormones in the body in response to stress, such as adrenaline.

back trouble? Maybe you are one of them. The second chakra is closely linked to the colon, and holding the colon increases the pressure within, causing some areas to swell and others to shrink—not the way our colons are meant to be! And once again, all this negative energy goes straight to the back. There's a reason we call it "holding *back!*"

Keeping both the front and back muscles strong and in motion will go a long way toward easing back problems and releasing this second chakra.

The colon is connected to the second chakra, and so are the kidneys, both organs of elimination. The glandular system for this chakra is the *adrenals*.

In yoga mudra you roll over the second chakra and your heels press into the second chakra.

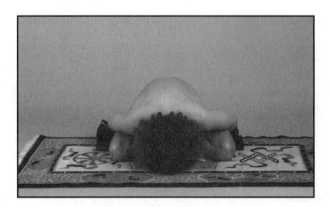

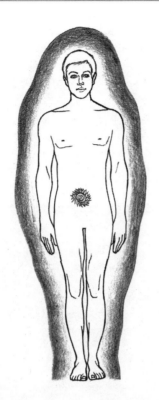

The area of the second chakra.

The Third Chakra: Are You Yellow?

The third chakra sits on your *solar plexus*, that area right below your rib cage. The solar plexus gets its name because this chakra is yellow, like the sun.

If you look at a healthy body, this is the first part of the body to touch the world around you, the leading edge of your body. This is where you bring in energy. The *diaphragm,* which is your primary breathing muscle, sits here, and every breath makes the diaphragm pull in air, then exhale and push out air. The third chakra affects the intake of life through air.

The third chakra is also behind the stomach, which takes in food and water. This is also the feeling center. You know those butterflies you get in your stomach before a big event? You're feeling that third chakra's response to what is happening to you. It is the source of your "gut feeling."

Power Words

The **solar plexus** is a network of nerves in the upper abdomen, behind the stomach. The **diaphragm** is a plate-shaped muscle that divides the chest from the abdominal cavity and *is* instrumental in breathing.

This chakra has its problems, too. We take in more than food and air—we take in experience. When we are very young and sensitive and easily scared, we can pull experiences in that frighten us, blocking this third chakra. We pull in, close off, block that center off so we won't be afraid anymore, so those butterflies—and worse—can't get in.

As we get older and stronger, we may be able to learn to trust our feelings so that we can begin to open this center again. But it means trusting your own intuition, which isn't easy if you aren't used to doing it. It also means toning this chakra by exercising the mechanisms that take in air, and by bringing pure, healthy, life-bestowing air, water, and food into the body.

The glandular center for the third chakra is the digestive glands—the pancreas, liver, and gallbladder.

In stomach lift, the stomach is drawn right up into the center of the third chakra.

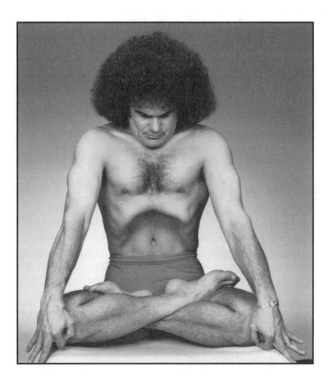

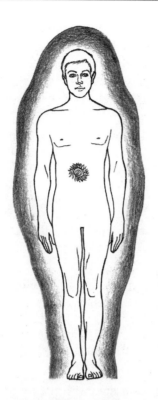

The area of the third chakra.

The Fourth Chakra: It's Easy Being Green

The fourth chakra is in the center of the body. The three chakras below are the earthly chakras, and the three chakras above are the mental chakras. But the fourth chakra sits squarely in the middle, the center of the whole system.

The fourth chakra is the heart center. Its color is green. It is our emotional center, and all of my yoga is built around it because these days, so many problems come from here.

Geo's Journey

Have you ever noticed how some people's shoulders hunch forward as if protecting the heart? Dr. Dean Ornish, who has done some pretty famous research into the nature of heart disease, worked with the International Association of Yoga Therapists, of which I am a charter member. When working with his team, we found that people with heart trouble actually reflected this condition in their posture. Subconsciously or not, these people's bodies curved in to protect their hearts.

Have you ever thought about the typical stance of a prizefighter? They roll in to protect the heart center. This center is so powerful, the slightest event can affect us our whole lives. You can even hear sounds in the womb that you'll carry with you your whole life—your parents arguing about you, for example. You can have a relationship and if it doesn't work out quite the way you want it to, all subsequent relationships suffer because you hold on to that event in your heart center.

Let me give you an example of what I mean. Recently I've been thinking about going back to Vietnam. I had plenty of negative experiences in Vietnam, and certainly didn't like the idea of going back. But then I realized that my spirit was telling me to go back so I could clear my slate. I have an understanding of Vietnam, but that goes back to 1968. Vietnam has changed, I've changed, the world has changed; so now I need a new experience of Vietnam, so I can erase or let go of the emotions and feelings I still hold in my heart chakra from 1968. I need to go back and replace the old, painful experiences with new ones, so that I may finally let go.

When we work with this heart center, we often need to go back, look at things again from a newer, more mature, more understanding point of view so we can move on. Sometimes after I do a yoga pose, I'll lie down and I'll unexpectedly drift back to an event from 20 or 30 years ago. It's like I'm experiencing a dream version of that same event. The yoga pose has tapped into a block in my heart chakra linked to that event, and I go back there and the block just disappears. My whole system clears out.

Power Words

The **thymus gland** is a gland near the heart linked with the effectiveness of the immune system, particularly in children.

The gland associated with the fourth chakra is the *thymus gland* of the immune system. The human immune system fights off all the little things that get into our body and try to make us sick. We live in a world where there are a lot of autoimmune diseases. This is the self attacking the self—the meaning of "autoimmune."

How evocative, the notion that turning on ourselves will literally make us sick! It doesn't just sound right—but has been proven. Beyond the level of our own cells attacking each other is the idea that emotional attacks on the self are similarly destructive.

We do a lot of muscle testing at the Ashram, and we like to use huge weightlifting guys to do our muscle tests. They are always shocked to find that, when I say really good things about them, their muscles test stronger, and when I say bad things, even when they know they aren't true, the muscles test weaker. (Of course we always bring back the good things so they go away strong!)

But the key is, if we carry thoughts and ideas that aren't good about us, it is very damaging. It is literally self attacking self. That goes deeper and reflects into the cells, organs, and glands of the body. So it's really important to carry a light in the heart, a very positive energy about ourselves, about our lives, to try and look for the best in everything.

Green is the color of the heart chakra, the color of balance. If you put it in a room, most everyone can sit and function well. Red in a room changes everything. Most bars are red and black because those colors incite passions and appetites. In a red bar, people will order a lot more drinks and food. A blue bar, on the other hand, would probably lose money. In fact, studies have shown that blue bars and restaurants don't do very well. People become too calm, perhaps too cerebral. They certainly don't get ravenously hungry.

Green is the color that strengthens a weak or blocked heart chakra. The goal of Power Yoga is to make this center as strong, powerful, understanding, and open as we can. Green is also the most healing of colors.

The Wrong Moves

They say that the only difference between an optimist and a pessimist is the optimist has a whole lot more fun. They both go through the same life. If we can look for all the best things in our lives, we create a positive energy. If we look for the bad things, the fearful things, the things that are going to get us, we'll always be protecting our heart chakra rather than opening it. We'll be on guard, and our bodies will settle and weaken.

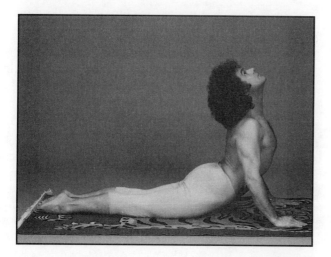

Cobra pose opens and powers the fourth chakra.

The area of the fourth chakra.

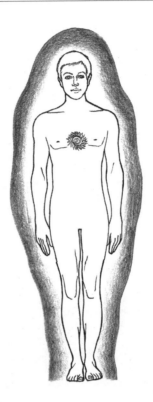

The Fifth Chakra: Light Blue

This chakra, with the light, sky-blue color, is just under the chin. It is our communication center. But this center isn't about talking. It's about *communication*.

Power Words

The **thyroid** is a gland in your throat responsible for regulating your metabolism, or the speed at which you use energy.

Some people actually talk too much to keep from communicating. I have an old friend who, every time I try to discuss personal issues, responds with a joke. If you touch a nerve somewhere, a joke comes out. It's a protective response designed to keep anyone from going deeper inside him.

After the first joke, there's another joke, and another joke, and pretty soon he's got you going in a completely different direction. It's a very powerful thing he does, repeating jokes until you're sidetracked from your original intention of getting to the meat of something. The problem is, nobody gets to know him very well. He can't communicate what's going on in his heart. And that's what this throat chakra is about—communicating what's going on in the heart.

The glandular center associated with the fifth chakra is the *thyroid*.

Geo's Journey

Today, approximately 40 percent of women over 40 in this country are diagnosed with hyperthyroid or low thyroid. Now, that's a pretty high number, and I'm not sure that there isn't something wrong with the testing system. We do know that stress causes a huge imbalance in the hypothalamus in the center of the brain, and that affects all the other chakras as well, so this could be a factor influencing the results. We get going too fast, we don't get enough rest, and our bodies get imbalanced.

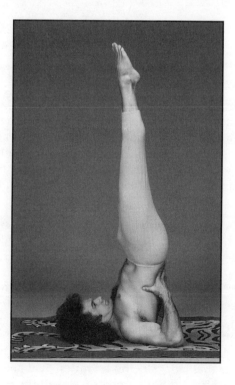

Shoulderstand drives the blood right into the thyroid and charges the fifth chakra in the throat.

The area of the fifth chakra.

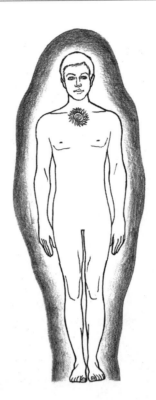

The Sixth Chakra: Your Third Eye Is Indigo

I love the sixth chakra. It's what we call the "third eye" in yoga. This chakra is located in your forehead, just above the place between your eyebrows, and it is the center for meditation, intuition, and imagination. Its color is indigo, like a bottomless ocean whose depths are superceded only by the boundless volume of your imagination. Remember your imagination, that childhood friend?

This chakra is very open and active when we are children. I remember being very focused on this center when I was a kid. Between the ages of approximately one and seven, we all spend a lot of time existing in this area. We call it daydreaming. We're always off in that subconscious mind. We have imaginary playmates, we act out scenarios, we live in a magical and limitless world that makes the ordinary, physical world drab by comparison. Colors are brighter, events more dramatic, fanciful creatures vivid and plentiful. We drift off into that other realm all the time. It is part of our everyday existence, to have visions and waking dreams, to see dragons and fairies and witches,

The Right Moves

In Power Yoga, you might be surprised to know that we spend a lot of time working on meditation and working here in the sixth chakra. Meditation and centering on the mind, the intuition, and the imagination are an important complement to the active physical movements of any workout.

128

pirates and elves, monsters and superheroes—or to be any of these things ourselves. Kids are imaginative because they're in that imagination side of the brain.

But something happens when we enter school. At about seven years old, I distinctly remember going to school and trying to get into the other side, the rational mind. At first, it wasn't easy. Do you remember first starting school? You'd have work to do, but you couldn't help drifting off, and the teacher would have to call your attention back to the task at hand. In first, second, and third grade, a teacher's job is to help us begin to move into our rational mind.

The rational mind isn't bad. In fact, it's necessary to function as adults. We have to come out of childhood a little bit to get along in the world. We have to become rational so we can make a living, have a place to live, buy food, create a family—do all those necessary things. I remember distinctly my third grade teacher finally being successful at introducing me to rational thought. She was a good teacher, and finally I understood what this new kind of thinking was all about, this 2 + 2 kind of thinking.

But, later on in life, when we are in our 30s, 40s, or 50s, many of us begin to get a longing to reclaim that dormant part of our minds. We go looking for our intuition and our imagination. We feel the need to become more spiritual. In some, that translates to wanting to go to church more (or to start going to church). Others might feel the urge to explore yoga, meditation, or other forms of self-exploration. We want to find out more about the other side of the mind. We know all about the rational mind, it's all set up and in good working order in most adults. But now, we want to re-open the huge, expansive side again, the side we knew so well as children.

This side of the mind has no limits. The rational mind has limits—it's a little box. It's 2 + 2, and we know how to work with it. The subconscious mind is limitless. It isn't constrained by 2 + 2. Anything is possible in that other side, and the chakra, where this other side is based, is our third eye.

The Right Moves

For people with an underdeveloped rational side, try creative visualization (imagining all the details of a desired scenario), mantra meditation (meditation centered around the repetition of a meaningful word or phrase), meditation on a saint, the sun, or anything else that focuses the concentration (see Chapter 26 for more meditation techniques). For people with an underdeveloped creative and intuitive side, try insight meditation (pure observation without attaching analysis), freewriting (writing without stopping whatever comes into mind for a set period of time), freeform dancing (dancing as the spirit moves you!), or meditation on the breath or heartbeat or any other meditation focusing on a rhythm or music.

But that isn't the whole story of the sixth chakra. The sixth chakra also has a rational component, or a masculine side (no, I'm not saying women are irrational—hear me out!). The feminine component of the sixth chakra is the intuitive, subconscious mind, the deep, limitless part of the self. Both aspects exist in our imaginations to balance each other.

Some people find, when they begin to explore and work with this chakra, that they actually need more work on the masculine side of that mind. Maybe you are an adult but you still have a well developed penchant for daydreaming. Maybe you are an artist who lives in the intuitive and subconscious part of your mind. For you, creative visualization is a great tool. Creative visualization is mental rehearsal. Before an event, you rehearse it in your mind, see it along the way, just the way you want it to be.

Amazingly enough, as you start this movement, things start to happen the way you want them to. It's a very powerful force, working with the rational mind in that way. It is structured practice, imagination rehearsal, the opposite of working with the imagination in an intuitive way, letting it go where it wants to go and create whatever it will create.

Power Words

The **pineal gland** is attached to the brain and is responsible for stimulating the adrenal cortex, which metabolizes carbohydrates, proteins, and fats and regulates electrolytes in the body.

The other side works exactly the opposite. Some of us oftentimes need to go back to the daydreaming self, relax, and let the mind drift and find its own way rather than always controlling it and focusing it. If your life is structured, disciplined, and low on the fanciful, if your job requires little free-form creativity, if you've forgotten how to daydream, then more open types of meditation and creativity exercises might be for you.

Either way, getting your third eye into balance is an important part of balancing your entire system. It is associated with the *pineal gland.*

Fish pose puts the focus directly into the third eye.

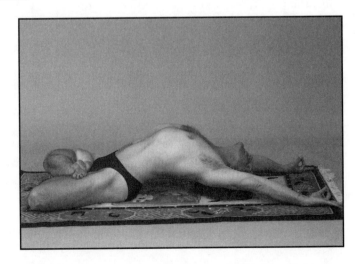

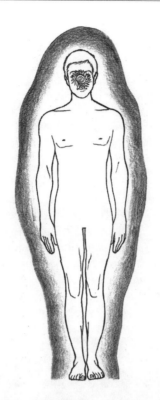

The area of the sixth chakra.

The Seventh Chakra: Violet

If you have children, you probably know that babies have a soft spot at the crown of their heads. As they grow older, the skull bones fuse around this spot and become harder, but the area where the soft spot was—and all of us had it at birth—is the area of the seventh chakra.

This is our connection to the universal "vine." It is our link to a higher existence and represents our coming down into the world, the place where we took on a physical form. The color of this chakra is violet—a deep, dark purple that I like to see as representing the highest spirituality. Perhaps it is the color of the universe itself—of space, of time transcendence, of our most perfect selves.

I don't like to teach that we are these gross beings that will one day leave our bodies and at last become wonderful spirits in some other place, in some heaven or other lifetime. Instead, I would rather think of us as beautiful and amazing spirits who have chosen this point in time to come down and experience humanity, right now, right here. Each of us is a spirit reflecting at this moment into this time, having come from some timeless place.

I like to think of our existence as if there is a big light—I'll call it God—beaming out into the universe. You and I are like little light particles out there, like nerve cells in the body of God reflecting right now, here in New York or Connecticut or Chicago or

Power Words

The **pituitary gland** is linked to the cerebral cortex via a small portion of the brain called the **hypothalamus.** The pituitary is a small gland that produces hormones that regulate many bodily functions, including the stimulation and regulation of other glands. For this reason, it is sometimes called the master gland.

Los Angeles or wherever you and I are at this moment. We are experiencing life as human beings, right now, today. And everything we do comes from there—the spirit is *right now* because it has chosen to be here now, to experience humanity the way each of us has chosen. What we do, what we eat and drink, where we work, our partners, our children, where we live, whom we love, all of these we have chosen to experience.

But that big light, that universal God light is still shining on us, and our seventh chakra is where the light beams in and radiates through us, all the way through the centers of our beings, through each of the other chakras and back up again into the light. This seventh chakra is our most spiritual of chakras, the chakra closest to our transcendent essence. It is associated with the *pituitary gland* and the *hypothalamus* region of the brain.

Headstand drives all the blood and energy right through the head and into the top chakra. In headstand, you actually stand on your seventh chakra.

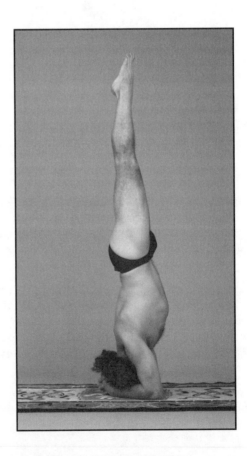

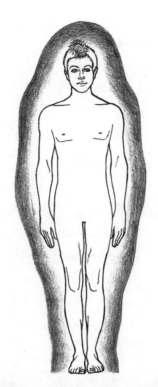

The area of the seventh chakra.

Powering Your Energy Centers

Now that you have an idea of what chakras are and what they do, you may think, sure Geo, that's really nice and interesting, but how do I feel the chakras? How do I know I really have them? How do I know which of my chakras are doing fine and which are blocked?

In the next chapter, I'll explain a system I have developed that will help you understand the condition of your own chakras, as a preparation for more targeted and personally effective Power Yoga practice.

The Least You Need to Know

➤ Chakras are energy centers in the body, each with a unique color, that are associated with certain glands or organ systems that can influence certain aspects of our existence.

➤ The first chakra is the center for our appetites and human urges. Associated with the sex glands, its color is red.

➤ The second chakra is the center for elimination and letting go. Associated with the kidneys, colon, and adrenal glands, its color is orange.

➤ The third chakra is the center for taking in—air, food, water, and emotions. Associated with the digestive glands, its color is yellow.

➤ The fourth chakra is the heart center. Associated with the thymus gland and the immune system, its color is green.

➤ The fifth chakra is the communication center. Associated with the thyroid gland and the throat, its color is light blue.

➤ The sixth chakra is the third eye or imagination center. Associated with the pineal gland, its color is indigo.

➤ The seventh chakra is the spiritual center. Associated with the pituitary gland and hypothalamus, its color is violet.

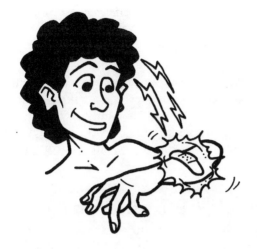

Chapter 10

Chakra Testing for Power Healing

In This Chapter

➤ What's wrong with you? The pendulum knows!

➤ Finding the chakras

➤ Reading the chakras

➤ Healing the chakras

Have you ever noticed that sometimes you can look at a person and know just where they are? Not physically, but where they are emotionally, or even spiritually? What exactly do you mean when you say, "She looks pretty down," or "Wow, he's happy today!" Such assertions come from more than the appearance of a smile or a frown. They come from body language, vocal tones, and a person's state of physical health, of course.

But there is more to it than that. Sometimes someone looks very bright, almost glowing. Other times, they may look dull and gray. What we're really seeing is the effect of the aura. Auras can be sparkling and alive or dull and depressed, or, of course, somewhere in between.

Learning to See

You might have been skeptical when you read, in the previous chapter, that most of us intuitively see chakras and auras. You don't think you've seen them? Are you sure?

Power Words

The **etheric body** is the part of our bodies extending beyond our physical bodies, consisting of energy. It is the energy that radiates beyond the limits of our skin. If you were a scientist and took a picture of Mars, you would see the actual rock, but cameras today can actually take pictures of the heat, light, and energy that radiates from Mars. People are the same way. Our energy doesn't stop at our skin.

Chakras, which reside in the *etheric body,* consist of electrical energy. But because chakras and auras are subtle, we don't see lightning bolts or sparks or pulsating neon halos.

Each of us has energy, like a battery. We have a right side that gives and sends energy and a left side that receives energy. A healer will lay hands over a person and send energy through the right hand and draw off the energy with the left hand to create a circuit. And you can do it, too.

The Healer Within You

We are all healers; it comes naturally. If someone we love gets hurt, what is one of the first things we do? We hug them. Parents know this impulse. A child falls down and skins a knee or stubs a toe, and the parent feels a strong urge to wrap his or her arms around the child. Or, a good friend has suffered an emotional hurt. Intuitively, we know they need a good, firm, supportive hug.

A hug is a very powerful gesture. If you hug someone, you close off your energy field. The giving right side and the receiving left side form a circuit. To enfold someone's energy field in your own is a magnificent gesture of love.

But we can heal ourselves, too. A familiar scenario to many is that trip to the bathroom in the middle of the night. As you walk through the living room, it seems that coffee table is always in your way, and you invariably smash your shinbone right into the corner. What do you do? It hurts so much! You grit your teeth for a moment, and then, sure enough, your hand goes down to rub the injured area. Finally, you proceed to the bathroom, then go back to bed. In the morning, you look down and ... there's nothing there! The injury has disappeared.

Sure, sometimes you'll see a bruise, but often you won't. Is it because the injury wasn't serious enough to cause a bruise? Or did you heal the bruise with your own, healing energy?

I've got another example for you. I have this huge, beautiful hybrid wolf dog named Koda. One day we were running together in the hills. Koda would usually run ahead of me a bit, then return. But on this day, she came back to me with her back leg hanging limp. My first thought was that she broke her leg. But I pushed that thought out of my mind, went over, put my hands on her leg, gave her a little rub, and concentrated on sending her some energy. About 30 seconds later, she got up, ran away—she was fine! I never saw any more sign of an injury. It was as if the event had never happened.

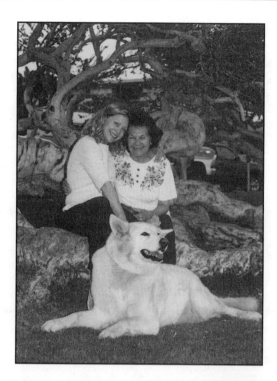

Katresha, Phyllis, and Koda. The female power in my life: my wife, my mom, and my she-wolf.

Geo's Journey

Healing is a kind of Power Yoga because it is a powerful use of one's energy. In fact, every powerful, positive movement and motion performed with attention and mindfulness, from hiking through beautiful scenery to washing the dishes, could be considered a form of yoga. My teacher, Indra Devi, used to say that there are over 8,000 yoga poses. To me, that means that almost anything I do with focus, breath, and grace is yoga.

Maybe there really was nothing wrong with my dog's leg. Maybe she hurt it, but just needed a few minutes to recover. But maybe it was broken and maybe I did heal it. It could be! I can't prove it either way, but I do know that the leg sure looked broken.

Of course, had my dog continued to limp or if she had expressed pain, I would have taken her to the vet. Humans, too, must seek medical attention from a qualified professional if they experience serious illness or injury. Luckily for humankind and

137

animalkind alike, medical care is evolving to embrace a more integrated, mind-body approach. More and more doctors and other healers are recognizing the benefits of alternative therapies, changes in lifestyle, and the effects of attitudes, both positive and negative, on health. Finding those enlightened healers and working with them to resolve your health issues from a whole-self standpoint is surely the best way to thrive.

But maybe, just maybe, we do heal ourselves and each other all the time. We can't always heal everything, of course, but perhaps we do so more often than we realize. Maybe we forget about our healing events. It's easy to forget about an event that doesn't end up impacting us for very long. If my dog's leg had been broken and I had taken her to the vet, she would have been recovering for weeks, maybe longer. But because she ran away happily, her leg intact and back to normal, it was easy for me to dismiss the event.

But I decided not to dismiss this one. I think we are constantly healing each other and when we give our energy to anyone—man, woman, dog, or whatever—it is always healing and always good.

Now that you understand a little more about chakras in general and my thoughts on healing, I'd like to show you how to experience your own chakras, and how to "read" the chakras of someone else so that healing can begin. Think you can do it? Anyone can! All it takes is an open mind, a pendulum, a handful of colored stones, and a friend.

Chakra Healing: The Color of Health

To really feel the chakras and to get a sense of how they work, you can try an exercise I originally developed with the Venerable Vera Dharmawara, and have used for a long time. To do it at home, you'll need some basic tools:

➤ **A pendulum.** While some progressive stores (such as those that sell crystals, New Age music, and meditation supplies) carry pendulums, it needn't be something manufactured as such. A pendant on a chain or a cord will work fine, too. A pendulum is anything that hangs. It could be a favorite necklace on a chain. My first pendulum was actually a contractor's pendulum used to level ground. My current pendulum is a beautiful piece of jade that hangs on a gold chain. It's best to use something close to you, or that you only use for healing.

➤ **Stones in the colors of the chakras.** These stones needn't be expensive. Inexpensive polished stones of many types are widely available. You'll need at least one stone that is primarily red, one that is orange, one that is yellow, one that is green, one that is light blue, one that is indigo, and one that is violet or purple (see Chapter 9, "Chakras and the Power of Color").

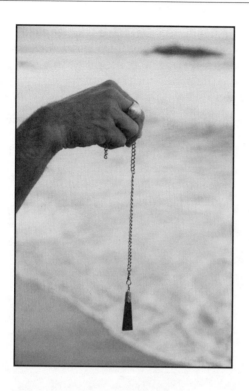

Geo holds his pendulum, jade on a gold chain.

➤ **A partner.** The only qualification necessary is that you and your partner feel comfortable and are able to open up to each other.

Now you are ready to try the exercise, which consists of four steps. First, you get to know your pendulum. Second, you find your partner's chakras. Third, you test the chakras to see which are blocked. Fourth, you test the blocked chakras using color, to see what each chakra needs to regain its balance. Let's take a closer look at each of these steps.

Know Thy Pendulum

Now that you've chosen an appropriate pendulum, you'll need to get acquainted. Really! Pendulums are like compasses, pointing us to where our energy is ebbing and flowing. But pendulums work differently for different people, and before you can read someone's chakras, you'll have to understand what your pendulum is telling you.

The Right Moves

If you don't have access to, or don't want to use, colored stones, other colored objects or even saying the names of the colors of the chakras will work, too. For an economical option, cut vividly colored pieces of paper into manageable shapes (a three-inch square or circle, for example).

139

Pendulums are funny things. I have a pendulum that has always worked for me. Some people think of a pendulum the same way they think of a Ouija® board—that you are really moving it yourself, consciously or subconsciously. In a way, you and the person you are testing *are* moving the pendulum, but not the way you might think. You aren't moving the pendulum with your muscles, but with your energy.

And that's not saying you *couldn't* move the pendulum with subtle movements of your arm or hand. Pendulums will lie to you if your ego gets involved, or if you already think you know an answer, so I only use a pendulum for healing work, and with a completely open mind, not assuming I know how it will move. (And I wouldn't dare go to the racetrack with this, or go to the stock market—I'd be in serious trouble!)

To get a true reading from your pendulum, you must first hang it down through the thumb and first finger of your right hand. Sometimes people are afraid of the pendulum and get too stiff. "It's not moving!" they'll announce, frantically. Just relax and let the pendulum go on its own.

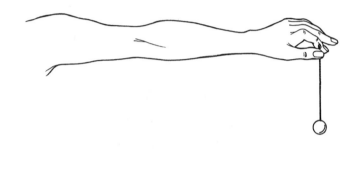

Once you feel relaxed, ask the pendulum which way it will move for "yes." Pretty soon you'll find it will start to move in a direction. For me, the pendulum crosses my body for yes, back and forth. If I ask what it will do for no, it starts to circle and goes the opposite direction. But you each have to ask the pendulum which way it will go for you. For some people, it will do the opposite of what it does for me. A pendulum can move in straight lines, in circles, or in an elliptical shape. You really have to talk to the pendulum and find out how it's going to work for you. When you know what the different movements mean, you'll be able to tell which chakras are strong and which aren't.

When you hold your left hand over a chakra, drawing the energy into the left hand while holding the pendulum to the side in your right hand, the strong, balanced chakras will move the pendulum in a positive way. We want to find those negative points, those chakras that are a little out of balance, so we can bring them into balance. We want to find out what brings us into balance, which will tell us a lot about what's going on in our system.

But first, we have to find the chakras.

Chakra Hunting

After you've determined how your pendulum will "speak" to you, have your partner lie on the floor on his or her back in an open, relaxed position. Your partner should not have his or her arms or legs crossed, which closes you off. The partner should concentrate on being very relaxed and allowing the energy to flow openly for you to read.

The next step is to try to locate the chakras. Sit on the left side of your partner. Then, place your left hand a few inches above the general area of your partner's heart. Let your hand relax and move slowly up and down above this area until you feel a slight change in the energy. It might feel like a tingle, heat, or a subtle ledge. It is the place where you feel the energy most intensely. That's the heart chakra! It's not at some particular point in the body, say 2 centimeters below this or that point. It's where you feel the energy the strongest.

Finding your partner's heart chakra.

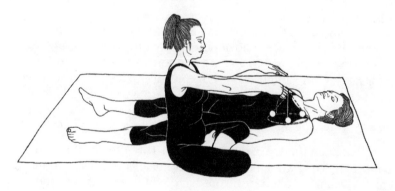

The heart chakra is a good chakra to begin with because it is the center of the system.

Feeling the electrical energy of the chakras.

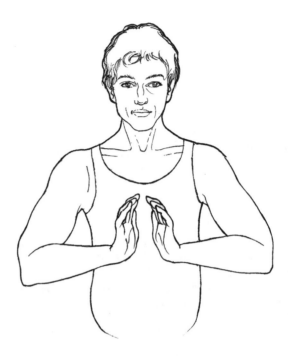

Now that you know where your partner's heart chakra is located—because people's chakras aren't all in exactly the same place—move slowly down the body, feeling for the first three earth chakras. You may need to go back and forth a few times until you feel them. As I said, it's a subtle thing and it takes some practice to feel. But you'll get it—keep trying. The third chakra will be in the area of the solar plexus at the base of the rib cage. The second chakra will be somewhere just below the navel. And the first chakra will be at the base of the body, in the area of the lower abdomen.

Now, return to the heart chakra and move back up the body. The fifth chakra will be in the area of the upper throat. The sixth chakra will be in the area of the forehead, and for the seventh chakra, you'll need to move your hand all the way back to the crown of your partner's head. You almost have to go to the floor to find it.

The person on the ground may or may not feel the chakras as you feel them, but if you are the one being read, it's nice to relax enough to feel where the person is reading, and to try to make yourself a little more sensitive to the energies you and your partner are communicating.

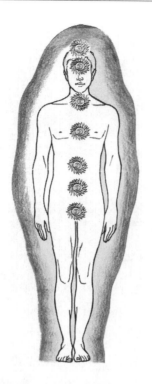

Use this body map to help you remember where each chakra is situated.

Chakra Testing

Once you've established where the chakras are, the next step is to determine the condition of each of the chakras. Some will be strong and balanced, others may be blocked and emitting less energy. Your pendulum will be your guide. When it responds to a chakra that is strong, it will tell you "yes." When it detects a blocked chakra or negative energy, it will tell you "no." The pendulum will change as soon as you hit the chakra.

Start at the heart. Feel again with your left hand for the location of the heart chakra. Once you've found it, hold the pendulum between the thumb and index finger of your right hand, to the side of the body. Imagine the energy flowing from your left hand (which is still over the chakra) through your body and into the pendulum. Now, watch the pendulum. If it moves in the direction that you previously determined to be "yes," great! That chakra is strong. You can move on. If it tells you "no," make a mental note of it, then try the pendulum over the third chakra.

The Wrong Moves

When you approach the fifth chakra, you're going to feel your partner's breath on your hand, and that can make finding the fifth chakra difficult. Don't mistake the feel of moving air for the feel of chakra energy. The chakra is located just below the chin.

Geo's Journey

Chakras aren't fixed. A strong chakra today could be weaker tomorrow, and vice versa. We are always changing, and a chakra's particular energies could be unique to today or to this week, this month, this year. Or, in some cases, a chakra will stay particularly strong over the course of your life. Continue to look at yourself and stay in touch with your energy state, because you are not fixed, either. You are like a pulsation and a vibration.

Continue on down the body, and then back up. If all the chakras are strong and balanced, you are in great shape! In most of us, however, one or two, or sometimes more, chakras will have a problem. These are the chakras that need some further work.

Color Healing

What we want is balance. We want pure white light. When our energies are imbalanced in one direction, we have to bring the opposite color in to help balance them.

When you find an imbalance in a chakra, the next step is to experiment by placing stones of different colors on the chakra to see what effect the colors have on the energy. For example, place a red or a green or a blue stone on a blocked fifth chakra (under the chin) and test to see which color makes the pendulum say "yes." Once you've found the healing color, you can take action (or stop taking action, depending on what color works).

How do you know which colors mean what? Red, orange, and yellow represent heat, fire, and activity. These are the living-in-the-world colors, the solar colors, and the rational mind colors. They ask you to take action.

The blues, indigos, and violets, however, are the daydreaming, intuitive side. These represent the lunar, feminine side and also the side that suggests you lessen activity. Each color group tells you whether you should do more of something or less of something. The chakra in question cues you to what area is the trouble spot. Green indicates balance and the need for more balance in our lives.

For example, if your throat chakra causes the pendulum to say "no," signaling a blockage, but turns positive when you place a red or orange stone on the chakra and try the pendulum again, you may need to speak out more. Perhaps you are prohibiting yourself from communicating necessary thoughts and feelings. If the chakra responds positively to indigo or violet, you may need to speak less and perhaps listen more, lessening your communication activity for the purpose of greater inner peace.

Green is the balance color, the center. If a chakra gets stronger with green, it needs balance. If your first chakra is out of balance but responds positively to green, you may typically never allow yourself to have fun and experience sensual pleasures. However, when you have repressed your inner desires for too long, you may go completely the other way, drinking too much, losing your temper, getting into trouble. You are swinging between extremes and need balance.

Let me give you another example. Perhaps the pendulum says "no" when reading your sixth chakra, the third eye chakra. The warm-colored stones don't seem to help, but a blue stone makes the pendulum swing to "yes." That may mean your mind is too engrossed in the rational, earthly world and you probably need to spend more time daydreaming, trusting your intuition, and watching your thoughts rather than directing them.

Once you've determined which chakras are positively altered by which colors, that information must, to some degree, be interpreted by your partner. What does he or she think it means that the fourth (heart) chakra responds favorably to red, or the second (letting go, elimination) chakra responds to light blue? A general guideline:

➤ Warmer colors (red, orange, yellow) represent varying degrees of need for more passion, intensity, externalizing, the rational mind, worldliness, the masculine side, as well as a more structured spiritual exploration.

➤ Cooler colors (indigos, blues) represent varying degrees of need for more daydreaming, intuition, creativity, internalizing, transcendence, the feminine side, and a less structured spiritual exploration.

➤ Green represents balance.

The Right Moves

Words have a very powerful effect on energy. Studies show that people who are prayed for, even when they don't know it, experience a greater degree of healing. So, in the absence of colored stones, use words! You can put your right hand (the hand that sends energy) on a chakra and say the word "red," and that word can take the place of a colored stone.

Now, of course, you and your partner should switch so you get a turn to be read, too. Then what do you do with the information? You make changes in your life, in your thinking, and in your actions. And one of the best changes you can make is to begin a Power Yoga practice. Power Yoga helps to balance all your chakras.

The Least You Need to Know

➤ Chakra healing consists of four simple steps: Finding a pendulum and determining which directions mean "yes" and "no"; finding a person's chakras; using the pendulum to determine which chakras are blocked; and using colored stones to see what the blocked chakras require to become unblocked.

➤ Warmer colors indicate that more passion, worldliness, heat, fire, masculinity, and rationality are required to balance a particular chakra.

➤ Cooler colors indicate that more daydreaming, internalizing, femininity, and intuition are required to balance a particular chakra.

➤ Green is the balancing color.

Part 3
Stand Up and Take a Bow

Now that your body is strengthened and ready, I'll take you into more advanced standing poses. We'll start with salute to the light within, my version of the traditional yoga sun salutation. We'll move on to warrior poses, a powerful series that builds strength in the legs and arms and powers your self-confidence and courage.

The warrior series flows easily into a series of powerful balance poses that strengthen your entire body as they work to keep you balanced on one foot in a variety of movements and positions. Finally, we'll really stretch out those sides and give your internal organs a nice workout, too, with triangle poses, angle poses, and the ultimate warrior pose, exalted warrior.

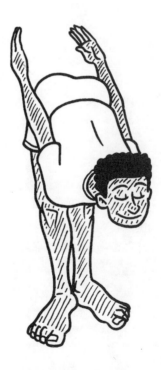

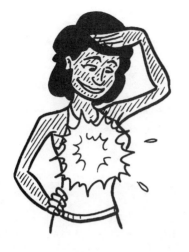

Salute to the Light Within

If you've ever taken a yoga class, read a yoga book, or even talked to anyone about yoga, you may have heard about a series of poses commonly called sun salutation. The series is called other things as well, and comes in many different forms, from very basic to advanced.

Finding Your Inner Light

Every yoga teacher seems to have his or her own version of the sun salutation series. Why? Because it's a great standing series that exercises your entire body while opening your heart and instilling your mind with a kind of reverence for the spiritual, as well as the physical, aspects of your workout.

Geo's Journey

My particular version of this pose series is called salute to the light within, because to me, the inner light is worth saluting at the start of each day. While you never know whether the sun will shine or not, your inner light is always with you. It is the light in your heart. It doesn't set at the end of the day.

This series of poses is a standing series, so we are picking up where we left off at the end of Chapter 6, "Stand for It." If you've been practicing your basic, developmental poses for a while, you are much stronger when you stand than you were before you picked up this book for the first time. Congratulations! Now it's time to develop your standing strength further.

Most people don't stand up straight. They slouch. Just look around you in any crowd, and notice peoples' postures. The head weighs about 15 pounds and if that head moves just slightly, it takes muscle energy to hold it in that unnatural position. Yet, many people—perhaps even you—walk around with their heads jutted forward, quite literally facing the day head-on.

But head-on isn't always the way to tackle something. Physically, it's a lot of stress on the entire body, particularly the spine, which has to round itself to support the head rather than straightening to provide a place for the head to balance. Eventually, spines misused in this way can develop osteoporosis or become rigid in that position, with the head hanging forward.

The first thing I'd like you to notice, even though you've been practicing standing poses for a while, is your posture. Make an effort to notice it often throughout the day until it becomes second nature. Keep your head up, keep your chin up (instead of pointing forward), and most importantly, keep your heart up. In other words, it's much healthier to face your day heart first than head first.

Heart problems are common these days. People are tied up emotionally in the heart so they hold the body in a way that shelters the heart, instead of leading with it. I can't stress enough how important it is to lift the heart, pushing it forward. Maybe you can't change your emotions or past experiences in a single day with a simple change of posture, but eventually you can alter your emotional and spiritual body through the manipulation of your physical body. I've seen it happen, and I've made it happen in myself. You have more power over your own state of mind than you might think!

Lift up your heart and notice the change it creates in you, both physically and spiritually!

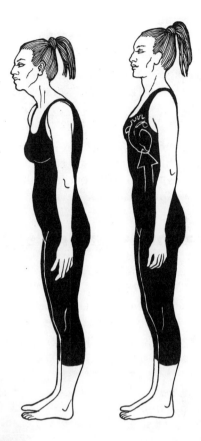

Geo's Journey

Most doctors will tell you that your emotional state can affect your physical state. Can you say "stress-induced illness"? Psychosomatic illness is an accepted medical fact, and we've probably all seen someone's health deteriorate after an emotional "injury." One of the great things about yoga is that our physical selves can begin to affect the spiritual and the emotional selves, balancing the two. When you shift your body into more confident, happy, content, strong, courageous movements, you'll find that, eventually, your emotions will begin to take on those characteristics. It's a miraculous, yet very real, process.

All the realms of the self are directly connected and mutually affected at all times. It can be difficult to alter the emotional or mental state and, for many people, it's difficult to even touch the spiritual, which is too bad—a symptom of the times, perhaps.

The good news is we can always start with the physical. We know where we stand with the body. There is no "what could be, should be, would be" with the physical body. There is only "what is." That leaves us with a very powerful tool with which to reshape our lives, our attitudes, and our personal power.

The salute to the light within is the perfect place to start. Its very name suggests that our physical movements are connected to our spiritual selves, and to honor one is to honor the other. Salute your inner light and begin the process of transformation with this powerful pose series.

The Marine with Prayer Pose

➤ *Difficulty Level:* I

➤ *Powers:* The legs, the back, and the self-esteem.

➤ *Caution:* After you have practiced the Marine pose for a long time, don't become lazy and forget how important it is to keep the body lifted and energized. Make the pose new, as if you were performing it for the first time each time you practice it.

In Marine pose, lead with your heart, letting it meet the world first. This pose opens the chest and spine, strengthens the legs and back, and reminds you what good posture feels like.

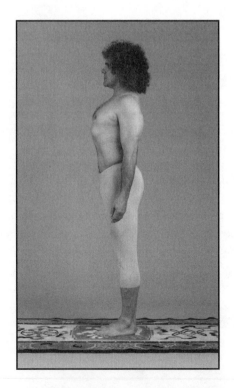

Scholliae

tense mid back rounded
body, voice, belly tap

irts with the basic Marine pose I showed you in
ieries of basic positions designed to energize and
vonderful way to begin the day. A few rounds of
rning will empower you with grace, strength, and

rolling the shoulders back and down to their natu-
iat sense of lifting with the head, the feeling of
the head toward the sky, almost as if the body is
her than collapsing into itself.

ily by your sides. Put your thumb and first finger
e Marine Corps.

t lifted, chin parallel to the floor. Look straight
and your big toes in line.

really the military attention pose. Stand up, get
ght and strong.

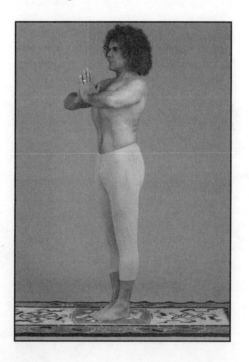

➤ Now, bring your hands together in front of your chest in prayer fashion. For
just a moment, get in touch with your heart. As your palms touch each other,

The Right Moves

Power Yoga makes a very strong and empowering workout. I advise my students to practice Power Yoga routines three times per week, really working hard. On the other days, take a good long hike or walk, do some gentle yoga postures, and work on areas where you need to increase your flexibility or strength.

fingers and thumbs together, feel the pulse in your thumbs, palms, down your arms, and into your heart. Feel your heart in the center of your chest. Try to feel its pulse, its rhythm.

➤ Stay here for five breaths at first, to get the feel of the position. Once you've mastered the series, you can spend one full breath per pose, or you can move more slowly, spending up to five breaths per pose. You may decide to vary your pace from day to day.

This movement puts you in touch with your heart. The movement is a dedication to your yoga, and your whole yoga practice is dedicated to the greatest good in you, the light in your own heart.

The Reed

➤ *Difficulty Level:* I

➤ *Powers:* The spine, the neck, and the arms.

➤ *Caution:* When looking up, don't throw your head back. That 15-pound weight could injure your spine. Look up with strength and control.

Inhale from prayer pose and lift the arms up to form the reed pose.

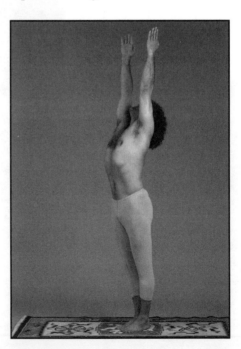

The reed pose moves from prayer pose quite naturally on the inhale.

➤ Inhale and lay your head back comfortably as you reach for the ceiling. Feel as if you are hanging from the ceiling by your fingertips.

➤ Let everything in your body reach and open, staying strong in the feet, strong in the legs, and strong in the buttocks. Reaching up is very strengthening for the back.

➤ Imagine you are a reed, growing and reaching for the light, for energy.

The Right Moves

The names of poses can help you to perform them correctly. Trying to capture the spirit of the pose name can help your body find the correct posture and flow gracefully through the movement. Your mind can also embrace the spirit of the movement if your imagination is engaged.

Standing Forward Bend

➤ *Difficulty Level:* II

➤ *Powers:* The entire back, spine, and hips.

➤ *Caution:* In standing forward bend, always bend the knees slightly. You can't see this in the photo, but the knees are bent slightly. Especially in the beginning, a bent knee is imperative. Without it, you risk a serious back injury. In yoga, people are most likely to injure their backs doing forward bends incorrectly.

Exhale and come forward into standing forward bend, with the eventual goal of resting against your upper thighs and grasping your ankles.

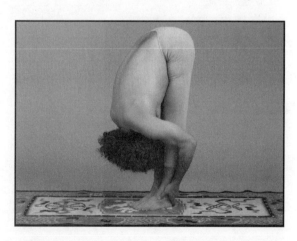

The next pose is a standing forward bend. The name describes the movement exactly. It is a rolling forward and reaching down over the thighs, the counterpose to reed pose, which reaches up.

➤ Exhale and roll forward toward the ground. Bend your knees just enough so you can drop your arms forward. Maybe your hands will touch the ground, maybe they won't. Find your flexibility edge and work there, not pushing over it, but working so you can make progress.

➤ Let your head hang out at the end of your spine and you'll feel a stretching and opening of your neck and your entire back.

➤ This pose squeezes all the lower glands and organs as you roll forward. The chest moves toward the thighs. You may not be able to reach your thighs, and your basic body build may have something to do with it. Someone with a long, thin body can reach the chest to the knees more easily than someone with a bigger, deeper chest or a short waist. Poses are always different for each individual. The goal is to move *toward* the legs.

➤ Stay in this position for the exhale, or as long as five breaths.

The Wrong Moves

Although in the photo of standing forward bend I've got my head to my knees, this may not be the way the pose will look for you. Don't force your body in an attempt to copy the photo exactly. I'm also gripping my heels, but if you can't do this, that's fine. For you, the pose will roll forward to the place where your back stops.

You'll repeat this pose frequently throughout this series of poses, so get used to it!

Dead Lift

➤ *Difficulty Level:* II

➤ *Powers:* The upper and lower back.

➤ *Caution:* Keep a strong, flat back in dead lift so your lower back isn't supporting your whole body by itself, but has the added strength of the entire spine.

With the inhale, move into dead lift.

➤ Inhale and, keeping your knees bent as you raise your head, flatten your back. A dead lift is lifting a weight with the lower back. We're lifting the weight of the upper body—the head, neck, and shoulders—with the back.

➤ Let the arms hang. As you raise your back with knees bent, concentrate on keeping the back, especially the lower back, flat.

➤ Exhale and drop your head back down into standing forward bend.

The Wrong Moves

Unlike a weightlifter's dead lift, a yoga dead lift is kinder to the body. Maintain more control and distribute the effort of lifting the upper body's weight across the whole spine rather than concentrating a sudden, uncontrolled force on the lower back.

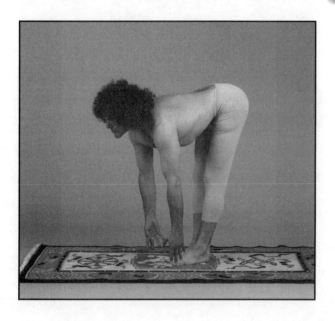

For dead lift, come out of standing forward bend by flattening the back and looking up with the head while keeping the arms lowered toward the floor.

Flat Back Pose

➤ *Difficulty Level:* III

➤ *Powers:* An even more powerful total back strengthener.

➤ *Caution:* At first, you'll find it helpful to do this pose next to a mirror to be sure you are maintaining a straight line from lower back to fingertips. Without a mirror, you may commit any number of positional errors that could unbalance your body and cause pain or injury.

Come out of a forward bend with the arms outstretched and hold them parallel with the floor for flat back pose.

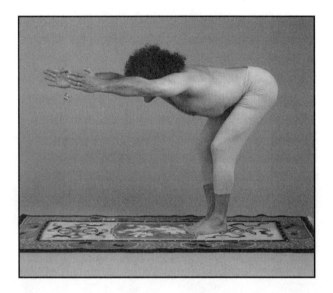

Flat back pose is a way out of forward bend, but it is also a pose in itself. You can move halfway up, as is shown in the photo, and hold. Or, you can move all the way back up into reed pose. We'll do both for this series.

➤ From standing forward bend, inhale and bend your knees even further, drop your hips down a little, and raise your head together with your outstretched arms.

➤ Let your body follow your head and arms up until your entire upper body is parallel to the floor.

➤ Exhale and drop back down to standing forward bend.

➤ Inhale and return to dead lift pose, keeping your arms hanging down to the floor.

➤ Exhale and come back down into standing forward bend.

➤ Inhale, bend your knees, drop your hips, raise your arms and head, and move back into flat back pose. This time, however, instead of stopping halfway up, continue up, into reed pose. Again, imagine you are hanging from the sky by your fingertips, allowing your entire body to open and stretch.

➤ Exhale and come back down into standing forward bend.

Back Arching Pose

➤ *Difficulty Level:* III

➤ *Powers:* The entire back, gluteal muscles, and abdominal muscles.

➤ *Caution:* Keep your gluteal muscles strong and tight when moving into back arching pose so your lower back and spine will be adequately supported.

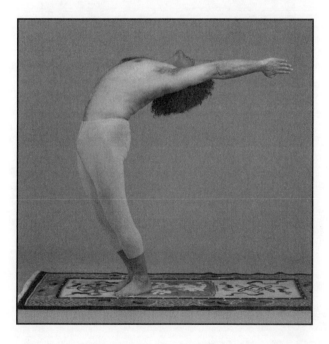

For back arching pose, move from reed pose into a graceful arch, extending your arms and head back over your body. Don't go back farther than your body can support, however.

Now you'll take the series even further, expanding the straight reed pose into a back arch.

➤ Inhale and move back through flat back pose into reed pose.

➤ Bend your knees to take the pressure off your lower back. Push your heels together and squeeze your gluteal muscles for back support.

➤ Lay your head back and reach back over your head, creating as much arch as your body can support. Focus on a spot behind you (you'll see it upside-down). Reach for that spot.

159

➤ Keep your knees bent slightly, hips forward, buns squeezed, and the whole upper body rolled back, squeezing kidneys and adrenals.

➤ Stretch out through the fingertips to open the back and work against compression in the vertebrae.

➤ Move back up through reed and back down into Marine pose with prayer position.

Finish salute to the light within with a final Marine prayer pose.

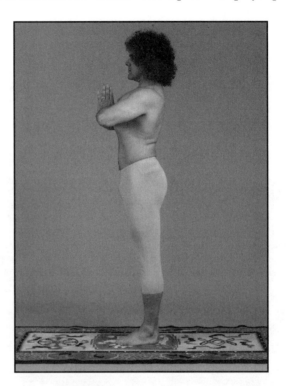

Geo's Journey

Once you know all the basic moves I've used to create the salute to the light within series, feel free to mix and match, change the order, and create a salute to your individual inner light that feels good and makes sense to your body. Just be sure you balance each pose with a counterpose: a bend with an arch, a stretch to one side with a stretch to the other side, and so on.

Variations: Add to the Mix

The basic routine of salute to the light within, as you've probably noticed, is to alternate up poses and down poses, stretching poses with bending poses.

You can easily add more poses into this routine. Two I like to add are chair pose and full squat.

After the flat back pose and accompanying standing forward bend, move into chair pose.

➤ On the inhale, move back through flat back pose, but continue up with your arms so they angle toward the sky.

➤ Draw your hips back and lower them into a seated position so that your knees form an angle of approximately 90 degrees and your thighs are approximately parallel to the ground.

> **The Wrong Moves**
>
> Bringing your hips all the way down to the ground in a squat isn't a good idea for people with bad knees or for anyone who is just beginning a fitness program. Most people's knees aren't strong enough to move past a 90-degree angle, so reserve the squat position until you are sure your knees and entire lower body are strong enough.

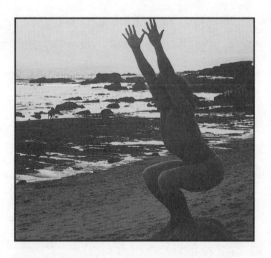

In chair pose, you squat to the point where you would sit in a chair if you had one, letting your muscles do the work in the absence of a chair's support.

➤ Exhale and lower your arms while raising your hips to return to standing forward bend.

➤ Inhale and move into dead lift position, then bend your knees to either side and squat all the way down, keeping your head raised.

➤ Bring your hands together in prayer pose in front of your heart.

➤ Exhale and bring your hips up while lowering your head, to return to standing forward bend.

➤ Continue on with the salute to the light within series, picking up with the reed pose, then on to the back arch.

Salute to the light within is a wonderful daily exercise series for anyone ready to move beyond the basic standing poses. The series is meant to be repeated, not just performed once. Move through it five or more times each morning. It tones the body and the attitude so that you'll be more likely to have a great day.

In full squat, your body is primarily upright while your knees are bent and your hips and buttocks are low to the ground. This position is a natural human position and in some other countries, people spend much of their day in this position. With practice, you may find it quite comfortable.

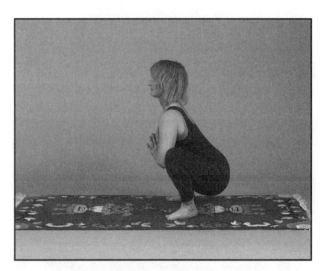

The Least You Need to Know

➤ Salute to the light within is one version of the popular yoga sun salutation.

➤ Salute to the light within is a series of standing poses for anyone who has mastered the basics of Marine, butterfly, and linebacker poses.

➤ Salute to the light within series consists of the Marine with prayer pose, the reed pose, the standing forward bend, the dead lift, the flat back, and for more advanced students, the chair pose and the full squat.

➤ Practice salute to the light within each morning, moving through the series five times or more, to add strength, power, and a reverent attitude to your day.

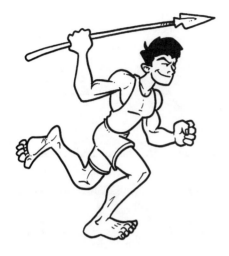

The Warrior Within

When you have strengthened your body with beginning standing poses and are warmed up and revved up for a really invigorating and empowering workout, the next step is to work with the lunge.

You see lunges in many fitness activities—karate, T'ai Chi, fencing, boxing, weight lifting, gymnastics, dancing, and skating. Lunges are great. They represent stepping out fearlessly into the universe, reaching out with the heart open and strong.

Warrior Strength

In yoga, we call the lunges the warrior series. These yoga poses probably originated with the movements of the ancient warriors. Some people say that *all* yoga evolved from the movements of the ancient warriors.

Warrior movements were designed for war. There are sword maneuvers, spear maneuvers, reaches and thrusts, movement and control of the body with force and direction.

Geo's Journey

Warrior movements involve a lot of leg, knee, and foot work. The shifting and centering of body weight strengthens every leg muscle, and the lunges these movements involve bring awareness to our knees and feet. The balance they require strengthens the foot's arches, bones, and muscles.

The Wrong Moves

Don't move into lunges, especially in the beginning, to an extreme angle, which could injure a knee that isn't yet strong. Move the knee no farther than over the middle of the foot, just past the ankle, but never past the toes. More extreme angles are safer in stretching positions. In strengthening positions and positions where the knee bears the weight of the body, take extra precautions not to overdo it.

Warrior movements also refine the balance. Unbalanced movements can cause injury. In the past, when I've done warrior poses improperly, the effects begin to show up through body pain, stress, and strain. Balance won't create pain or strain. To keep your body aligned and balanced, follow a few cardinal rules:

➤ Never move your knee past your toes.

➤ Always keep your knee in line with the middle of your foot. Don't let it roll inward or outward.

➤ Have someone check your foot for proper alignment and weight distribution by getting down on the floor and examining your foot's position. If you are rolling outward, your weight will move to the outside of your foot creating an arch, and your big toe will come off the ground. If you are rolling inward, your arch will be collapsed and the weight will come off the outside of the foot so that your little toe rolls off the ground.

Warrior series has three primary movements. Many yoga teachers call these movements warrior I, warrior II, and warrior III. I like to look at these movements from the warrior's point of view and give them more evocative names. The warrior movements suggest throwing and thrusting spears, lunging with foils, and pulling back with javelins. The front foot faces the direction of the target, and the focus and concentration is on one point in space, the mark.

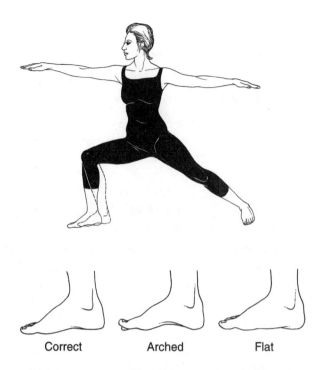

Correct placement of the knee and foot for warrior pose.

Correct   Arched   Flat

In my warrior series, I start with what is tradition-ally called warrior II because, to me, it is the most basic of poses. I've already introduced you to this pose in Chapter 6, "Stand for It," but in this chap-ter, I'll go over it in a little more detail, then move on to the other warrior poses (from here on out, I'll just refer to the poses with the Power Yoga names, not the traditional names).

You can choose to move in and out of each war-rior pose individually, or string them together as I have them here in a warrior series which you can run through five or more times in a row. Keep your movements fluid and graceful, and never for-get to coordinate your movements with your breathing! The warrior knows how to breathe—it is the secret of his courage.

The Wrong Moves

In warrior poses, the legs are about four feet apart, but each individual body will have a place that feels most natural. If your feet are too widely spread, your knee will feel strained even before it hits that right angle. If the feet are too close together, the knee will want to bend out past the toes. Work on finding the positioning of the feet that feels strong, cen-tered, and balanced for you.

Geo's Journey

Warrior movements do more than strengthen the body. They also represent the proper mental state of the warrior. In these movements, we're stepping onto the front foot, but at the same time, we're pushing off on the back foot. The weight is centered over both feet, strong in the back leg, foot solid on the ground, and strong in the front leg, foot placed courageously forward into the unknown. The back leg is like the foundation for the pose, a big tree trunk that carries us as we reach forward into this pose. We're grounded in two worlds when we move into warrior poses: the world we know, and the world ahead of us.

The Spear Thrower

➤ *Difficulty Level:* I

➤ *Powers:* The quadriceps, torso, and arms; also, a great emotion strengthener.

➤ *Caution:* Watch the knee; keep it in line with the foot and do not extend past the middle of the foot.

In Chapter 6, you practiced moving in and out of the spear thrower; but before we use it as a beginning movement in a longer series, let's check your positioning and make sure everything is in the right place.

Line It Up

Stand in front of a mirror or have a friend help you line up for this movement so you can get the feel of the proper positioning.

➤ To get into position, first stand straight and tall in Marine pose, then spread your feet so they are approximately four feet apart. Find the distance that is comfortable for you.

➤ Roll your right foot so that it opens, toes pointing to the right. Keep your left foot facing forward. Your feet will now be at right angles, the heel of your right foot in line with the arch of your left foot.

➤ Raise your arms out to your sides so that your right arm extends over the right leg and the left arm extends back over the left leg. Look to the right. Notice how it feels to have everything lined up correctly. You can even use a mirror (or a buddy) to check your position.

➤ Lower your arms again in preparation for the lunge movement.

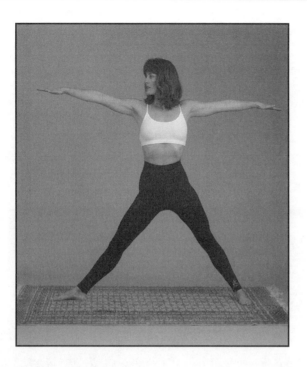

When setting up the spear thrower pose, line up your feet, arms, and legs before moving into the lunge.

The Movement

Now you are ready to begin the actual movement series with the lunges.

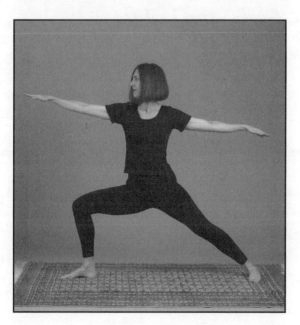

In spear thrower, imagine lining up your target with your forward hand and foot, then reaching back with your back hand to throw the spear.

➤ Inhale and bend the knee until it moves over the middle of the foot.

➤ As you lunge, reach out in opposite directions with the arms, the direction the foot is pointing with one arm and behind you with the other.

➤ Exhale, straighten your legs, and lower your arms to your sides again.

➤ Repeat five times.

➤ Switch sides, turning to your left, and repeat five more times.

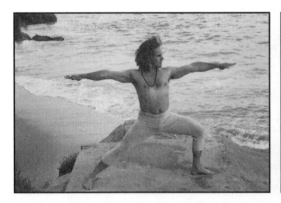 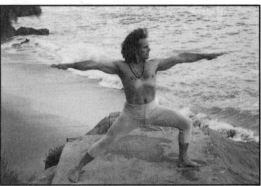

Geo inhales fully and deeply to move into the pose. At right, Geo exhales fully and deeply before straightening his legs to move out of the pose.

Variations: Rotations, Curls, and Holds

Once you've mastered spear thrower, you can add interest to the movement and gain some additional physical benefits.

The Right Moves

Don't get so caught up in the effort that you forget to envision yourself as a courageous warrior. Feel the power and strength of your movements.

➤ Extend the arms with palms facing up rather than down. This movement puts a nice rotation in the shoulder carriage and strengthens the biceps.

➤ From spear thrower with hands up, squeeze the fingertips together.

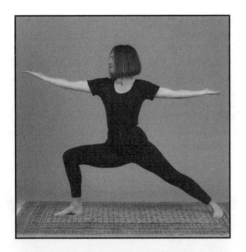

Rotate the arms so the palms face upward for spear thrower with hands up. This position works the shoulder joints and strengthens the biceps.

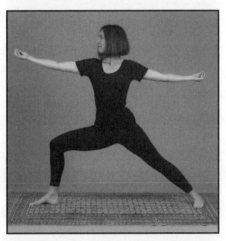

From spear thrower with hands up, bring the fingers together and squeeze for further biceps strengthening.

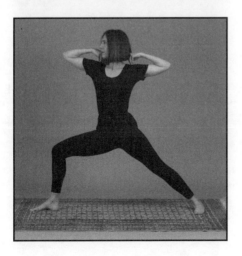

From spear thrower with finger squeeze, move into spear thrower with biceps curl by flexing your elbow joint and bringing your fingers to your shoulders.

➤ From spear thrower with finger squeeze, flex your biceps and bring your fingers to your shoulders in a biceps curl.

➤ Combine the above three movements into one continuous flow. Step into the spear thrower lunge on the inhale, extending the arms outward with hands up. On the exhale, squeeze the fingers. On the inhale, flex the elbows and bring the hands to the shoulders for the curl. On the exhale, straighten the arms. On the inhale, flatten the hands, and on the exhale, come out of the lunge and drop the arms.

➤ Once you are strong in this movement and your body is warm, try holding spear thrower for five breaths or longer before moving back out and dropping the arms. You'll still be moving as you hold the position, of course, creating and expanding with the inhale, rounding and deflating as you exhale. You can hold for even longer periods of time as you get stronger.

Geo's Journey

I think it's best to work in and out of poses at first, then gradually start to hold the poses longer as you get stronger and more balanced. Five to 10 breaths for each pose is adequate, even for an advanced student. Ten breaths in a pose with a slow breath gets to be close to a minute long, and that's usually quite a long time to hold a pose. Five breaths is probably more appropriate for most of the holding poses.

The Swordsman

➤ *Difficulty Level:* II

➤ *Powers:* The legs, the shoulders; stretches the torso, adds space in the spine.

➤ *Caution:* Adding your arms to the weight of your head can put an additional strain on your lower back. Stay strong in the gluteal muscles in this lunge to stabilize the back.

This pose flows naturally from spear thrower but takes just a little more flexibility in the arms. Swordsman imitates the movement of raising a sword above your head. The arms are lifted, and the goal is to get as much energy into the movement as possible.

This exercise is excellent for the heart, opening and lifting the chest.

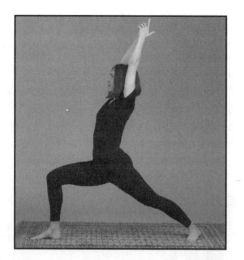

In swordsman, the entire body faces the lunging leg with both arms raised overhead as if grasping a sword in readiness for battle.

Geo's Journey

The swordsman pose creates a gentle arching of the back. There's actually an arc of energy going from the heel of the back foot through the leg, up the buttocks and lower back, right up the spine and through the arms and out through the fingertips. Extend that energy out past the fingertips like a beacon of light.

➤ Begin as in spear thrower with the feet about four feet apart. Remember, you can always adjust the distance if you find your feet are too close together or too far apart for a strong and solid base.

➤ Turn the right foot out to the right so your feet are perpendicular to each other, the right heel lined up with the center of the left foot.

➤ Turn your hips toward the "target" so they face the same direction as your right foot.

➤ Inhale and lunge forward on your right leg, bringing your knee no farther than over the middle of your right foot.

➤ At the same time, bring both arms over your head, clasping your fingers together with first fingers and thumbs extended.

➤ Stay strong in the back leg, but also be careful not to hyperextend the knee. Don't press your knee so far back that you feel pain.

The Right Moves

As you move into the lunge for swordsman, you may feel it is too difficult to keep your feet exactly perpendicular. Don't force your body into an unnatural position. Instead, press the heel of your back foot back a little farther so it feels like you are actually pushing off the back foot onto the front. This also puts a nice stretch in the back calf and Achilles tendon.

➤ Stay in the pose long enough to get centered and feel in control, not too far extended in the pose, both feet solid on the ground with feet and toes opened, weight spread evenly across all foot bones. Feel the lift in the chest and heart, the opening in the belly. Look straight ahead and keep your palms lifted, extending through your fingertips.

➤ Exhale and come up from the lunge, lowering the arms back to your sides.

➤ Move in and out of the position on the inhale and exhale, gently back and forth. Inhale, raise arms, press heel back; then exhale, straighten front leg, bring arms down, and relax back leg.

➤ Repeat five times.

➤ Turn the other way, lunging to the left, and repeat five times.

➤ Variations: Try bending the arms and bringing the elbows together, or keeping the hands apart with palms facing each other when overhead.

Swordsman with elbows together adds an extra stretch to the neck and strength to the upper back and chest.

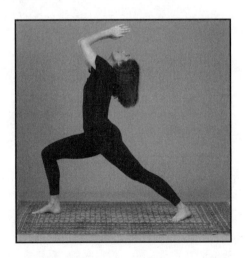

➤ As time goes on and you get stronger and want to build more heat, move into the position and hold for about five breaths, up to about a minute. As we hold the pose, too, we can start to refine it a little, see where we're strong and where we're not, and find the areas we need to work on.

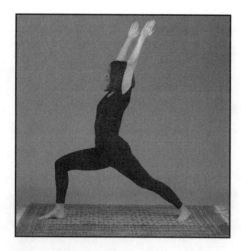

Swordsman with hands apart is a more powerful arm position.

Extended Warrior

➤ *Difficulty Level:* III

➤ *Powers:* The quadriceps, hamstrings, shoulders, arms, and entire back.

➤ *Caution:* Keep the weight centered on both feet even when your body is moving out over your front foot, to lessen strain on the knee.

Extended warrior is a natural extension of swordsman and a great strengthener for the entire back.

➤ With the inhale, move into swordsman with hands apart (one of the above variations; see photo earlier in the chapter), then lean out over the front knee.

The Right Moves

On the days when you don't do a full-blown Power Yoga practice, spend some time working on refining your position in different yoga poses by holding the poses and making adjustments.

➤ Lift the chest and reach out with your arms to create an extended angle from the heel of the back leg right up through the leg, buttocks, torso, and out past the fingertips. Keep your chest, heart, and head up using the muscles of the back.

➤ Exhale as you come out of the lunge and lower the arms.

➤ Repeat five times to each side.

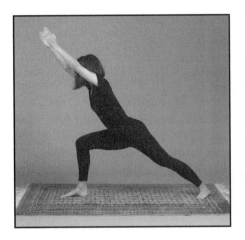
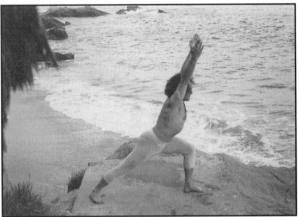

For extended warrior, move into swordsman with hands apart, then angle the body over the front leg to create a straight line from the back heel up through the fingertips.

Bent Knee Forward Bend in Warrior

➤ *Difficulty Level:* II

➤ *Powers:* Great counterpose for warrior balances the back, stretches the hamstrings, and sends blood to the brain for clarity of thinking.

➤ *Caution:* Be very careful coming out of this pose. Don't stretch your arms over your head at first. Instead, start with your hands on your hips so you don't have too much weight over your head for your lower back to lift.

Bent knee forward bend is the counterpose to extended warrior, bringing the body down rather than up. The arms can be held behind the back, with hands on hips, or extended over the head toward the floor.

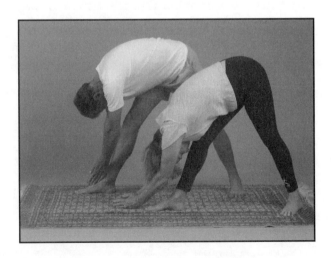

We have yet to insert a counterpose in our warrior series, and your body is ready for one right about now. After extended warrior, balance your warrior movements with bent knee forward bend. This is a great stretch for the back and the hips.

➤ From extended warrior, lower the arms and bring them either behind your back, on your hips, or toward the floor.

➤ Maintaining the front-leg lunge, exhale and bend forward and lay the body over the thigh, head down, spine rounded.

➤ Inhale and come back up carefully with back leg straight and strong, feet solid on the ground. Lift your chest and head together, then let your body follow to move you back into extended warrior or swordsman with a strong, flat back.

➤ You can also rest in bent knee forward bend for five breaths or longer. A full minute in this position becomes a very comfortable, nice stretch for the back. Play with this movement and see how comfortable the bent knee forward bend can be for you.

T-Balance

➤ *Difficulty Level:* III

➤ *Powers:* All the muscles in the standing leg, the back, the arms, the gluteal muscles, the neck, and the sense of balance. Becoming skilled in this pose is also great for the self-esteem.

➤ *Caution:* Don't attempt this pose until you are comfortable balancing on one foot in a less extreme position. Practice with tree pose (see Chapter 13, "Power Balances"), and also practice the pose first without extending the arms.

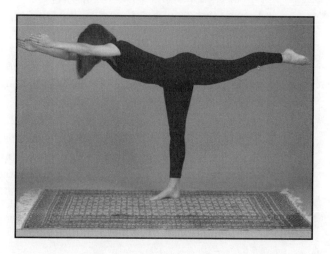

In T-balance, the body forms the shape of the letter "T." This challenging balance pose is the culmination of the warrior series.

The final pose in the warrior series I like to call the T-balance. This balance pose involves standing on one leg, which isn't easy for some people and takes a lot of practice and a lot of leg strength. But don't let this keep you from trying it!

The Wrong Moves

When first trying T-balance, don't keep your leg straight as in the photo. Instead, maintain a good bend in the knee for steadiness. When you become stronger, you can gradually straighten the knee of the base leg, but don't hyperextend the knee or you will lose control over your balance. A slight bend is always best.

The Right Moves

Focusing on one small spot ahead in T-balance is important for maintaining your balance and concentration because the body tends to follow the eyes. If you start looking around, you won't be able to stay up because your body will be trying to move in whatever direction you are looking. It's like driving a car. If you look down the road in front of you, you'll find your car will just follow along. In hiking, if you look down the trail in front of you, you'll find that you'll naturally just walk along the trail and never trip.

Our warrior series has accomplished a progression thus far. First, we started by standing in one place with Marine pose. Then we moved one foot forward into the world while keeping the other foot firmly in place.

The last of the warrior movements removes that back foot, symbolically plunging us forward into the unknown universe. A move like that takes courage, but you've built up a lot of courage through the basic warrior movements, so you're ready!

➤ From extended warrior, step onto the front foot, shifting your weight forward over the front leg. This foot has to be opened up, not gripping the floor. Lay your weight on the foot bones.

➤ Reach out with the arms, extending them to the right and lifting the back foot off the floor behind you.

➤ Keep absolute control as you shift your weight onto one foot. Remain focused on a point in front of you to help keep your balance.

➤ This pose is centered in the hips, so it's important to keep the hips in line. If you roll the hips open, the left hip above the right hip, it will throw your weight to the right side and you'll fall in the direction the hips are moving. Let everything reach outward from the hips so that energy radiates back through the back leg and toes, and forward through the body, head, and fingertips.

➤ Variations: If extending the arms and back leg all the way up to a position parallel with the floor is too challenging, practice this position at first with the back leg raised just a foot or so off the floor, and/or with the arms hanging straight down toward the floor.

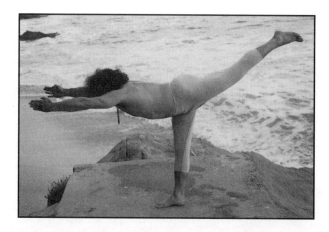

Whether your back leg is just a foot off the ground, parallel with the ground, or even higher as Geo demonstrates, find your place of comfort in the pose and start there. Concentrate!

T-balance isn't an easy pose, but it is incredibly strengthening for the leg and for the entire side of the body holding your weight. Because of the difficulty of the balance, T-balance is also a great tool for improving focus and concentration.

The Least You Need to Know

➤ Warrior poses build physical and emotional strength and courage.

➤ Warrior poses, and possibly all yoga poses, originated from the fighting moves of ancient warriors.

➤ The basic warrior poses are spear thrower, swordsman, extended warrior, and T-balance.

➤ A good warrior counterpose to balance the body is bent knee forward bend.

➤ Balance poses are excellent for strengthening both the body and the concentration.

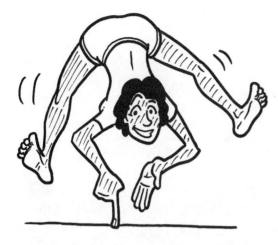

Power Balances

I can't emphasize enough the importance of balance poses. Balance poses are truly yoga for the body and the mind. They bring incredible strengthening, power, and fine-tuning to the muscles of the feet, calves, and thighs. They work the foot bones, the ankles, the knees, and the hip joints. And, they give your mind a workout, too. They focus and refine the concentration, giving you many of the benefits of a meditation session right in the middle of your Power Yoga workout!

The Power of Balance

Balance poses are accomplished by maintaining a tiny point of focus. A spot on the wall, a leaf on a tree, a meaningful object on a table, anything can serve as your point of focus. When moving into a balance pose, your eyes fix on this point of focus and don't move. Because your body tends to go in the direction your eyes are looking, a fixed gaze will help to fix the body.

Holding a point of focus helps to channel our energy, one of the greatest skills you can have, one that will serve you in all aspects of your life. In addition, channeling and controlling your energy will increase your awareness. Yoga in general increases awareness of the world around us, but balance poses super-charge awareness—yoga's fast track to greater sensitivity!

Geo's Journey

When yoga first became popular in the West, back in the 1970s, people tended to think one of yoga's features was the obliteration of awareness, tuning out in favor of some more esoteric or universal consciousness. Things have changed. Now, people realize that yoga is really about increasing awareness in order to more fully live in and experience each moment.

Other than that, balance poses are very powerful strengtheners for the entire standing leg, including the knee, ankle, and foot.

The Wrong Moves

If you haven't done balance poses before, you might feel like your ankle is on fire after holding a bal-ance pose for any length of time. Don't let that discourage you! This reaction in your body shows how much your body needs this kind of work, so keep it up! You'll quickly get stronger.

These days, most of the areas in which people live consist of nice, even surfaces. In reality, our feet aren't designed for even surfaces. In the normal, natural world, surfaces are uneven. Our feet are designed to roll, move, and function over uneven surfaces which then massage, work out, and strengthen the feet.

Now, we all wear big, padded tennis shoes and walk around on perfectly flat surfaces. Then we get to be 50 and wonder why we have bunions and arthritis in our ankles and feet!

As we hold a balance pose, we're forced to work that foot all over, developing, creating, and strengthening the arches. You work all the little bones in the foot, because the strength of the leg starts in the foot. Mov-ing up the leg, balance poses shape the calf, stabilize the knee, tone the thigh, and even strengthen and open up the joints of the hip.

T-Balance

➤ *Difficulty Level:* III

➤ *Powers:* The arches, bones, and muscles of the foot, ankles, calves, and knees; all back muscles; deltoids; hip joints.

➤ *Caution:* Don't try to hold T-balance for very long at first. When you gain strength, you can practice this balance for five breaths. Holding this pose longer would be extremely challenging.

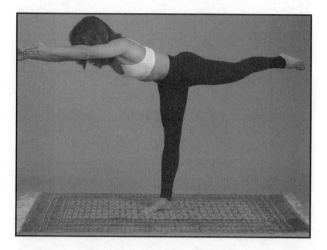

T-balance is a great starting position for the following series of balance poses.

I already walked you through T-balance in the last chapter, as the final pose in the warrior series. For balance poses, it is a beginning rather than an ending.

You may find it difficult to bring your body into a true T position. Lifting and holding your arms, upper body, and leg so they remain parallel to the floor takes quite a lot of strength and stability. You'll get it with practice, but be patient with yourself.

If you are having a hard time with this position, try it in stages. First, practice how it feels to extend the upper body and arms in a true right angle to the leg, without the balance.

Then, practice extending the leg in a true right angle to the standing leg without extending the arms.

Once you've got the feel of each side, you can work on putting them together. This is a good project for those Power Yoga days off, when you take a walk and then spend some time working on particular poses rather than moving through an entire routine.

The Wrong Moves

If you have bad knees, work very slowly with balance poses and don't lock the knee of your standing leg. It is perfectly okay to do balance poses with a bent knee. You'll have more control over your balance and won't risk injury.

Half Moon Pose

> ➤ *Difficulty Level:* III

> ➤ *Powers:* The hip joints; the muscles of the limbs, both the limbs bearing the body's weight and the lifted limbs; the neck and chest.

> ➤ *Caution:* Don't move into half moon pose unless you are very comfortable and secure in T-balance.

Half moon pose takes T-balance, rotates the body to one side, and extends one arm to the ground.

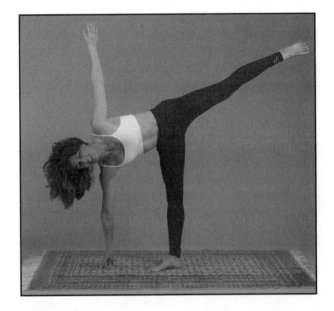

From T-balance, it doesn't take much effort to fall forward a bit and turn your body into half moon pose.

> ➤ From T-balance, move forward and let your hands drop to the floor.

> ➤ When on your right foot, leave the fingertips of your right hand—not the palm, not the bones, just the fingertips—for a little bit of balance. Line up the place where your fingertips touch the floor with the line extending straight out from your little toe.

> ➤ Look to the left and focus on a spot. Lock into that spot, then slowly roll your body open to the left, lifting your left hip above your right hip.

> ➤ Lift your left leg and stretch it straight out, also lifting your chest and heart. Try not to roll forward on the hand. Let all your weight remain over your base leg.

> ➤ Hold for one to five breaths, then rotate your body back toward the ground, lower your extended leg, lower your raised arm, and raise yourself back up to a standing position.

> ➤ Repeat on the opposite side.

Geo's Journey

When practicing balance poses to each side, you'll probably notice that one side is easier to balance upon than the other. This tells you which side of your brain is more dominant, and this may even change from day to day or throughout different periods of your life. Remember, one side of the brain controls the opposite side of the body. So, if you are stronger in your right side, your left brain is dominant and you tend to be more rational. If your left side is stronger, your intuitive right brain is in control. Because in yoga, balance is key, try to work out a little more on the side that feels less strong.

Half Moon Head Down

➤ *Difficulty Level:* III

➤ *Powers:* The neck muscles and vertebrae, in addition to the muscles working in half moon pose.

➤ *Caution:* Be sure to choose a point of focus on the floor when turning the head down, or you'll lose your balance.

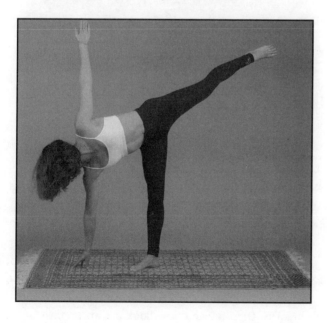

For half moon head down, get into half moon, then rotate your head to look at the floor.

Half moon head down pose adds a nice stretch in the neck and further challenges your balance.

➤ From half moon pose, slowly rotate the head down.

➤ Find a spot on the floor for focus instead of on the wall to maintain your position.

➤ Hold for one to five full breaths.

➤ Come back up to standing, then repeat to the other side.

Revolving Half Moon

➤ *Difficulty Level:* III

➤ *Powers:* Your internal organs through a torso twist; also strengthens and stretches your obliques, the muscles along the sides of your torso.

➤ *Caution:* You don't want to fall when switching arms for this "balance with a twist." Move slowly and carefully, keeping your eyes fixed on a point on the floor for balance.

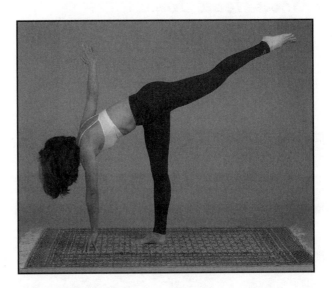

For revolving half moon, the arms switch position and the focus moves to the floor.

Revolving half moon puts a nice twist in your torso, adding a challenge to the balance of half moon.

➤ Get into half moon position, then slowly bring your raised arm (your left arm if you are standing on your right leg) to the floor.

➤ Looking down, find a point of focus on the floor, then carefully raise your other arm (your right arm if you are standing on your right leg) so the fingers point toward the ceiling.

➤ Hold for one to five full breaths, then lower, come back up, and repeat on the other side.

Single Leg Split

➤ *Difficulty Level:* II

➤ *Powers:* All the muscles of the standing leg: heel, calf, hamstrings, gluteal muscles. Weight of the head stretches the spine. Opens hips.

➤ *Caution:* Don't come out of this pose too quickly or you'll get dizzy. Come up slowly with hands raised above your head.

The Right Moves

When performing half moon pose on the right leg, you'll get stronger on your masculine side. When performing half moon pose on your left leg, your feminine nature will strengthen.

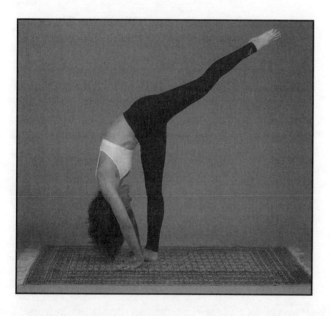

Single leg split offers the benefits of the forward bend and balance poses all in one.

From half moon (or any of its variations), balance the body by releasing some of the pressure on the standing leg and shifting it forward with a nice balancing standing forward bend.

➤ From half moon, exhale and bring both hands to the ground as you rotate your torso so you are facing the ground. Leave your extended leg up.

➤ As you bring your hands to the ground, move into a nice forward bend, bending your knees a little bit. This forward bend is deeper than the bend required for half moon.

185

➤ Lay the body forward, walking the hands back until they are on either side of the foot.

➤ Keep your back leg stretched toward the ceiling. Let your head hang down toward your front foot.

➤ Feel as if you are a ballet dancer in a graceful split position. Feel the huge stretch from the heel of the standing foot all the way up through the calf, back of the leg, gluteal muscle, and as the body hangs over that thigh, the nice stretch in the back as the 10 to 15 pound head hangs from the spine.

➤ Feel the opening of the hips as you reach with the back foot as far back and up as you can.

➤ Hold for one to five full breaths, then move up into tree balance.

Power Words

Lactic acid is a product of anaerobic respiration, the process that takes over when the lungs and circulatory system are no longer able to supply muscles with enough ready oxygen and nutrients during strenuous activities. In anaerobic respiration, lactic acid is produced and accumulates in muscle tissue, causing the burning sensation people call "sore muscles."

When in balance positions, when the muscles and tissues aren't yet strong enough to hold a position, they may begin to shake. *Lactic acid* is building up in the tissue because you aren't getting enough oxygen into those muscles. As you practice these poses, the shaking will eventually disappear as you get stronger. Meanwhile, don't let yourself shake so much that you fall over or hurt yourself! Honor your weak places until they become strong.

Once you feel strong and confident with the single leg split, return to an upright position and be a tree!

Tree Balance

➤ *Difficulty Level:* II

➤ *Powers:* Strengthens the legs, opens the torso and spine, stretches the shoulders, and hones the sense of balance.

➤ *Caution:* All yoga should be practiced in bare feet on a non-slip surface. Tree balance is easiest if you make your leg non-slip by wearing shorts so that your bare foot is held against your bare leg, skin on skin. Slippery clothing makes it more difficult to hold your foot in place.

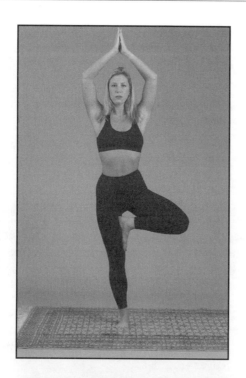

Tree balance imitates the proud height and flexible strength of a tree.

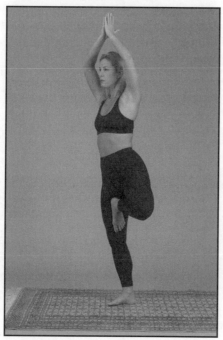

Fixing your eyes on a point in front of you will help you to keep your balance in tree balance.

This beautiful pose is relatively easy to accomplish, but after warrior series and a few more challenging balance poses like T-balance and half moon, your muscles are more fatigued and tree balance becomes a greater challenge. And we're always up for a challenge!

Tree pose is standing on one leg at a time, working one side of the body at a time, like most balance poses. As usual, let's start on the right foot.

➤ Inhale as you come out of single leg split to stand upright, staying balanced on the same base leg (we'll say the right leg). If you need to steady yourself, you can touch your left leg to the ground before bringing it up again. Keep your hands on your hips for now.

➤ Bring the left foot off the ground and put it either on the side of your calf in the beginning (touching the floor when necessary for balance), or eventually up to the inside of the thigh. Your ultimate goal is to place your heel at the root of your thigh where it connects with the hip, rolling your left knee open to open the hip and leg.

➤ Lift your chest and heart, open your belly, breathing nice and easy.

The Right Moves

Very advanced students can take forward bend in tree balance once step farther by moving into a tree balance squat. Not for the beginner!

➤ Now, inhale and bring your hands in prayer fashion in front of your heart, then raise them over your head.

➤ Stand in this position as if you are the god or goddess of the trees looking out over the forest. Imagine standing in the air like this, floating above the forest.

➤ Hold this position for as long as you comfortably can. This is more of a pose to hold while breathing than to move in and out of with the breath. A minute in tree pose is a long time. Five breaths is a good start.

➤ To counter the lifting of the arms and body with tree balance, bring the arms down, move the raised foot to the front of the opposite hip, then bend down toward the floor in a standing forward bend, squeezing the foot between your hip and upper body. This pose is difficult at first, but you'll get the feel of it with practice. Go only as far as you are comfortable with. Hold for one to five breaths.

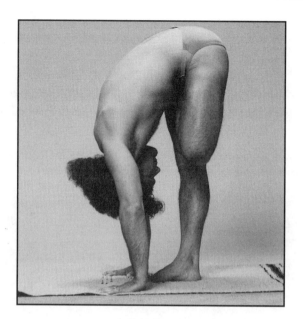

Forward bend in tree balance is a challenging pose for balance and flexibility in the hip and knee. You might try this pose in a sitting position before attempting it while standing.

➤ Be careful coming out of this forward bend. Bend your knee more deeply and look at the floor. Then, slowly come up until you're standing back on one foot. Gradually bring your hands above your head again to be back into tree balance.

➤ Hold for one to five more breaths, then bring your leg and arms down to the floor. Repeat on the opposite side.

Geo's Journey

The ideal way to accomplish difficult poses is to move in and out of them with such strength and grace that they look effortless. It's much more difficult to go slowly into and out of yoga positions. It's easy to just fall into poses, but be careful of that kind of loss of control. That's how we get hurt.

After this series of balance poses, your legs should be thoroughly worked and in absolute need of stretching and opening. Now is the perfect time for the triangle series.

The Least You Need to Know

➤ Balance poses strengthen all the leg muscles and work to tone and strengthen the bones, muscles, and joints of the foot, ankle, knee, and hip.

➤ T-balance is a challenging balance pose and a good starting point for a series of balance poses.

➤ Half moon pose and its variations are challenging balance poses that open the front of the body and strengthen the limbs.

➤ Single leg split is a graceful counterpose to T-balance and half moon.

➤ Tree balance is an easier pose than the previous balance poses, but it is still challenging after a balance series.

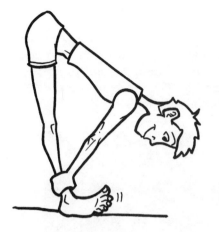

Chapter 14

Angling

In This Chapter

➤ Stretch out your sides with triangles

➤ Experience a deeper stretch with angle poses

➤ When you have gained enough strength, you can be an exalted warrior

Athletes, and anyone else working to be more fit, sometimes forget about the sides of their bodies. We work the stomach, the back, the legs, the arms, the chest, the shoulders, even the wrists, calves, neck ... but the sides of the body remain unchallenged.

But working the sides of the body—more precisely, the external oblique muscles along the waistline, the latissimus dorsi, which wraps around the upper body from front to back, and several smaller muscles that wrap around the sides of the hips, is important for maintaining a body that is truly in balance, injury-resistant, and flexible.

Power Yoga, and more traditional Hatha Yoga, for that matter, spends a lot of time on the sides of the body, unlike many other forms of exercise. In addition to stretching and strengthening the muscles on the sides of the body, the triangle and angle poses help to alternately compress and open the internal organs of the torso, including the heart, pancreas, spleen, liver, and gallbladder.

Angle poses reshape the back, remind the spine of its proper place (which is *not* hunched, but straight and strong), and even help to open and release the fourth or heart chakra, the center of your emotional life and the center of your entire body. These are truly balancing poses and movements.

Can You Angle This?

Balance poses flow nicely into angle poses, which take a sense of balance themselves, but aren't quite as difficult to maintain. Instead, these poses concentrate on opening and releasing the sides of the body. All the chapters in Part 3, "Stand Up and Take a Bow," are meant to create one long flow of poses. This chapter represents the final group in that continuous series of power stands, so keep moving!

Triangle can be adjusted for any body type and fitness level. Positions can be gentle or highly challenging.

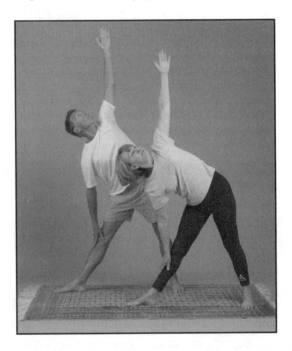

Angle poses make wonderful counterposes for the warrior series. While warrior movements work the quadriceps and hips by mostly keeping the body upright, angle poses work the obliques and other muscles of the torso by sending the upper body down toward the ground.

Triangle

➤ *Difficulty Level:* II

➤ *Powers:* The external obliques, latissimus dorsi, pectoral muscles; opens and stretches the hip joints; also gives a nice twist to the neck.

➤ *Caution:* If your body doesn't let you bend all the way to the ground in triangle, don't push it. Put your lower hand on your leg and slide it down gradually toward the floor, working at the edge of your flexibility.

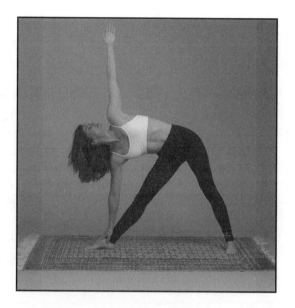

Triangle pose is a beautiful pose that forms several triangles: between the legs, under the lower arm, and the implied triangles formed by the upper arm and the top edge of the body.

Begin your triangle series directly from tree balance.

➤ Step back with the leg that was raised in tree balance (we'll say your left leg) and set your foot down into warrior pose. Have your feet about four feet apart, your left foot in back, your right foot pointing forward and perpendicular to the back foot.

➤ Once you feel that your feet are solid, straighten both legs, inhale, and stretch up with your right arm.

➤ As you reach up, look up at your right hand. This movement creates an arch in the left side of your back and a powerful effect in the left kidney and adrenal areas. Pause here before reaching out over the right leg and dropping your hand down. This pause at the top of the reaching-up movement is an important part of the pose.

➤ Exhale and reach over your right leg until you come to the place where your leg muscles stop you. This is your edge.

The Wrong Moves

If you have to bend your knee or can't flatten your body to the left in this pose, you're going too far. The left hip should roll open, belly and heart should be flat to the left, and left arm should be reaching up as if God were pulling on your fingertips. If your hand drops too far down the leg, you won't get the benefit in the upper back. You want the chest and heart to be up, not rolling forward.

The Right Moves

Triangle poses are great for women. One reason is that triangle pose works against the forces that worsen osteoporosis. I call it the "anti-osteoporosis pose." Triangle pose reshapes the upper back, where osteoporosis often sets in. Just be sure to keep your upper back flat and your chest up when practicing the pose.

➤ Drop your torso and stretch your right arm toward your right foot, sliding your hand down your leg if you can't make it all the way to the ground.

➤ Hold the pose long enough to feel the great stretch down the leg and the heart opening, for one to five full breaths. Your upper back will also feel the stretch. Don't let your head hang. Keep your neck straight and strong, in line with your spine. Be strong and active with your neck, head, and eyes.

➤ Slide your hand back up your leg to come upright again as you exhale, then repeat to the other side.

Extended Triangle

➤ *Difficulty Level:* III

➤ *Powers:* Opens the external obliques, the shoulder, ribs, latissimus dorsi, heart, pancreas, and down into the intercostal muscles, helping to open up space for deeper breathing. When extending to the left, you'll get an added stretch in the left hip and spleen. When extending to the right, you'll open and stimulate the liver and gallbladder.

➤ *Caution:* Keep your weight evenly centered over your feet. Some people tend to roll toward the outside of the foot, bringing the big toe off the ground, which puts an unnecessary strain on the side of the knee.

Extended triangle takes triangle to the extreme, giving the side of the torso a magnificent stretch.

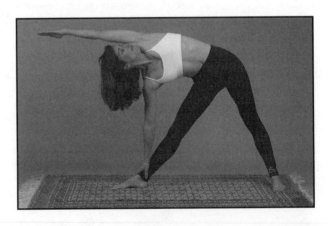

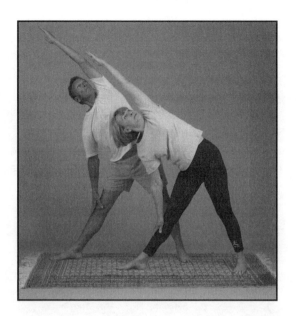

Even extended triangle can be modified for a less extreme angle, to match any fitness level.

After coming up from triangle on each side, go back down into extended triangle for an even greater stretch.

➤ Keeping your feet in warrior position, inhale and reach up over your head with your right hand and over to the side. Feel your whole side, waist, ribs, shoulder, and outside of your hip open up as you stretch over your head. You'll still feel the nice stretch in the right leg from the hip through the heel. Extend as far overhead as your body will allow.

➤ At the same time, slide your lower hand back down your leg toward the floor.

➤ Look up toward the ceiling from underneath your upper arm. Hold for one to five full breaths.

➤ Exhale and come back up to a standing position, then repeat on the other side.

The Right Moves

You should be able to look at a spot on the ceiling when doing triangle poses, and you should feel the pressure in your upper back. Look at a spot on the ceiling and line up everything with that spot. If you don't feel pressure in your upper back, you're rolling forward too much. Keep your right shoulder stacked over your left shoulder, and always keep in mind the feeling of hanging from the sky by your fingertips (or, in the case of extended triangle, from your elbow) to help line you up correctly.

Twisted Triangle

➤ *Difficulty Level:* II

➤ *Powers:* The spine, hip joints, and muscles of the torso. Very powerful in the heart as the front of the chest opens. Also a great stretch for the lower glands and organs, including the pancreas, diaphragm, intestines, kidneys, adrenals; opens the lung on the open side.

➤ *Caution:* Again, don't roll your foot open on this pose or you'll strain your knee. Keep your weight evenly distributed over your foot and your big toe firmly on the ground.

Twisted triangle is the counterpose to triangle, stretching the body in the opposite direction.

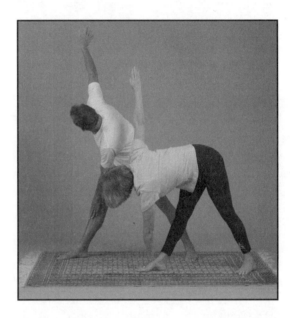

Twisted triangle moves the body in the opposite direction as triangle and so makes for a great counterpose.

➤ Move into triangle again.

➤ Turn your head and look down toward the floor.

➤ Bring your left hand down to the floor or to your leg, at the same time rotating your right arm (which was down in triangle) upward, opening your chest and heart to the right (your masculine side).

➤ Hold for one to five breaths. Even though you aren't balancing on one foot in twisted triangle, it is a good balance pose and excellent for focus and concentration. The twisting adds a challenge to the sense of balance.

➤ Bring both arms down to the ground, keeping the torso lowered.

➤ Exhale and turn the torso toward the leg, moving into a bent knee forward bend, and hold for one to five breaths.

➤ Inhale and come back up to standing, then repeat on the other side.

Angle Series

This series follows the series of triangle poses, stretching and extending and lunging the triangle further down to the ground.

Angle Pose

➤ *Difficulty Level:* III

➤ *Powers:* The hip sockets, external obliques, quadriceps, inner thighs, knee, shoulder, neck. Also stimulates the turning point of the colon.

➤ *Caution:* Don't extend the knee past the middle of the supporting foot.

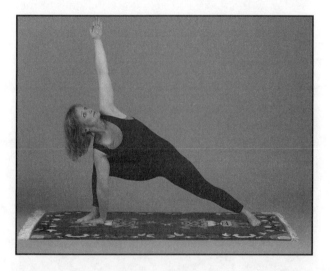

Angle pose moves the body from triangle into a side lunge to create a beautiful, sweeping angle from fingertip to toe.

Angle pose is a great pose for the hips, the obliques, and the muscles of the supporting leg and arm. It stretches the inner thigh and really opens up the side of the body.

➤ After finishing twisted triangle, inhale and bend back down to the right side into triangle.

➤ Slowly lunge with the right knee until the knee is at a right angle, resting your right elbow on your right thigh for support.

➤ Stretch your arm over your head, reaching for the sky.

➤ As you get stronger, take your right elbow from your right knee and slide your right hand inside the right ankle. Set your palm on the floor inside your right ankle. This position deepens the angle of the hip, but don't try it before you are ready.

➤ Keep your back foot solid, feet perpendicular. Roll and twist in the waist and lower back, reaching straight up with your hand to open your shoulder joint.

➤ Look up under your left arm. Hold for one to five breaths.

➤ Bring your raised arm down and slowly lift your body up again.

➤ Come out of the lunge on the exhale.

➤ Repeat to the other side.

Extended Angle Pose

➤ *Difficulty Level:* III

➤ *Powers:* Just like angle pose, but with an extra stretch along the sides of the body.

➤ *Caution:* Keep the knee at a right angle and don't overextend the upper arm so much that you strain your shoulder.

Extended angle pose creates a straight line with the body from fingertip to toe.

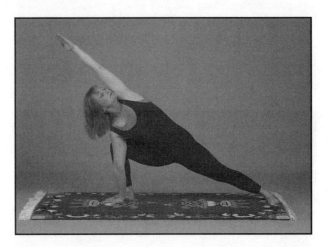

Just as in triangle, we can take this pose farther. After angle pose on each side, move back into angle pose again as you inhale. You can still leave your elbow on your supporting thigh if reaching the floor is too difficult.

➤ This time, extend your arm even farther over your head to create a straight plane from your fingertips to your toes.

➤ Feel the stretch along the entire side of your body as you look up under your extended arm.

➤ Hold for one to five full breaths, then come up and repeat to the other side.

➤ Variation: Some people like to move their right hand to the outside of the foot, which bends the knee a little more. I actually prefer to keep the hand inside the ankle. I feel the effects are better and don't believe this deeper pose necessarily has a better effect.

Twisted Angle Pose

➤ *Difficulty Level:* III

➤ *Powers:* Puts a nice twist in the torso and puts a great stretch in the hip, in the direction you are twisting. Also opens the lung of your open side.

➤ *Caution:* Move into the twist slowly to protect your lower back. Keep your body controlled.

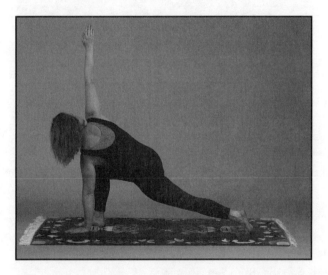

Twisted angle pose revolves angle pose so the opposite hand extends upward.

Twisted angle pose is the counterpose to angle pose, just like twisted triangle is the counterpose to triangle.

➤ From extended angle, bring your left hand down and put it where the right hand was, inside the ankle.

➤ Twist to the right, roll the right arm up, and take the back heel off the ground, up onto the ball of the foot.

➤ Reach straight to the ceiling and look up toward your raised palm.

➤ Hold for one to five full breaths, then come down and repeat to the other side.

Extended Twisted Angle Pose

➤ *Difficulty Level:* III

➤ *Powers:* Again, a nice twist in the torso and a great stretch in the hip, in the direction you are twisting. Strengthens the back of the leg and the knee. Gently squeezes the kidneys and adrenals on the side being twisted.

➤ *Caution:* Move into the twist slowly to protect your lower back. Keep your body controlled and stay strong in the shoulder.

Extended twisted angle pose extends the arm farther over the head from twisted angle pose.

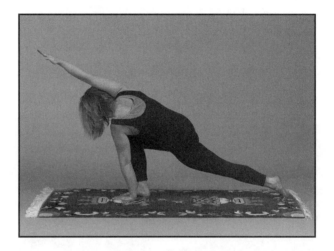

From twisted angle pose, simply extend the arm again to create a straight line from fingertip to heel.

➤ Feel the line of energy from the ball of your back foot out through your fingertips.

➤ Feel your foot pushing off your toes.

➤ Hold for one to five full breaths, then repeat on the other side.

This completes our series of standing poses. While I've suggested repeating each pose to the opposite side as you go, you could also complete the entire series of standing poses to the right, then go back, start over, and do them all to the left. It's your choice. You could also alternate methods with each workout for a change of pace and better all-over conditioning. Keep your body surprised!

Extended twisted angle pose is also a great segue into animal poses because you can easily move down onto all fours. See Part 4, "Your Animal Nature," for the animal series.

Or, if you are feeling really strong, you can add one more pose to the mix that flows out of the angle series: exalted warrior.

Exalted Warrior

➤ *Difficulty Level:* IV

➤ *Powers:* The quadriceps, knees, ankles, and feet; opens the chest, stretches the neck, opens the hips, and gives you a great sense of personal power.

➤ *Caution:* Don't try this pose before you have gained sufficient strength. Also, if you have bad knees, this pose may create too much of a strain, unless you have the leg strength to properly support the knees.

Exalted warrior flows nicely from extended twisted angle pose.

➤ Bring both hands to your front knee, lift your chest and heart, roll your shoulders back, and feel the great stretch in your back leg and back hip.

➤ When you feel solid and balanced, gradually bring your hands off your knee and reach them overhead with palms shoulder-width apart or palms together in prayer position.

➤ Slowly lay the head back and look up. Focus on something to stabilize your position, such as a spot on the ceiling or the area of your third eye (the center of your forehead).

The Right Moves

Twisted angle pose is great for all your internal organs. It especially stimulates the turning point of the colon, the heart, diaphragm, back, and pancreas. However, you have to do it correctly. Make sure you keep your foot solid and your knee in. People have a tendency to roll the knee out to the side. You can also do this pose with your elbow on your knee, if this variation will help you to have more control over the pose and keep your body in better alignment.

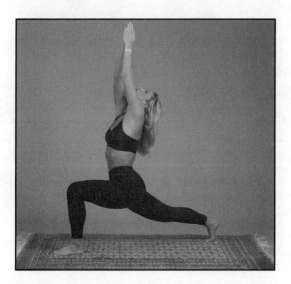

Exalted warrior is a difficult pose that takes a lot of leg and knee strength as well as a keen sense of balance.

➤ Hold only as long as is comfortable—this may be only half a breath, which is fine as long as your positioning was strong and straight for that half-breath.

➤ Bring your arms back down, stand up, and repeat on the other side.

Geo's Journey

I love exalted warrior pose. It is both physically and symbolically empowering. The pose gets your head out of the way and shifts your body in such a way that you lead with your heart instead. As you hold the pose, imagine your heart is like a beacon in your chest, radiating, celebrating your warrior power.

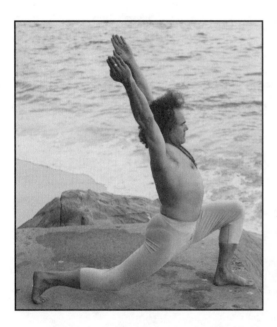 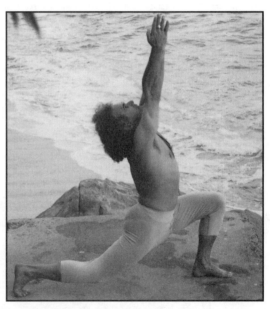

Geo moves into the exalted warrior pose. Feel the warrior power!

Exalted warrior, the ultimate warrior pose, is very powerful. All the other warrior poses work up to this one, which takes the most strength of any warrior pose, but is perhaps the most beautiful and empowering.

Because all standing movements lead to this pose, from exalted warrior you can move to any other series. I suggest exploring your animal nature. (In other words, move on to the next chapter!)

The Least You Need to Know

➤ Triangle poses and angle poses are good counterposes to the warrior series.

➤ Twisting the triangle and angle poses stretches the body in still another direction.

➤ Exalted warrior is the ultimate challenging warrior position, which comes naturally out of angle poses once you are sufficiently strong.

Part 4

Your Animal Nature

This section focuses on the four-legged poses, each of which evokes a different animal form or movement. The first series flows out of exalted warrior into monkey and pigeon poses and a challenging yoga split. Then, you'll get down on all fours for a rigorous series of lunges, push-ups, squat thrusts, and dog poses. Four-legged poses are strenuous, so you'll get a great aerobic workout with this series, in addition to the spine-aligning and muscle-strengthening benefits.

At the end of this section, I'll spend a full chapter on my 13 steps for natural living. Learn how you are sabotaging your body's natural efforts to be healthy; then, one by one, change your habits to create more vitality, energy, and health. From simple living and following some traditional yoga abstentions and observances to meditation, an improved diet, and cultivating a positive attitude, you'll be feeling better fast.

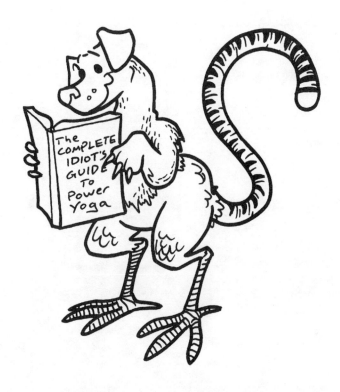

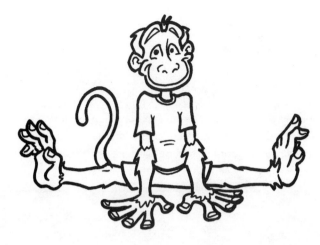

Chapter 15

Primates and Pigeons

In This Chapter

➤ From exalted warrior to monkey

➤ For every arch there is a bend

➤ Doing the pigeon

➤ You can do the splits!

This first chapter of animal poses has a little of everything—primates, pigeons, bends, and splits. The next chapter will concentrate on the four-legged animal poses, but for this chapter, I want to move straight from exalted warrior into a position that is a lot like exalted warrior: monkey pose.

The Wild Kingdom

Although it may seem to you like moving from the sublime to the ridiculous in a sort of de-evolution (after all, what is a monkey compared to an exalted warrior?), monkey pose is actually a challenging and highly effective pose for opening and stretching the hips, chest, shoulders, and neck. Give it a try, and start getting in touch with your animal nature!

Geo's Journey

For the poses in this chapter, I suggest you do the entire series on one side, then repeat the entire series on the other side. In other chapters, I recommend alternating sides after each pose or small group of poses. However, your method of balancing your routine is up to you. Feel free to alternate sides with each pose if that feels more comfortable.

Monkey Pose

➤ *Difficulty Level:* III

➤ *Powers:* The hips, chest, shoulders, arms, and neck. Also gives a great stretch to your back foot. Squeezes the kidneys and adrenals and opens the colon.

➤ *Caution:* Keep your hips straight and steady and your spine straight in this pose. A strong base in the hips is necessary to keep the lower back supported.

Monkey pose is like exalted warrior, but the lunge is deeper and the arms are behind the back for an even greater opening of the chest.

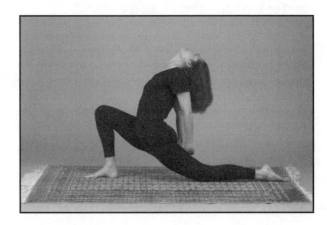

You can begin the monkey series straight from exalted warrior.

➤ From exalted warrior, let your hands come down slowly as you drop your back knee to the floor.

➤ Point the toes of your back foot straight behind you, resting the entire top of your foot against the floor.

➤ Without moving your front foot, let your right knee slide forward over your toes. You can move past the right angle here without straining the knee because you aren't really using the muscles, you're stretching them.

➤ Reach your hands behind you and interlock your fingers. Reach back toward your back knee, opening and expanding your chest.

➤ Keep your back foot extended straight back, knee touching the floor. You should feel almost as if you are dragging your back foot behind you, pulling the weight off your back foot onto your front foot.

➤ Hold for one to five breaths, then bring arms forward, come up, and do single leg forward bend as a counterpose before repeating on the opposite side.

The Wrong Moves

In monkey pose, keep your front foot solid on the ground. If your heel starts coming off the ground, then your foot is too far under you.

Single Leg Forward Bend

➤ *Difficulty Level:* II

➤ *Powers:* A great stretch for the hamstrings, quadriceps, and back.

➤ *Caution:* Don't bend farther forward than your body will allow. Feel the stretch, but don't cause yourself pain. Everyone has a different level of flexibility. Find yours. Also, it isn't easy for everybody to sit on the heel. If it isn't comfortable, slide your foot under your thigh. Bend your knee if you need to. Don't hyperextend your knee.

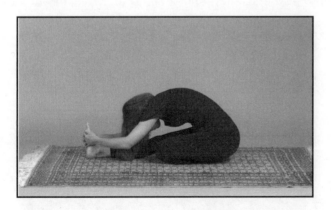

Single leg forward bend balances the spine with a nice bend after the arching movements in monkey pose and exalted warrior.

Go straight into this pose from monkey pose without standing up. Your spine will thank you for this relaxing and balancing counterpose.

➤ From monkey pose, bring the body upright, then shift the hips back until you are sitting on the heel of the leg that was extended behind you.

➤ Extend your front leg in front of you.

➤ Slowly stretch toward your front leg, reaching for your foot and letting your spine bend.

➤ Hold for one to five full breaths. Repeat after monkey pose on the other side.

Geo's Journey

Counterposes offer you a great opportunity to get better acquainted with your body. Learn to feel the effect of a bend or an arch on your body, and then experiment to find the degree of opposite movement and length of time to hold the counterpose in order to achieve balance.

Pigeon Pose

➤ *Difficulty Level:* III

➤ *Powers:* Opens the chest, heart, ribs, and hips. Squeezes the kidneys and the adrenals.

➤ *Caution:* Be gentle on your knees in pigeon pose. If your knees feel strained, come a little higher off the ground, and/or put a pillow under your front knee.

Pigeon pose is similar to monkey pose, except the front knee rests on the floor and the hands extend to the floor.

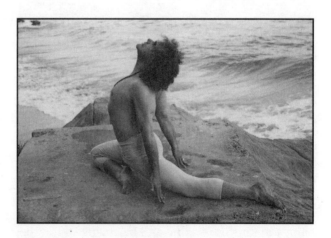

Now you are ready for an even deeper hip and quadriceps stretch. After monkey pose and single leg forward bend on one side, go straight into pigeon pose on the same side. You'll repeat the entire series on the other side later.

➤ From single leg forward bend, rise back up onto your knees, extending your back leg behind you as it was for monkey pose. Point the toes straight back behind you.

➤ Ease your front leg forward so your bent knee comes to the floor and the entire front of your lower leg rests on the floor with your heel under your hips.

➤ Bring your fingertips to the floor and slowly walk your hands back as far as you can until you feel your shoulders rolling back, your chest and heart opening.

➤ Lay your head back and lift and open with your heart. Let the weight of your head assist in the opening of the front of your body.

➤ Stay strong in the gluteal muscles and push on the fingertips to alleviate the pressure on the lower back and to continue to lift the front of the body.

➤ Hold for one to five full breaths.

Geo's Journey

If you've ever seen a pigeon puff up its chest, you've seen pigeon pose. Maybe it's part of the mating process. I've seen weightlifters do the same thing! A man comes into a room with a straight, strong chest, and all the other guys in the room puff their chests out as well! That's what we want with pigeon pose—a sense of puffing out the chest and reaching out with the heart.

Pigeon Hip Stretch

➤ *Difficulty Level:* III

➤ *Powers:* A strong, deep stretch into the hip joints.

➤ *Caution:* Be careful as you rest your weight over your bent knee. If you feel any strain in the knee, ease up and center your weight over your shoulders, leaving a little space over the knee.

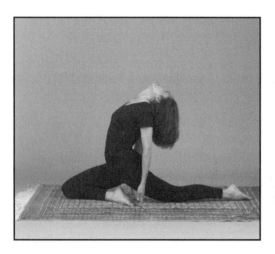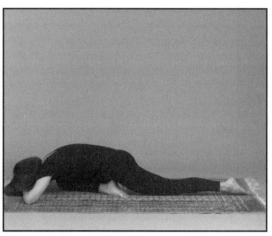

Pigeon hip stretch (right) counters pigeon pose (left) by moving the spine in the opposite direction and giving the body a brief rest after the strenuous hold required for pigeon pose.

After pigeon pose, your body is ready for another counterpose. Give your body what it needs with a pigeon hip stretch.

➤ From pigeon pose, raise your head, then ease your body forward over the front bent knee.

➤ Bring the arms forward, elbows bent, to rest on the floor. Let your forehead rest on your arms.

➤ Feel the weight of the body sinking down into the hips and let your spine bend forward over your knee.

➤ Rest here for one to five breaths, or longer if it feels really great.

Geo's Journey

Twenty seconds is about as long as you would need (or want) to stay in poses like monkey pose and pigeon pose. The forward bends, however, like single leg stretch and pigeon hip stretch are resting poses designed to be held for much longer, if you so desire.

Pigeon Pose with Shoulder and Quad Stretch

➤ *Difficulty Level:* IV

➤ *Powers:* The shoulders, hips, quadriceps, knee, and the lower back; a magical way to relieve tension and tightness in the hips.

➤ *Caution:* People with knee problems shouldn't attempt this pose, or should do so with extreme caution and a very gradual knee bend, slowly working up to the degree of bend in the photograph over a period of weeks or months.

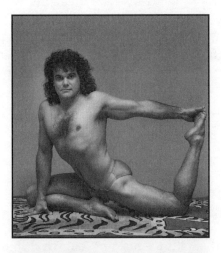

Pigeon pose with shoulder stretch opens the shoulder and readies the quadriceps for a deeper stretch.

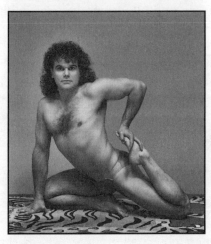

Pigeon pose with quad stretch takes the position one step farther, adding a deep stretch to the quadriceps.

For the advanced and/or very flexible student, try this final variation of pigeon pose. Move into this pose straight from pigeon hip stretch.

➤ From pigeon hip stretch, lift the torso back to an upright position and return to pigeon pose, but keep the head upright rather than letting it drop backward.

➤ Slowly lift the foot of your back leg and reach back with your back arm. Grasp your foot with your hand. Move your opposite hand in front of the hip you are turning toward, for support.

➤ Inhale and pull the foot out slightly to give your shoulder a gentle stretch. Your arm should be straight so the shoulder can really stretch.

➤ Exhale and ease your foot toward your lower back, bending the elbow and pulling gently with the hand to create a deep stretch in the quadriceps muscles. Don't stretch so far that you feel strain in the knee, however.

➤ Keep the chest lifted and your body twisted just enough so that your back shoulder is pulled back. Look straight ahead. Your bent heel should be under your body and your hips lifted slightly off the ground.

➤ Hold for one to five full breaths.

Split Forward Bend

➤ *Difficulty Level:* IV

➤ *Powers:* A fantastic stretch of the inner thigh muscles and hips; a nice counter-movement for the spine.

➤ *Caution:* Most people can't do the splits the first time out. Wait until your flexibility allows it. If this position is too difficult, do another pigeon hip stretch at this point in the series.

Split forward bend is a pose to challenge even the most flexible.

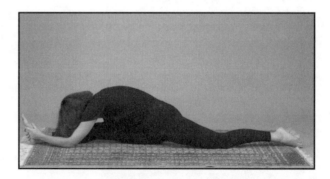

Move into split forward bend as a counterpose to pigeon pose with heel to hip stretch.

➤ From pigeon pose with heel to hip stretch, slowly lower your back foot so your back leg is once again extended behind you.

➤ Return your hands to the floor on either side of your hips, and twist to both sides, preparing your body for the split.

➤ Lift your body up slightly, allowing your front leg to unfold in front of you.

➤ Settle your weight into your hips so you feel centered and balanced in this split position. Your back leg and front leg should be approximately in a straight line.

➤ Stretch your back toes straight back, front toes straight out. The stretching of the toes actually helps to move the body into the split. People tend to turn their toes inward in a split, which rolls the hip in the wrong way. Work for a really big stretch down the center of the hip. It doesn't matter how far apart your legs are, as long as you are getting that deep stretch.

➤ Inhale and reach as high overhead as you can.

➤ Exhale and bend your torso over your front leg, reaching for your foot.

➤ Variations: If you aren't yet flexible enough for a full split, you have several options. You can keep your front leg bent, as in pigeon hip stretch, repeating that pose here. Or, you can bend your back leg and stretch out over your extended front leg, as in alternate leg stretch (see Chapter 18, "Sitting Series").

The Right Moves

The splits can be hard on the knee joints. Keep your knees slightly bent, even in split poses, to lessen the strain on this delicate joint. In general, in almost every straight-legged pose, you will lessen your risk of injury if you keep your knees slightly bent.

The Wrong Moves

Don't force your body over your extended front leg for split forward bend. If you can only come down a little way toward your front leg, that's fine. Again, find your edge and work with it. The limit of your flexibility isn't fixed. The more you work on it, the more it moves.

➤ Hold for one to five full breaths before coming up into a yoga split.

Yoga Split

➤ *Difficulty Level:* IV

➤ *Powers:* Stretches the inner thigh muscles, opens the chest, loosens the shoulders and neck. A very empowering position.

➤ *Caution:* If you can't do a full split, don't force it. For beginners, keep either the front or back leg bent as you bring the body up.

The yoga split is another challenging pose which, when performed correctly, creates a beautiful and energized shape with the body.

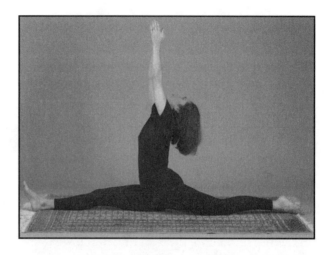

The Right Moves

Some people will never get into a full split. That's okay. Just find your edge, expand it a little, and work with your individual flexibility. But you may be surprised! Sharon, a student who was never able to do a full split, even as a teenager, finally reached a point of flexibility on her sixty-fifth birthday, after three years of yoga, by achieving a full split.

Come up into a yoga split for the final pose in this series.

➤ Lift your torso, with arms outstretched, to an upright position from split forward bend.

➤ Reach straight up and bring your palms together in prayer position.

➤ Gently lower your head back to look toward your hands.

➤ Let your body settle into the split and, once again, feel as if you are hanging from the sky by your fingertips. Let your body fall into the position it would if you were suspended.

➤ Feel the energy flowing out of each outstretched limb—down both legs and out the ends of your toes, and up your arms, out the ends of your fingertips.

➤ Variation: If the full split is too difficult, you can keep either your front or back leg bent, bringing your heel in to your body as you reach up.

➤ Hold for one to five full breaths, then exhale and bring your arms down.

➤ If you find it difficult to raise your arms, walk them out next to the front leg instead, walking yourself down.

Pendulum

➤ *Difficulty Level:* II

➤ *Powers:* The hips, hamstrings, spine, and neck.

➤ *Caution:* To avoid pulling a hamstring muscle, only come down as far as your body will let you. Don't let the weight of your upper body overextend muscles that aren't ready.

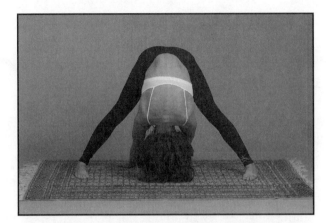

Pendulum pose brings the body gradually out of the yoga split.

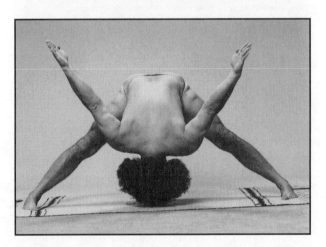

For an extra stretch in pendulum pose, raise the arms on the diagonal so they cross the legs making two Xs.

Pendulum pose is a lovely and gentle way to come out of the full split.

➤ From the split, put a hand on the floor on either side of your body, tuck your toes under, and walk your feet toward each other.

➤ When your feet are about four feet apart, push up on your hands, turning your feet in so you are pigeon-toed.

➤ Come up off the floor with your knees bent.

➤ Keeping your knees bent slightly, lower your body and let it hang like a pendulum.

➤ Slide your hands along the floor between your legs and really feel the stretch in the back, legs, and hips.

➤ Variation: For an added challenge, instead of sliding your arms along the floor, lift them up so each arm crosses in front of each thigh, making an X shape. Rest your head on the floor as the third point of a tripod you make with your body.

➤ Hold for one to five breaths.

➤ Bring your hands to the floor underneath your body and slowly push your body upright.

➤ Turn to the left and move into exalted warrior.

➤ Repeat the entire series (exalted warrior, monkey pose, single leg forward bend, pigeon pose, pigeon hip stretch, pigeon pose with shoulder and quad stretch, split forward bend, yoga split, pendulum) on the other side.

That's the end of the beginning of the animal poses, but also the end to a possible longer series of poses including the warrior poses, angle poses, and those described in this chapter. You can do this entire longer series all on one side and then repeat them all on the other side in the following order:

➤ Spear thrower

➤ Swordsman

➤ Extended warrior

➤ T-balance

➤ Half moon

➤ Standing forward bend

➤ Tree pose

➤ Forward bend in tree

➤ Triangle

➤ Extended triangle

➤ Twisted triangle

➤ Angle

➤ Extended angle

➤ Twisted angle

➤ Extended twisted angle

➤ Exalted warrior

➤ Monkey

➤ Single leg forward bend

➤ Pigeon

➤ Pigeon hip stretch

➤ Pigeon pose with shoulder and quad stretch

➤ Split forward bend

➤ Yoga split

➤ Pendulum

If you do nothing else, this routine would make you much more powerful in your everyday life. You would probably never have back pain, your legs would be stronger, your breathing more controlled, your mind more focused in stressful situations, with better concentration, having activated all the chakras, awakened, aligned, and lengthened the spine, with just this series.

You can do this entire series in about 20 to 30 minutes. I recommend this to most of my students—15 to 30 minutes of yoga every day, rather than yoga once or twice a week for 90 minutes. Then maybe take a class or two during the week to add to your repertoire and tone your body in new ways.

The Least You Need to Know

➤ Monkey pose and pigeon pose are both similar to the previous chapter's exalted warrior, and make good transition poses into a series of animal poses.

➤ Counter every pose with a pose that moves the body in the opposite direction. For example, move from monkey pose to single leg forward bend; from pigeon pose to pigeon hip stretch; and from split forward bend to yoga split.

➤ Any difficult pose, such as the full split, can be modified for beginners and people whose flexibility isn't developed enough for a particular pose's standard form.

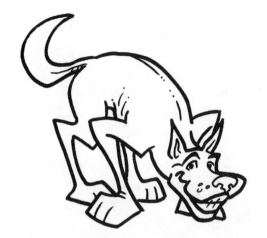

Chapter 16

Down on All Fours

In This Chapter

➤ On the prowl again

➤ The strength of the alligator

➤ The power of the dog

➤ A miscellaneous menagerie of movements

I like to start in the standing positions and move toward relaxation. I think most of us come to yoga from a busy position, a point of activity, so I like to go from activity and move gradually toward the ground, where relaxation takes place.

Now we are moving closer to the ground by getting down on all fours with the animal poses. But don't think the most exhausting part of the workout is over. On the contrary—the four-legged animal poses are the most strenuous part of the Power Yoga routine (though not the most complicated), so get ready to sweat!

On the Prowl

The four-legged poses produce the most heat and physical strength in the upper body because we begin to really use this area. In the lunges and warrior series, we created tremendous strength in the legs, knees, hips, and lower back. We need to start there and get our foundation. Once we're safe, strong, and comfortable there, we'll move down onto the hands and feet to strengthen the upper body.

Normally, I don't do the four-legged poses in my Level I classes. I begin them in Level II classes and emphasize them in Level III classes because a lot of beginners have problems and weaknesses in their upper body, especially in the wrists, shoulders, and back. Movements that really work these areas can be a little too much for the beginner.

Build up plenty of strength and confidence with the poses in Parts 2 and 3 of this book before tackling this chapter. But when you are ready, go for it!

Prowling Tiger Warm-Up

➤ *Difficulty Level:* II

➤ *Powers:* Adds strength and flexibility to the spine, strengthens the muscles of the entire back, and increases neuromuscular coordination.

➤ *Caution:* Don't skip the warm-up for this strenuous workout. Start into the warm-up slowly and give your body time to adjust, especially if you are beginning your workout this way and aren't already warm.

Inhale and raise the opposite arm and leg for prowling tiger.

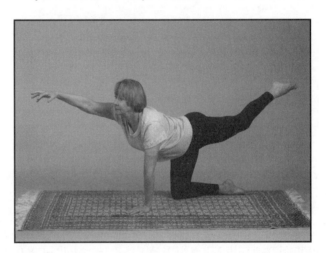

Remember the prowling tiger series from Chapter 8, "Prowling Tiger Series," in the section on developmental poses? That was a great beginning for four-legged poses, and at this point in the book, we'll make it our warm-up. If you've been following along as I suggested, this series will be very familiar and should make a great beginning to more advanced animal poses.

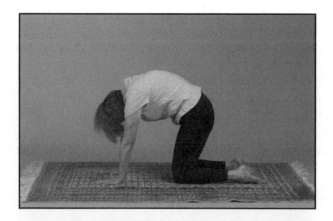

Exhale between prowling tiger extensions with a good cat pose back bend.

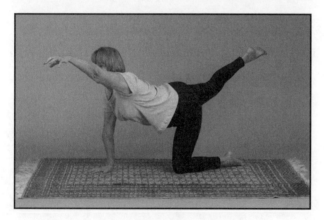

Inhale and extend the opposite arm and opposite leg for the final prowling tiger movement.

Prowling tiger series puts your body through a basic four-legged movement, working the entire back and neck. Remember to move with the breath, and don't worry about holding any of the four-legged poses for very long. They are meant for movement. Especially in the beginning, just hold each pose for half a breath and then move into the next pose and then the next. Inhale on one pose, exhale on the next, always expanding the body and arching on the inhale, contracting as you exhale, arching as you inhale, bending as you exhale.

➤ Sit in Japanese sitting pose, move into worship to the supreme, and then into prowling tiger movement, as described in Chapter 8.

➤ Repeat the prowling tiger movement gently 10 times until you feel warm and limber.

Alligator Series

Now you are ready for a more vigorous workout. Come back up to a standing position. In this group, which includes several series, I'll give you a series of poses, then I'll keep adding in new poses to increase the length of the series. In other words, you'll keep doing the series again and again, each time adding a new step.

In alligator series, we'll start much as we did for salute to the light within (see Chapter 11, "Salute to the Light Within"). At the floor, however, we'll add in some vigorous movements that will build strength fast. Practice this series every day and you'll get noticeably stronger in a few weeks.

Reed

> ➤ *Difficulty Level:* I

> ➤ *Powers:* The back, legs, and arms. Opens the chest and lengthens the spine.

> ➤ *Caution:* Keep your body in a straight line and keep your gluteal muscles tight to prevent an uncontrolled swaying of the lower back.

Begin this series as you began many others, standing straight and strong in Marine pose.

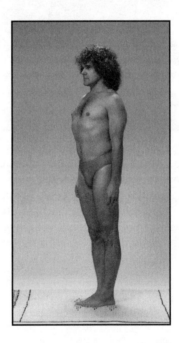

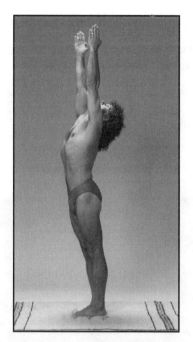

Reach up into reed pose for a powerful beginning to a powerful series of exercises.

From a standing position, begin the alligator series with reed pose.

➤ Stand up straight in Marine pose and find your balance. Breathe normally.

➤ Inhale and bring your arms straight above your head, palms facing each other.

➤ Keep your entire body strong and energized.

➤ Gently let your head drop back and lead with your heart.

Standing Forward Bend

➤ *Difficulty Level:* II

➤ *Powers:* The hamstrings, the lower back, and stretches the spine using the weight of the head. Also brings a lot of blood to the brain.

➤ *Caution:* Come down carefully, keeping your lower back straight and your arms overhead. Bend your knees slightly.

The Right Moves

To this day, I still bend my knees in standing forward bend. Bent knees aren't just for beginners! Be kind to your knees and lower back and keep energy and flexibility in those legs with a slightly bent knee.

225

Now move into a standing forward bend, to bring all four limbs to the ground.

➤ From reed pose, slowly lower the body down to the floor. Keep the arms in place above the head and keep the back straight. Bend your knees as much as you need.

➤ Bring the hands to the floor. If you can't reach, bend your knees a little more.

➤ Let the weight of your head hang down, opening and stretching your spine.

➤ Let your body lie over your knees, hands toward the ground.

➤ Walk your hands back so your palms are on the ground next to your feet.

Standing forward bend is the first true four-legged pose, bringing all four limbs to the ground.

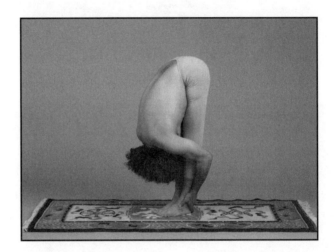

Lunge

➤ *Difficulty Level:* II

➤ *Powers:* The hip joints, muscles of the inner thigh, and arms.

➤ *Caution:* Keep your front foot directly between your palms to align this position correctly.

The lunge puts a nice stretch in your inner thighs and begins the upper-body workout.

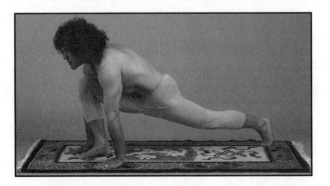

I like to think of lunge as a little like a four-legged warrior pose.

➤ From standing forward bend, inhale and step back with your right foot.

➤ Come up onto the ball of your back foot, and keep your front foot between your hands.

➤ Look in front of you.

Board

➤ *Difficulty Level:* III

➤ *Powers:* An incredible strengthener of the entire torso and arms, especially when held for any length of time.

➤ *Caution:* Keep your abdominal and gluteal muscles very strong in this pose to keep the strain off the back.

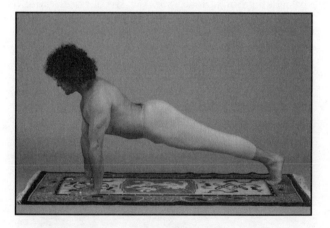

Board pose is a super-powered torso strengthener.

This pose is like the upward end of a push-up.

➤ From lunge pose, exhale and bring the front (left) leg back next to the back (right) leg.

➤ Stand on the balls and toes of your feet, keeping your body straight as a board. Keep your arms straight and strong.

➤ Inhale, and raise your head up, stretching the arms, squeezing the thighs and buns, and creating a very slight, supported arch in the back.

➤ Exhale and drop your head back down.

➤ Inhale, then bring your right leg to the front again, placing your feet between your two hands to return to the lunge.

➤ Exhale, drop your head to the floor, and bring your back leg forward, raising your hips to return to the standing forward bend.

➤ Inhale and return to lunge, but this time, bring your left leg back behind you.

➤ Exhale and bring your right leg back so you return to board pose.

➤ Inhale, and raise your head up, stretching the arms, squeezing the thighs and buns, and creating a very slight, supported arch in the back.

➤ Exhale and drop your head back down.

➤ Inhale and bring your left leg forward, returning to lunge.

➤ Exhale, bringing your right leg forward and raising your hips to return to standing forward bend.

➤ Inhale and come back up into reed pose with arms extended over head.

➤ Exhale and lower the arms back into Marine pose.

This completes the first, very basic, alligator series. Note how we did both sides to balance and complete the series. But we haven't inserted the alligator pose yet, so keep reading. This is only the beginning.

Board pose is a great strengthener on its own, outside of a series of poses. Got a few extra minutes? Get down on all fours and hold board pose for as long as you can.

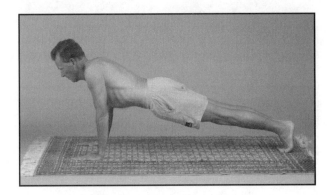

Geo's Journey

We get tremendous power from upper-body strength. A strong upper body simply looks better. The chest and shoulders, arms, triceps, and back get bigger, or more shapely, and strong enough to move us through life with ease and grace. Using your arms helps straighten the back, helping to prevent osteoporosis by pushing the back toward an arching rather than a rounding shape.

Push-Up

➤ *Difficulty Level:* III

➤ *Powers:* The entire body—a super-powered movement.

➤ *Caution:* Not everyone is strong enough (yet!) to do a push-up. Rather than starting with knee push-ups, as many workout instructors recommend, stick with board pose and come down even just an inch or two. The more you work, the stronger you'll get.

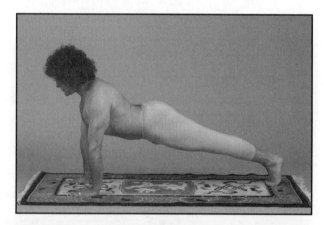

Start your push-up with board pose, keeping the body straight and strong.

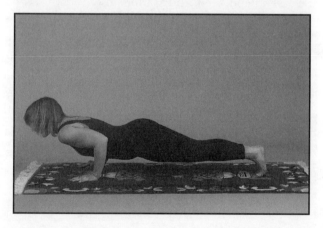

Lower your body down to about six inches from the floor for a push-up. If you can't go that low, start by lowering just a few inches.

The next movement to add to alligator series is a familiar and very powerful one. Before adding it, make sure you feel strong and confident with the basic series of Marine, reed, standing forward bend, lunge, board, and then back up.

From there, when you feel stronger moving your feet back and forth, down and back up, you'll be ready to work into the super-strengthening push-up.

229

The Wrong Moves

People with lower-back problems may find moving back and forth from standing forward bend to lunge to board pose and back difficult and even painful. If these movements put a strain on your lower back, "back off" and stick to back-strengthening basics for a while, such as the developmental routines in Chapter 6 and the salute to the light within series in Chapter 11. No need to be in a hurry. You can keep practicing yoga into your old, old age.

The Right Moves

Push-ups are wonderful strength training. They strengthen the back, shoulders, arms, stomach, legs, and gluteal muscles. They literally strengthen the whole body and should be included in any Power Yoga routine.

➤ Repeat the series as above, beginning with Marine, moving into reed, standing forward bend, lunge stepping back with the right foot, and board pose.

➤ From board pose, inhale and lower the body down to about six inches from the ground.

➤ Exhale and raise the body back up.

➤ Inhale and step forward with the right foot into lunge.

➤ Exhale and step forward with the left foot, raising into standing forward bend.

➤ Inhale and stand up into reed pose.

➤ Exhale and lower back into standing forward bend.

➤ Inhale and step back with the left foot into lunge.

➤ Exhale and step back with the right foot into board, lower into the push-up, and come back up as before, through lunge, standing forward bend, reed, and Marine pose.

➤ Repeat on both sides. Work up to 50 repetitions (25 on each side) over the course of a couple of weeks and you'll find yourself much stronger than you were before. If you can do 50 repetitions, you'll be doing 25 lunges on each side and 50 push-ups. Quite an accomplishment!

But we aren't done yet. Still waiting for that alligator pose!

Alligator

➤ *Difficulty Level:* IV

➤ *Powers:* The muscles of the torso and the arms. A difficult and incredibly strengthening pose.

➤ *Caution:* It takes money to make money, and it takes strength to make strength! This pose is quite difficult, so don't worry if you can't do it yet. Keep working and building strength, and you'll get there.

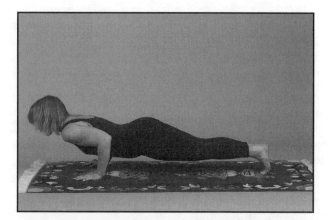

Alligator pose, also called chataranga or four-legged staff in traditional yoga, is a highly challenging and strengthening four-legged pose.

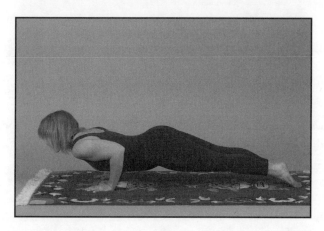

To add an additional challenge to alligator pose, point the toes and let the tops of your feet, rather than the balls of your feet, share the weight with your hands.

The alligator, also called chataranga, is the next step in this routine. Just as board pose is the beginning of a push-up, chataranga is the end of the pushup, where we drop down and stop about six inches from the ground and see if we can hold this, for a breath in the beginning, and eventually for about five breaths. You can actually work up to a minute, but I prefer to keep moving in this pose, and five breaths is more than enough time to spend in alligator pose, as you'll soon see.

➤ Repeat the series as above, but when you get to the push-up, lower your body, and hold for one full breath.

➤ Lift your body and continue with the series, doing both sides.

➤ Eventually work up to holding alligator pose for five full breaths.

Holding alligator for five breaths, then pushing back up will be the most difficult push-up you ever attempted. It doesn't take many alligator push-ups to start building strength, heat in the body, and power in your arms, shoulders, back, and belly.

Dog Series

Once we've accomplished alligator series, we can add the dog series to the routine. If you watch a dog, you'll see the upward stretching dog pose and the downward stretching dog pose any time the dog gets up off the ground. Dogs stretch in these ways to get their hips and legs back into place.

We can gain phenomenal benefits from these poses. They strengthen the whole body, move the upper back into an arch instead of a forward bend, and add power to the shoulders, wrists, lower back, and the entire body.

Geo's Journey

Sliding back and forth between upward stretching and downward stretching dog positions is the movement some of the new workouts call seal push-ups. When we were kids, we would do a similar movement and put our noses between our hands on the downside.

This series can follow straight out of the alligator series. Pick up from board pose.

Bear Pose

➤ *Difficulty Level:* II

➤ *Powers:* The entire torso, especially around the abdominal area; also strengthens the quadriceps.

➤ *Caution:* If your knees feel strained in this position, you can begin working on this pose with less of a bend in the knee and hips raised, keeping your knees higher off the ground. As your legs and knees get stronger, you can gradually lower the knees closer to the floor.

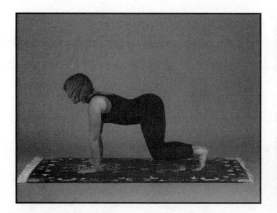 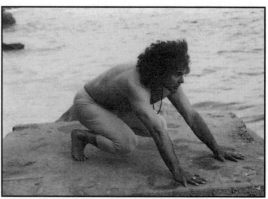

Bear pose imitates the movements of a bear cub, or of a small child developing its crawl. Inhale into the position at left, then exhale as you move.

Bear pose is like a dog series warm-up, moving the body in a less extreme but similar way to the dog poses. It makes a great transition into downward stretching dog, being a kind of combination between downward and upward stretching dog poses.

This is the defensive lineman position in football practice. It's basically running around on the hands and feet. Kids do it, too. It's the next step up from crawling.

➤ From board pose, bend your knees until they are about six inches off the ground. Keep the arms straight. Your weight should be balanced on your hands and the balls of your feet and toes.

➤ Imagine your feet and hands are bear paws. Turn your tailbone up slightly to create just a slight arch in the lower back and look up.

➤ Inhale and roll forward slightly, keeping the knees off the ground and arching the lower back while looking up.

➤ Exhale and, while keeping the knees about six inches above the ground, move the hips toward the heel to create a four-legged squat.

➤ Continue inhaling forward while pushing off toes, then exhaling back. This movement is very powerful for the knees and legs.

The Wrong Moves

When you inhale and roll forward in bear, stop your shoulders just above your hands. Don't extend all the way into upward dog.

Downward Stretching Dog

➤ *Difficulty Level:* III

➤ *Powers:* The hamstrings, spine, and shoulders; also aligns hips and increases blood flow to the brain.

➤ *Caution:* This pose really stretches hamstrings and calf muscles. Don't try it until your body is well warmed up or you could pull or strain a muscle.

Downward stretching dog has the same benefits for dogs and humans. It's a great way to open and align the hips and spine.

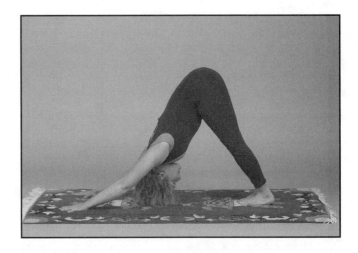

When you feel comfortable with the bear movement, you can let it evolve into a movement between downward stretching dog and upward stretching dog. Begin with downward stretching dog, which is easy to accomplish from bear pose.

➤ From the basic bear position, push your tailbone toward the ceiling, push your buns up, drop your head, straighten your legs, and push your heels down.

➤ Flatten your palms, keeping your fingers pointing straight ahead, heels toward the floor for a great stretch in the calves.

➤ Keep your legs straight and press on the balls of your feet to pull the weight back off your arms and onto your legs. You want your legs to do most of the work.

➤ Turn your tailbone up so your back flattens.

➤ Feel the breath move into the belly and create a little arch as you inhale. Roll your elbows out a little to farther and roll your shoulder blades toward each other to open the chest farther.

You can also incorporate the dog series into the alligator series. From the board pose, lift the hips, drop the head, and move into downward stretching dog. Then slide back down into alligator, stopping just above the ground with the body straight like a board, about six inches above the ground, legs straight, head up. Then move into upward stretching dog and back through the rest of the series.

Upward Stretching Dog

➤ *Difficulty Level:* III

➤ *Powers:* Stretches the spine, opens the chest, and strengthens the arms.

➤ *Caution:* Don't arch the spine beyond your flexibility or you could injure your lower back. Keep your thighs strong and your buns squeezed together to support the lower back in this position.

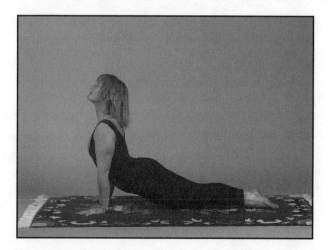

Upward stretching dog is the counterpose to downward stretching dog, moving the entire body in the opposite direction.

When incorporating this pose into alligator series along with downward stretching dog, start from alligator pose. Or, as a stand-alone routine, do 10 repetitions of bear pose, then 10 repetitions of downward stretching dog to upward stretching dog and back. Work up to 50 repetitions for a really vigorous workout.

➤ From alligator or downward stretching dog, move to upward stretching dog by pointing the toes and rolling the heels toward each other so the front of the hips open and the back of the hips squeeze.

➤ Press on the hands, straighten the arms, raise the head and chest, and create an arching movement. The only parts of your body that should be touching the ground are your palms, fingers, the tops of your feet, and your toes.

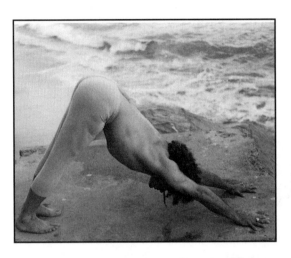 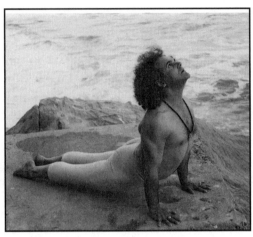

Geo moves from downward stretching dog (left) to upward stretching dog (right).

➤ Feel the arch from the toes to the top of the head. Keep the heels rolled toward each other and pressed together, the thighs strong, and the buns squeezed to protect the lower back.

➤ As you push up with your chest, feel as if you are pulling your upper body up and back, out of your hip sockets.

➤ Now, move back either to alligator and back through alligator series, or back and forth with downward stretching dog. You can also put alligator pose in between these two poses each time without incorporating the rest of alligator series, for an extra power punch.

Geo's Journey

My wonderful Samoyed, Teko, I told you about earlier on in this book, had bad hips. Teko was always going into his own doggy version of upward stretching dog. He used his upper body a lot, trying to take over for his hips. When Teko would stretch his chin up in this pose, I could see how this pose was meant to stretch and expand the area around the heart.

You can vary your combination of four-legged poses in many ways. When you become very advanced, you might try the following. Repeat each pose, up to 50 times.

➤ Marine pose

➤ Reed pose

➤ Standing forward bend

➤ Lunge

➤ Board pose

➤ Bear movement

➤ Downward stretching dog

➤ Alligator pose

➤ Upward stretching dog

➤ Strong press back to downward stretching dog

➤ Back to bear movement

➤ Move into lunge

➤ Standing forward bend

➤ Reed pose

➤ Marine pose

Burpees

➤ *Difficulty Level:* II

➤ *Powers:* The arms, legs, abdominal muscles, back, and heart.

➤ *Caution:* If jumping back isn't comfortable, stick with the step-back of the lunge.

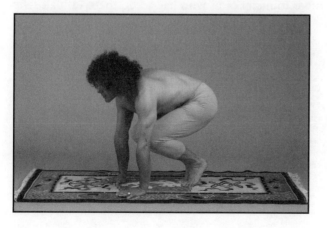

Burpees begin with a squat pose.

Continue the burpee by jumping back with both legs.

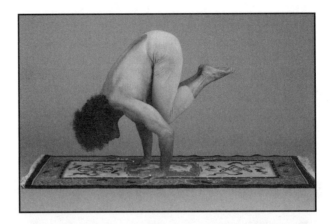

Land in board pose.

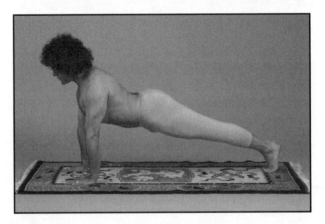

The final movement in this series is burpees. We called this movement burpees in the Marine Corps, but I've also heard it called a squat thrust. These movements are traditional to yoga, but also familiar to many of us who had to do them in high school gym class when we were kids, and everyone who has been in the service. They are very powerful exercise.

Insert this series between the alligator and dog series, as follows:

➤ Begin with alligator series in Marine pose, inhale and stretch up into reed, exhale to standing forward bend.

➤ Inhale and drop into a squat, putting the weight on the hands. Lift your feet off the ground, and hop straight back into board pose.

➤ From here, continue with pushups or the rest of the alligator series, or pick up the dog series here, moving through bear, downward stretching dog, upward stretching dog, and so on.

➤ Hop the feet back into a squat, then come back up.

In the beginning, just do a series of burpees:

➤ Begin in Marine pose.

➤ Squat, jump the legs back into board, then forward into a squat.

➤ Stand back up in Marine pose.

➤ Repeat up to 50 times.

Geo's Journey

Burpees are great for your cardiovascular system because the squat cuts off the blood flow at the hips, then the jump-back into board opens the flow of blood, so the heart really has to work to keep up. Also, when you come down, you are on all fours again. This is very powerful for the upper body, and strengthens the back and heart. The jump-up creates strength in the back, the belly, and the gut muscles deep inside your body, including your entire network of lower abdominal muscles. Burpees are very powerful, really working the whole body. They are a great way to get your heart pounding.

Animal poses are very stressful, strengthening, exhausting poses that create a lot of body heat. From here we need to back off a little bit. In my classes, we're usually at 45 minutes to an hour here and people are pretty sweaty and tired.

So we drop to the ground at this point, and move into sitting poses. In the next section, we'll get down onto the ground and work with sitting poses, stomach and back strengthening poses, and some more advanced arches, wheels, and twists, then on to some very advanced poses. But before we wrap up this section, read on in the next chapter for some tips on how to make the most out of your workout by living in the most healthful way you can.

The Least You Need to Know

➤ Four-legged poses, or animal poses, move our bodies back to their primal roots, into positions in which we are no longer very strong.

➤ Animal poses build incredible strength and endurance.

➤ Our four-legged series begins with prowling tiger for a warm-up.

➤ The four-legged series continues with the alligator series, incorporates bear pose and dog series, and ends with some vigorous burpees, or squat thrusts.

➤ All the animal series can be combined in different ways and with many of the other series in this book.

➤ Animal poses are the most strenuous part of the Power Yoga workout. After these series, the body will be ready to wind down with some floor work.

Chapter 17

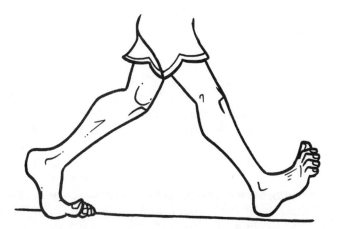

Thirteen Steps to Natural Living

In This Chapter

➤ Do you live naturally?

➤ My personal transformation to more natural living

➤ Change your life in 13 steps

I'm walking along, and it's a beautiful day. I feel absolutely fabulous. I feel stronger and healthier than I've ever felt in my life, and I wonder why people think that achieving this state is such a difficult process. I feel the gentle breeze on my face, and I am completely connected to the life process. Then I realize, that's really what it is: The path of Power Yoga means getting into life, as it really, naturally is—living as close to natural as possible.

As I walk along this trail, eating a piece of fruit at the height of its season, like every other animal in the area, I think about the coyotes. Their species seems ageless. Once they mature to adulthood, a two-year old coyote is indistinguishable from the eight-year-old coyote. In some sense, the natural spirit of the coyote keeps the body ageless.

Humanity should follow the coyote's example. If we live our lives as naturally as possible, which means eating properly and exercising in a natural way, then we can live agelessly until the end of our days, with no real concern for that time when our lives on earth end. But what does it mean to live naturally? We have come so far from our natural state that sometimes it's hard to remember what it is we are supposed to do. How are we supposed to move? What are we supposed to eat? In this chapter, I'll talk a little about what I have come to understand as the natural way for humans to live.

This natural way of life will do more than prolong our lives, although it has a significant effect. It will also enrich the quality of our lives, making us vital and full of energy well into what people call "old age."

If Geo Can Do It...

When I first decided to change my life, it happened in an instant. During the summer of 1974, I was the bar manager of the Crown House restaurant in Laguna Beach, California. It was one of the first places in south Orange County with an elite clientele. Standing behind the bar one day, I noticed that most of my customers didn't smile much until they had had a few drinks, and I also realized that at that time in my life, *I* didn't smile much either until I'd had a couple of drinks.

This observation haunted me for a few days, and at some point, I came to the awareness that it took energy to smile. My energy wasn't what it used to be. I realized that I couldn't even muster the energy for a smile without the crutch of a few drinks! I decided this was a condition that would worsen if I didn't change my life immediately.

I started by reading all about natural eating and fasting. Then, I took some time off and went up to the mountains for four days. I fasted on water and lemons. Because I'm of Greek and Italian descent, and I grew up in the restaurant business, the first day without food almost killed me. The second day was a little bit better. On the third day, to my amazement, I woke up with more energy than I'd had in years. I couldn't sit still, so I climbed up to the top of San Jacinto, the mountain where I camped. When I got to the top, I sat and meditated.

At that point, I had a spiritual experience like I've never had since. I saw myself doing exactly what I do now, spending my days teaching yoga and hiking outdoors. At the time, I didn't know what a *vision quest* was, but the spirit in me knew, and drove me instinctively into the vision I needed at the time.

The next day, I felt fantastic. After four days without food, I went home to Laguna and changed my life. I threw out all the processed food and drink, all white sugar, white bread, even the white rice. I bought all the fresh vegetables and fruit I could carry. (I was

The Wrong Moves

Fasting can be a great way to purify the system, and there are many types to choose from. Juice fasts, juice and broth fasts, or water and lemon fasts are all popular. However, never fast if you are pregnant, nursing, suffering from a serious medical condition, or if your doctor advises against it. Also, before you fast, read as much as you can on the subject so you can fast safely—improving, and not destroying, your health.

Power Words

A **vision quest** is a personal spiritual journey that can take many forms. Typically, the questor goes into nature alone for a few days, fasts, and meditates until he or she experiences a spiritual revelation.

working up a pretty good appetite by this time, still not having eaten.) I broke my fast with stewed tomatoes and I felt great.

Then I registered for a yoga class and started the next day.

The yoga class was difficult for me. As an ex-athlete and ex-Marine, everything in my body was tight. However, I felt something different in this movement than I had in any other—something wonderful. By the end of the workout, I had more energy than when I started.

I also loved the non-competitive aspect of yoga. I took classes every day with different teachers and in three months, I was in a different body and a different mind. I was a completely different person—still me, yet transformed. I lost 30 pounds, developed strength and flexibility I'd never known before, and for the first time in years, I had enough energy to smile easily.

I've never looked back. At 53, I have more energy than I've ever had and do things with my body and mind that I used to read about but had no real concept of.

The Right Moves

You must decide for yourself whether the time is right to change your life. Either your life is working, or it isn't. You're either becoming more full of life, or you are feeling as if your life is out of control, or even non-existent. If you need to feel more full of life, surround yourself with the tools that can help build energy and a healthy life: good food, pure water, clean air, positive thoughts and feelings, and movement!

A lot of my clients today are in the same place in their lives. They've come to realize the need for change. Are you at that point, too? The longer they, and you, put off the change, the harder it gets to actually do it. It's never too late, though. You are never too old to begin a change.

Geo's Lucky Thirteen

If you thought 13 was an unlucky number, you may soon change your mind after you read about the 13 steps to change your life. Of course, luck has nothing to do with it. You are taking your life into your own hands, and who is more capable to change your life than you?

Work on one step at a time, or even one sub-step at a time, and if you are committed and persistent, you can be a healthier, happier, more energetic person. I did it in three months. How long will it take you?

Some of these steps are pretty basic, while others are more complex. You don't need to follow them in order, and you don't even need to follow the steps that you don't think will work for you. It's your body, your mind, and your life. These are my guidelines, and you can do with them what you will. But if you follow them, I guarantee your life will improve.

Step One: Where Are You Now?

The first thing to do is some serious soul searching. Sit down alone in a quiet place and make a list of all the things in your life you do that feel good, natural, and right. These are the things that give you more energy, greater zest for living, and make you happier. Write them here:

_____

_____

_____

_____

_____

Now think about the things you do in your life that aren't good, natural, or right. These are the things that sap your energy, drain your zest for living, and detract from your happiness—even if they give you momentary pleasure. Write them here:

_____

_____

_____

_____

_____

Spend some time thinking about and meditating on how you can move and live in a more natural and exuberant existence.

Step Two: Live the Simple Life

Keep it simple. Simple living helps to eliminate distractions, materialistic thinking, and putting priorities on things that aren't rewarding, lasting, or healthy. Eat simply, move simply, dress simply, live in a simple environment. Speak simply. That doesn't mean speak as if you aren't intelligent. It means that you should say what you mean, and spend more time listening than talking.

Step Three: Yoga Abstentions

Observe the traditional yoga abstentions. Also called *yamas*, these five principles are guidelines for things to avoid in order to be happier and healthier. These principles will mean different things to different people, so think about what each principle could mean for your life:

➤ **Do no harm.** When you harm anything, you harm yourself because we are all connected.

➤ **Don't lie to yourself.** Be true to your spirit and be true to your life.

➤ **Don't steal.** That means everything from dime store candy to someone's attention.

➤ **Don't waste your essence.** Have respect for yourself and anyone you sleep with. Sex is a powerful expenditure of energy and not to be taken lightly.

➤ **Don't be greedy.** This means simplifying your life by minimizing material possessions and sensual pleasures. Don't waste your energy buying everything, eating everything, drinking everything. You can have everything in life, but knowing that, you don't need to have it all. You only need what will make your life better and happier, not what will weigh it down.

Power Words

Yamas are the traditional yoga abstentions: Don't harm others, don't lie, don't steal, don't waste your essence, and don't be greedy.

Step Four: Yoga Observances

The next step also involves traditional yoga advice, also called *niyamas,* but these five principles involve what to do, rather than what not to do, in order to live a happier, healthier life. Again, these principles will mean different things to different people. Reflect on what they could mean for your life:

➤ **Be pure.** Purity means respecting yourself; eating pure, natural foods; drinking pure water; maintaining good hygiene; and thinking positive thoughts.

➤ **Be content.** This step has to do with accepting that what is, is. Learning to be happy with the life you've been given and doing the best with what you have is a great skill to cultivate. It's like that old Irish blessing about accepting what you can't change, changing what you can, and having the wisdom to know the difference.

➤ **Be disciplined.** This means having a schedule and setting up personal rituals for yourself—a daily Power Yoga practice, a daily hike in the fresh air, a daily personal care routine, a daily salad of fresh vegetables, and so on—and *doing them every day,* not just when you feel like it.

Power Words

Niyamas are the traditional yoga observances: Be pure, be content, be disciplined, be studious, and be devoted.

➤ **Be studious.** This doesn't mean going back to school. It means studying yourself, your life, and your God. Never stop learning!

➤ **Be devoted.** You don't need to belong to a church to focus on your idea of what is divine. Talk to God (in whatever form God exists for you), meditate on God, thank God, and love God. Also, love the perfect, lovely world that was created for you, and of which you are an important part.

Step Five: Move It!

Exercise is the crux of this step. Find a routine and stick to it *every day* (see the previous step about discipline). I prefer a yoga-based routine because it is closest to our natural tendencies toward movement. My recommendation:

➤ Do a Power Yoga routine from this book or from my CD, *Geo's Power Yoga*, *every day*. (See the back of this book for instructions on how to order my CD.)

➤ Do 50 squat thrusts *every day* (you'll work up to this number, of course, or find a number that is better suited to your fitness level—be kind to yourself while being disciplined!).

➤ Do 50 push-ups *every day*. Or, if you can't do 50, no problem. Do as many as you can and keep adding as you get stronger—eventually you'll be at 50, but there's no rush as long as you are really keeping those muscles working.

➤ Take a walk after dinner *every day*.

You can certainly overdo this step. Exercise isn't meant to be a stress on your system. Back in the '80s, there was a huge movement toward health clubs. People would work hard all day, running around at a crazy pace, then they would leave work and go to some health club and get on a machine and just go crazy, running or pedaling or lifting weights. Then they'd go home, pass out, wake up in the morning, and do it all again!

I am certainly an advocate of getting outside and moving, but when it becomes obsessive, it's like we're always running nowhere, pushing ourselves way past our limits. You have to get back in touch with your body so your movement and exercise routine is based on natural cues.

Geo's Journey

I remember studying with an old friend back in the '70s when the whole health craze and jogging fad were beginning. We were driving through Laguna Beach at the time, where we had some classes, and he just looked at me with a very puzzled expression on his face and said, "Geo, why is everybody running nowhere?" That stuck with me all this time.

Step Six: Breath of Life

Breathing is an important part of increasing energy and making the most of every movement (see Chapter 24, "Breath of Life"). Every day, practice the breath of fire exercise in Chapter 24 and do 50 deep breaths.

Step Seven: Become the Watcher

While many of these steps involve doing, this step involves standing back and watching. You can gain a new and helpful perspective on your self and your life if you learn to spend some time each day in objective observation. Look at yourself in the mirror and be aware of your movements, voice, and posture as if you were looking at a stranger. Notice what that new person, you, likes and dislikes, fears and loves. What do you think of this person? Do you have any helpful suggestions for how this person could improve his or her life? Tell yourself!

Step Eight: Concentrate, Meditate

While there are many different ways to practice concentration and meditation, the most important thing is that you pay attention to both of these disciplines and keep at them. Try looking in a mirror, focusing deep into your left eye, for five full minutes. It isn't easy now, but with practice it will be.

Step Nine: We Are One

Know, and continue to remind yourself when you forget, that we are all brothers and sisters, we are all part of one universe. Everything we see is part of us, and we are part of everything we see.

Step Ten: Eat Well

This is tough for a lot of people because our society is so food-oriented, but I'm telling you, what you eat can have a huge effect on how you feel. Although you can modify these guidelines when you are in better shape, I suggest you start with the following:

The Right Moves

Here's another meditation exercise to try. Sit in a comfortable spot and focus on an object that has spiritual significance for you, whether a statue, a crystal, a religious picture, or an object from nature. Focus on the object and either pray or feel a line of communication opening up between you and your God.

➤ No meat (meaning beef, pork, poultry, and the rest). I don't count fish, which I include in my diet.

➤ Focus your diet primarily on fish and vegetables, and an occasional fruit snack before 4 P.M.

➤ No booze. Yes, yes, I've heard that wine is good for your heart and all that, but for now, let's work on purifying the body. I'm not saying you can never again enjoy a Cabernet with dinner— although you may find that eventually, you won't want to.

➤ Water, water, water! Drink water all day long. Your body needs hydration to function.

➤ Geo's Favorite Breakfast: One egg, one slice of whole-wheat toast.

➤ Geo's Favorite Lunch: Salad and fish.

➤ Geo's Favorite Dinner: Vegetables and fish.

➤ Don't eat after 6 P.M. Not anything. Water only. Let your body rest from the effort of digestion for at least 12 to 14 hours.

➤ Don't eat much bread, pasta, or pizza, except for that morning slice of toast. Too much yeast and refined flour products are bad for your colon and your digestion.

➤ No sugar. Not only can sugar activate and encourage the growth of yeast in our systems (see the following Geo's Journey sidebar), but it also gets into our bloodstream very quickly. The body likes to process things, and is meant to spend a lot of energy processing food. If you eat already processed and highly refined foods like white sugar, white flour, and bread, the body gets robbed and confused. Many bodily functions are involved in the process of moving food through the body. The body doesn't know what to do when it gets refined sugar. It receives all this energy suddenly, without working for it. Our whole system gets imbalanced.

➤ No soda. See above note about sugar. Diet soda is out, too. The new artificial sweeteners haven't been out there long enough to be proven truly safe, and as long as you are eating naturally, you'll want to avoid artificial anything.

➤ No coffee or tea, except certain herbal teas. This is also very difficult for many people, who feel as if caffeine fuels their very existences. A lot of that is psychological, but caffeine is addictive and if you are addicted, you'll probably get a nasty headache when you first give it up. Within a week or two, you should be over it completely, if you persevere. For some, it only takes a day or two. On the other hand, for some, their morning or afternoon cup of coffee or tea is an important ritual. I've switched to naturally decaffeinated coffee and get the best of both worlds. Green tea can be great, too. It has caffeine, but not as much as black tea, and recent research shows that it may contain certain cancer-prevention properties.

➤ No high-sugar, high-fat desserts. See above on sugar. Yes, that three-layer chocolate truffle torte looks delectable, but you *know* your body doesn't need it or even want it. You'll feel so much better if you pass it up. Dessert is a nice ritual, too, however. Why not order a fruit cup with just a dab of whipped cream?

➤ Limit your milk consumption. An occasional splash in your decaf coffee or a very occasional glass of milk should be fine. The best milk product for your system is natural yogurt. To counteract the yeast in our systems, yogurt is a wonderful dietary addition, fabulous for the colon. I don't mean the frozen or sugary sweet stuff, but pure, natural yogurt, perhaps with blueberries or blackberries mixed in. Don't eat yogurt that lists sugar and high fructose corn syrup among its ingredients. Get a good quality plain yogurt. Buttermilk works, too. People who live very long lives, over 100 or 120 years, almost all regularly eat some form of clabbered dairy product like yogurt or buttermilk. Soy milk is a healthy milk substitute and is especially good mixed in things like coffee or oatmeal. Some people do well on it, while others don't tolerate it.

➤ I'll say it again because it is so important: Drink water, all day long! Carry a container of water with you wherever you go.

> **The Right Moves**
>
> Why should you give up your beloved cup of java? Because you are searching for your internal energy, your natural source of life. Our lives today are so busy and stressful that we tend to expend most of our energy by about 3 P.M. What do we do? We go right to the caffeine to keep our energy up for another six hours or so. It is, of course, far better, healthier, and less stressful on our bodies to generate energy naturally, and not to wear ourselves down to the point of collapse in the first place. If you really love your coffee, try a naturally decaffeinated organic brand. You may not even notice the difference.

Geo's Journey

I grew up in the restaurant business, where we baked lots of bread. Do you know how to make bread? You take a bowl and throw in flour, water, a little salt, a little oil, and yeast. You mix it all together, then you put it up in a nice, warm place. Pretty soon the heat activates the ingredients and it all starts rising. Have you noticed how many people have pouchy, swollen stomachs? Some of it is fat, but some of it is yeast. What do we put in our stomachs? Probably a lot of bread, oil and grease, salt, a little bit of water, and sugar. All that stuff starts to ferment in the colon. It's like a little bread machine down there. Soon, the colon starts expanding, literally getting dammed up. If you're going to eat bread, eat the really heavily grained bread so your body has something to process.

Step Eleven: Early to Rise...

There is something spiritual about the early morning. It represents a fresh start, a new beginning, purity. Get up early every morning—I like to say around sunrise—and meditate to get your mind in the right mode for the day. While getting enough sleep is perhaps most crucial, I've always felt that we are meant to wake with the sunrise and fall asleep with the sunset. We are creatures of light, and we sleep best in darkness. We are so affected by the light that it makes sense to me to coordinate the sleep cycle with darkness.

Step Twelve: Early to Bed...

Go to bed by 10 P.M. I know, you aren't 12 years old, but being an adult doesn't mean you are obligated to stay up past midnight, just because you *can*. Your body has important repair work to do, your dreams are waiting, and you can't possibly function at your best or experience peak energy when you are sleep-deprived. And again, we all sleep best when the world around us is in darkness. If your schedule prohibits you from sleeping at night, at least take steps to sufficiently darken your sleeping quarters.

Step Thirteen: Be Positively Radiant!

Be positive, see the good, radiate the good, believe in life, the spiritual, yourself, and your fellow humans.

I've spent many years working on finding balance, and these 13 steps are what I have discovered really works. If I eat too much, I have to exercise too much to get rid of extra food, then I need to rest more because I'm more tired, I feel less positive, and the next day the whole cycle starts again. However, if I regulate my diet, so that I don't eat too much but just enough to get by feeling good, then I don't have to exercise as hard or as much to keep my body tuned and strong. I have a lot more energy so I don't have to sleep as much, and I feel clear-headed when I get up.

Following these 13 steps, or modifications of them that work best for you, will give you greater energy and a sense of self-control, too. I have a lot more energy when I live this way, and if I can do it, so can you!

The Least You Need to Know

➤ Living naturally will give you better health, a higher energy level, and greater personal happiness.

➤ Examine your life to see where you need improvement; keep life simple; and follow the traditional yoga abstentions and observances such as contentment, discipline, studiousness, and devotion.

➤ Exercise consistently in a natural way.

➤ Practice daily deep breathing, self–observation, concentration and meditation, and an awareness of the oneness of the universe.

➤ Eliminate meat, alcohol, most bread, sugar, soda, coffee and tea, desserts, and milk products other than yogurt from your diet. Instead, eat a pure, natural diet based on fish, vegetables, and plenty of pure water.

➤ Get up early and go to bed early.

➤ Maintain a positive and loving outlook toward yourself, life, the spiritual, and your fellow human beings.

Part 5

Get Down

Even though we'll get down on the floor in this next section, the hard work isn't over yet. I'll challenge you with a series of sitting poses; a series of poses to strengthen your stomach muscles; more advanced arches, wheels, and tilts; and a great workout for your back, an area too often ignored and infamous for causing pain.

I'll end the section with some super-powered inversions that send blood out of your extremities and into your head, flushing your brain with nutrients for clearer thinking and a boost of brain power. From the easiest half shoulderstand to the super-challenging feathered peacock and scorpion poses, you'll work hard, teach your heart how to pump against gravity, and see the world in a whole new way—upside-down!

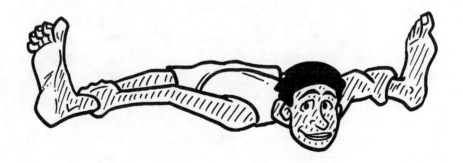

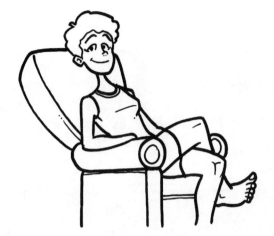

Chapter 18

Sitting Series

In This Chapter

➤ Slow things down by taking a seat

➤ Rock the boat

➤ Sitting stretches

➤ Winding down to the ground

Sitting poses begin the relaxation process in our Power Yoga workout. That doesn't mean they are easy, but they are less strenuous, in a cardiovascular sense, than the four-legged poses in the previous section.

Many people aren't comfortable with sitting on the ground, even though it is very natural for the human body. Have a seat, but don't get too relaxed. We aren't finished yet.

Sitting Reach

➤ *Difficulty Level:* II

➤ *Powers:* The hips, quadriceps, back, and shoulders.

➤ *Caution:* Some people can get a little dizzy or nervous when they lay their heads back. Take it slow and lower your head back slowly as you reach up.

Make your body into a living "L" and remember to keep your heart lifted (top figure). Reach up and lay your head back (bottom figure) in a seated version of reed pose, the sitting reach.

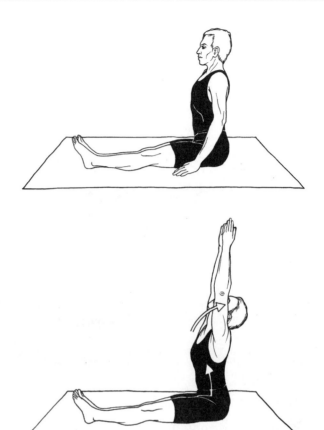

The sitting poses begin with a sitting reach, and the sitting reach begins with a basic, L-shaped sit. All the sitting poses move from this pose. It is for the sitting series what the Marine pose is for the standing series.

➤ Sit comfortably on the floor with your legs straight out in front of you, forming the letter "L."

➤ Inhale and reach your arms straight up overhead, stretch up out of the hips, and look up.

➤ Lay your head back and reach straight up, as high as you can, creating a slight arch in the back. This is a lot like the reed pose, except that you are in a sitting position.

➤ Hold for one to five breaths.

Boat Pose

➤ *Difficulty Level:* III

➤ *Powers:* The abdominal muscles, the quadriceps, and the lower back. Great for defining those washboard abs.

➤ *Caution:* If you have lower back problems, don't try this pose until your abdominal muscles are very strong and can properly support the lower back.

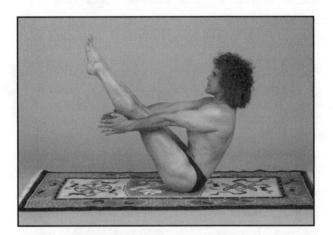

Boat pose imitates a little boat rocking on the water. For added effect and extra muscle control, try rocking your body in this position.

Boat pose is both a sitting pose and a stomach-strengthening pose, and could go just as easily in the next chapter with the tummy series.

➤ From sitting reach, bend your knees and sit back a little so you are balanced on your tailbone.

➤ Keep your chest up and raise your feet off the ground with your knees bent.

➤ Raise your hands up and bring them next to your knees with palms facing toward each other. Your arms should be parallel to the floor.

➤ Play with this position for a little while. Work to find a strong balance.

➤ As you gain strength in the abdominal muscles (over a period of workouts), start to straighten your legs so your body takes the shape of a "V" with your head looking up. If you are already strong in the abdominal muscles, you may be able to straighten the legs right away, but don't rush it. Keep working to raise the legs. The higher the legs in this pose, the better.

➤ Lift your chest, keep your back straight and strong, don't round your lower back, and push the breath low into the belly.

Geo's Journey

Boat pose channels a lot of blood into the lower abdominal region just by the sheer effect of gravity. Everything is channeled into the lower abdominal region in this posture, activating the first chakra and all the lower glands and organs.

Sun Pose

➤ *Difficulty Level:* III

➤ *Powers:* The hamstrings, back, shoulders; hones focus and concentration.

➤ *Caution:* This pose is a more challenging balance pose than boat pose, but easier on the abdominal muscles. It's better to gain the strength required for boat pose first. Then you'll be strong enough to handle the added balance challenge.

Sun pose is a variation of boat pose in which the body makes a more extreme V-shape and the hands grasp the heels.

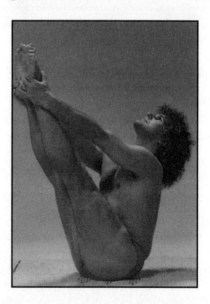

The sun pose is a nice-looking, fun pose that can flow right out of boat pose without coming back down. You can look at the body in sun pose and see how gravity would draw blood into the hip area, so that all the lower glands and organs and the hip joints are toned.

Of course, it is also a balance pose, so it's a wonderful pose for focus and concentration. Holding onto the legs creates a nice stretch in the back of the legs. As you lift your head back and keep your arms straight, it opens the shoulders and back. The heart lifts, and laying back the head helps to relieve the neck.

➤ From boat pose, raise your legs just a little higher and bring your torso closer to your thighs.

➤ Grab your heels.

➤ Slowly lay your head back and look up. Focus on a point above you in order to balance.

The Right Moves

One of the great things about sun pose is that it allows you to let the head drop back gently. So much in the world today causes the head to push forward, you may not even be aware of how often. Sun pose is a gentle way to ease the head back, releasing that tension in a backward direction.

Back Stretching Pose

➤ *Difficulty Level:* II

➤ *Powers:* A great stretch for the entire back and the backs of the legs. Also concentrates energy into the first chakra.

➤ *Caution:* Forcing yourself down farther than your body wants to go could injure your back. Take it slowly and ease yourself down, working on the edge of your flexibility.

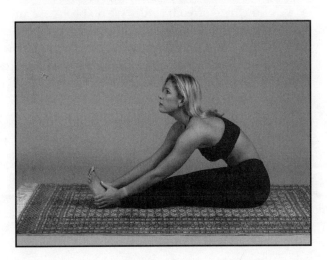

Inhale and raise the head before lowering the torso toward the legs in back stretching pose.

Back stretching pose stretches and lengthens the muscles of the back.

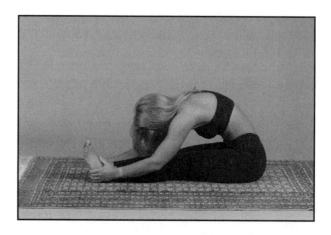

From sun pose, we move right into a seated forward bend I call back stretching pose.

The Right Moves

For back stretching pose, you almost want your body to lie as if you just passed out. You want to be so comfortable that you could fall asleep in this position. I've held this pose for 30 or 40 minutes with no trouble at all. You go off into a dream world. It may seem difficult at first, but the more flexible you get, the more this will be a very restful pose.

➤ From sun pose, let go of the ankles and slowly lower the legs back into the L-shaped sit.

➤ Inhale, stretch up into sitting reach, then exhale and roll forward over the legs. In the beginning, bend the knees as much as you need to, until you get really strong and warm in this pose.

➤ Lie forward, folding the whole body over the legs.

➤ Now, focus all your energy and concentration at the base of your spine. We do boat pose and sun pose right before back stretching pose because they draw energy into that area. This is what we call a first chakra pose because it concentrates energy into the base of the spine, where the first chakra lies.

➤ Lie in this pose and pay attention to your breathing. Every time you inhale, feel the expansion of the breath creating a stretch in the back. The inhaling expands the spine, puts space between all the vertebrae, stretches the hips, stretches the hamstrings, and expands the whole back of the body from the heel right out through the top of the head.

➤ Hold for 5 to 10 breaths, then gently come up.

Plank Pose

➤ *Difficulty Level:* II

➤ *Powers:* The shoulders, arms, and wrists; also a great stomach strengthener.

➤ *Caution:* Don't let the hands move too far into the body, or the bend in the wrists will be too extreme. Keep the hands about a foot back from the shoulders, fingers pointed toward the body.

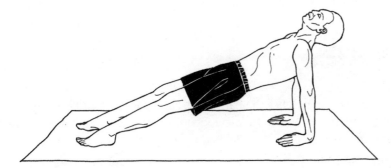

Plank pose is similar to an inverted board pose.

Now that you've stretched the back forward, a counterpose is in order. Plank pose is a great counterpose to back stretching pose, and a super strengthener for the stomach and arms, too.

➤ From your L-sit, gently drop your head back and slide your hands back behind your hips about one foot, with the fingers pointing back toward your body.

➤ Push yourself up on your hands and feet, keep your head back, and lift your chest and hips so your body forms a straight line. This is like an inverted board pose.

➤ This is a difficult pose normally held for no more than five breaths. One breath is great for a start.

➤ Variation: Table pose is a good alternate pose if plank pose is a little too strenuous for your current fitness level. In table pose, come up on your hands as in plank pose, but bend your knees and lift your hips so that your body forms the shape of a table, with your stomach and chest as the table-top. Hold for one to five breaths.

The Wrong Moves

Be careful not to pull the toes back too far in back stretching pose. At first, point your toes. If you do pull toes back for an extra stretch once you've gained flexibility, keep your heels on the ground. If your heels come off the ground, you'll begin to hyperextend your knees, which will weaken them. You don't want to loosen your knees too much, or they may give out on you when you least expect it.

*Support the table by lift-
ing with the gluts and
abdominal muscles.*

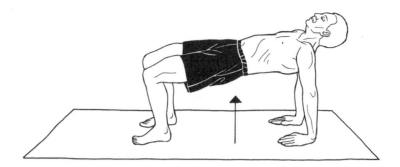

Alternate Leg Stretch

➤ *Difficulty Level:* II

➤ *Powers:* Opens the hip joints, stretches the hamstrings, and energizes and activates
all the lower glands and organs, including the appendix, colon, liver, gallbladder,
pancreas, intestinal tract on the bending side, and the ovaries in women.

➤ *Caution:* Don't put your foot up on the opposite thigh until your hip flexibility
allows it. Keep your foot on the floor against your body at first.

*For alternate leg stretch,
bring the heel of the left
foot all the way in to the
body so it presses on the
center of the pelvic area;
fold the body over the
extended right leg.*

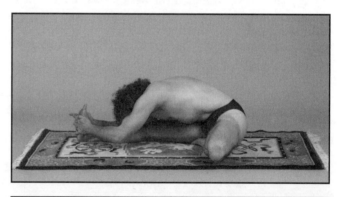

*For more flexible students,
bring the left foot on top of
the right thigh in alternate
leg stretch. On the inhale,
stretch the body up.*

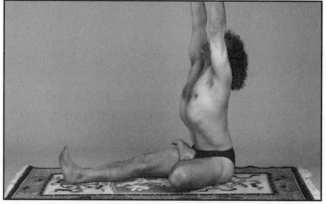

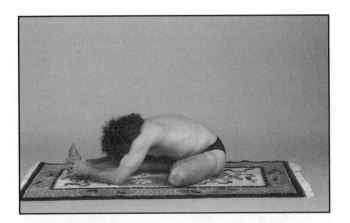

On the exhale, fold the body over the thigh of the extended leg in alternate leg stretch.

So far, everything we have done in this series has been forward and back. Now it's time to work the sides of the body separately again, with alternate leg stretch.

Alternate leg stretch is a pose that lessens the blood flow into the extended leg when we bend over, like a restricting bandage that slows circulation in the leg. This pose creates a damming effect in the top of the thigh, putting a lot of pressure on the lower glands and organs—the appendix, colon, liver, gallbladder, pancreas, intestinal tract, and ovaries.

Blood pressure increases in every organ in the lower-right side of the body (and in the lower-left side when you reverse the pose). Alternate leg stretch dams up the blood flow and squeezes the entire lower abdominal area, pressing and concentrating energy through all the glands and organs, right to their outer fibers. It's a great stretch in the hips, too, and a good practice pose for yoga split.

The Wrong Moves

Plank pose and table pose are great strengtheners for the wrists, shoulders, and upper back, but they can be especially hard on the wrists. If you have problems with your wrists, you may want to skip this pose. Or, be sure to keep the arms at least a foot back from the hips before lifting your body weight. The closer your hands are to your body, the more extreme the angle of your wrists.

➤ Lower your body from plank or table pose, back into the L-sit.

➤ Inhale, reach forward, and take the left foot by its ankle. Draw it up next to the right thigh, pressing the heel into the center of the pelvic area. This position is great for men because it draws energy into the prostate. More advanced students can bring the foot all the way onto the opposite thigh, right at the root of the thigh in the crease where the thigh meets the hip.

263

➤ Keep your extended leg straight, with the knee slightly bent and rolled slightly out.

➤ Roll forward over the right leg. If your foot is on top of the base of the opposite thigh, you'll create a damming effect in the right leg because the foot is lying across the femoral artery and slowing the blood flow and energy to the leg, causing it to collect and concentrate in the lower abdominal area.

➤ Hold for 5 to 10 breaths.

Geo's Journey

I recommend bending over the extended right leg first in alternate leg stretch because of the way the colon works. The ascending colon starts in the right side of the body and moves upward, against gravity, then makes a turn to the left across the transverse colon, then down the sigmoid colon and out the rectum. Bending over the right side first works the colon the same way the body naturally does. Think of the colon like that trap underneath your sink. Things can sometimes get slowed a little bit right at that upward bend, since everything is moving against gravity. A little pressure on the base of the ascending colon really helps get things moving.

Side Stretch

➤ *Difficulty Level:* II

➤ *Powers:* The leg muscles, especially after alternate leg stretch, because the blood rushes back to the leg muscles in this pose. Also opens up the side of the body.

➤ *Caution:* Watch your knees in this pose. If you need to put a pillow under the knee holding your weight, do so.

Side stretch opens the side of the body, creating a flow of energy from feet to fingertips.

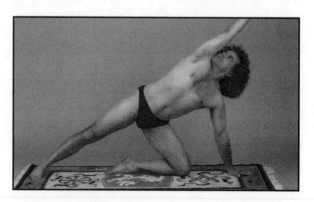

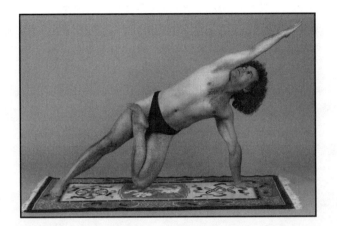

For the advanced student, vary side stretch by keeping the foot on top of the opposite thigh after alternate leg stretch, then lifting the entire body off the floor.

This pose rolls right out of alternate leg stretch.

➤ From alternate leg stretch, roll up onto your left knee and bring your left hand back behind your right hip to support your body weight.

➤ Twist slightly around to the left side.

➤ Stretch out your right leg to open the leg and hip. Press your hips up and out.

➤ Stretch your arm over your head to form a straight line from fingertips to toes. Feel the whole right side of your body opening and the blood and all the energy concentrated in alternate leg stretch flowing through the body.

➤ Variation: If you placed the foot on top of the thigh in alternate leg stretch, you can keep it there for a more advanced version of side stretch, lifting the entire body off the ground so the knee doesn't help to support the weight. This variation takes a lot of strength.

➤ Hold for about five breaths.

Gate Latch Pose

➤ *Difficulty Level:* II

➤ *Powers:* Opens the opposite side of the body from side stretch; opens the hips; stretches the hamstrings.

➤ *Caution:* Again, watch the knee and cushion with a pillow if necessary.

Gate latch pose is the counterpose to side stretch, moving the body in the opposite direction.

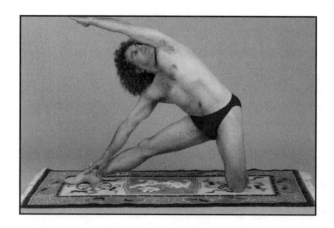

Gate latch pose is really side stretch for the opposite side.

The Right Moves

I tell my students to hold most poses for about five breaths, or to work up to five breaths. It takes your body about 20 seconds to adjust to a pose or movement, so once you are strong enough to move in and out of the poses comfortably with the breath, then your goal should be to try holding the poses for about five breaths to really increase your strength.

➤ From side stretch, flatten the foot of the extended leg to the floor as if you were preparing to stand on it.

➤ Shift your bodyweight to the bent (left) knee. If your left foot was on your right thigh, gently remove it so your lower leg extends behind you on the floor.

➤ Move your body in the opposite direction, stretching to the right over the extended leg.

➤ Reach overhead with your left arm and look up under your arm toward the ceiling. Keep your head and neck strong. Feel the entire left side of the body opening and stretching.

➤ Hold for about five breaths.

➤ Come back down into the L-sit and repeat the entire routine on the left side, beginning with alternate leg stretch, left leg extended, and ending with gate latch pose extending over the left leg.

Back and Side Stretch with Legs Apart

➤ *Difficulty Level:* IV

➤ *Powers:* The inner thigh muscles, hips, and sides of the body.

➤ *Caution:* If you don't want to pull a groin muscle, take it easy in this pose. Don't bend down farther than your body can handle. If you feel pain, you've gone too far.

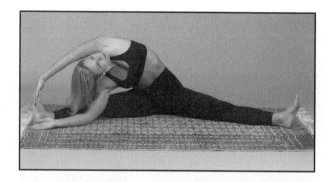

Side stretch with legs apart opens the entire side of the body and puts a great stretch in the inner thighs and hips.

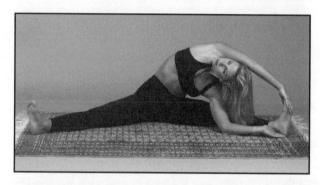

Always counter a side stretch to one side with a side stretch to the other side for balance.

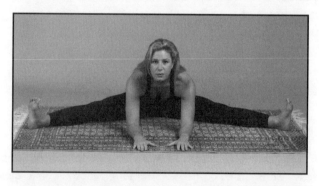

Inhale and raise the head before lowering the body into the full stretch for back stretch with legs apart.

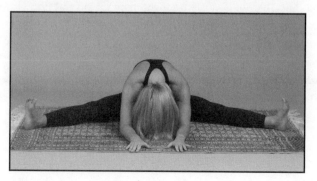

Exhale into back stretch with legs apart, a challenging flexibility pose.

Now that you've worked both sides of the body, the final group of poses will challenge the flexibility of your hips and inner thighs.

➤ Come back down from gate latch pose into a seated position. Sit up straight and separate your legs on the floor as wide as you can.

➤ Inhale and stretch your arms overhead.

➤ Exhale and lie out over your right leg, face down. Hold for five breaths.

➤ Inhale and stretch up again, then exhale and move down over your left leg. Hold for five breaths.

➤ Inhale and stretch up, then exhale and twist your body toward the front. Drop the right elbow down inside your right knee and look up under your arm, twisting your left arm overhead, as in the photograph. Lie out over your right leg with your side toward your thigh.

➤ Inhale and stretch up, then exhale and twist the other way, bringing your left elbow down inside your left knee, reaching with your right arm overhead to open the right side of the body.

➤ Inhale and stretch up, then exhale as you lower your body straight down the middle. Slide your hands forward on the floor until your body is about a foot off the ground (or almost to the edge of your flexibility).

➤ Inhale and lift your head up, then exhale and reach forward on the floor as far as you can. Let your head drop so the weight of your head can help to pull your body toward the floor.

Geo's Journey

The final movement of back stretch with legs apart is a common stretch for dancers, who often get to the point where they can just lie on the floor for long periods of time, their bodies resting between a full split. This position can be frightening for guys, at first. However, it really is almost a necessary pose to counteract all the sitting we do. We need to stretch and lengthen those muscles that get shortened and weakened. People carry a lot of tension in their hips, and this stretch really helps to eliminate it.

Relaxation Pose

➤ *Difficulty Level:* I

➤ *Powers:* The entire body by relaxing the body and letting it feel the effects of the workout.

➤ *Caution:* Don't fall asleep!

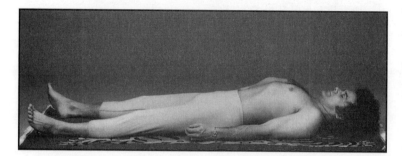

Relaxation pose allows you to lie quietly and feel what your body has done during the workout and what is happening internally.

All this work we've been doing has been moving us toward a goal you might not have expected: to strengthen our bodies enough so that they can sit strongly in a meditation pose with a straight back, strong hips, and knees rolled outward, sitting squarely on the tailbone.

But every effort requires a rest period. From here, we move down to the back.

➤ Come up out of the back stretch with legs apart and bring the legs and arms up again into a brief boat pose.

➤ Now lower the body, rolling down until you are lying flat on your back.

➤ Lie here for a moment and focus on your breath. Notice how it pulses a little stronger because of the effort of boat pose, how the heart's a little quicker, and the breath a little shorter. Feel your body literally pulsate from the breath and the blood flow, the energy that you've created moving through it, brought in from outside you and also merged and mixed with the life-force energy innate in you.

Don't be in any rush to get up out of relaxation pose. So many people these days are in a hurry. They get into this position, take three breaths, then jump right back up. Take your time. Relax. Enjoy the rest. You've earned it!

From here, you are in the perfect position to work on the stomach, which is the subject of the next chapter.

> ### The Least You Need to Know
>
> ➤ Sitting poses bring the body to the floor, beginning the process of slowing down.
>
> ➤ Sitting poses also prepare the body for the rigors of sitting meditation.
>
> ➤ Sitting poses consist of sitting reach, boat pose and sun pose, a series of sitting forward bends, side stretches, and split stretches.
>
> ➤ The sitting series ends by bringing the body all the way to the ground in relaxation pose, in preparation for stomach work.

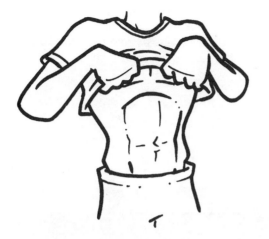

Chapter 19

Tummy Series

> ## In This Chapter
>
> ➤ The center of the body
>
> ➤ Pelvic tilts for any occasion
>
> ➤ Work those abs!
>
> ➤ Sit-ups with a twist

In this chapter, we'll work the belly. Stomach, "abs," tummy, whatever you want to call it, it is the body's center, so strength here affects strength throughout the body.

Many people carry around a little pouch over their lower abdomens, which doesn't want to go away. Those of you pushing 40, 50, or 60 probably know what I mean, unless you have been in great shape your entire life. Women who have given birth may find that the stomach still hangs down, long after those first postpartum weeks, stubbornly resisting all dieting efforts.

The truth is, the only way to firm up that stomach is by working with it. You've got to use those muscles so they don't go slack, and the more you use them, the tighter and more flexible they'll be.

Strong stomach muscles also give your body a sense of stability and inner strength. They support your back, lessening the chance of suffering back pain. You'll move with more grace and less effort if your belly is strong and tight, not to mention the fact that a strong stomach looks a lot better!

It's never too late to strengthen your stomach. Need proof? Take a look at my 68-year-old student Bill. Bill is one of the models in this book, who demonstrates push knee breath later in this chapter. He started yoga with me about six months ago and is gaining incredible strength and flexibility. If Bill can do it, so can you.

Pelvic Tilts Revisited

➤ *Difficulty Level:* I

➤ *Powers:* Strengthens and aligns the spine.

➤ *Caution:* Pelvic tilt is a very small movement. Don't exaggerate the arch or you could strain your lower back.

Inhale in pelvic tilt and arch the back as the belly fills with breath.

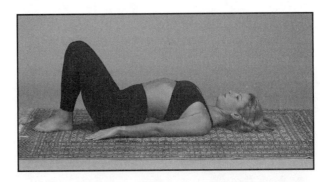

Exhale in pelvic tilt and press the lower back against the floor while pressing the belly in to push out the breath.

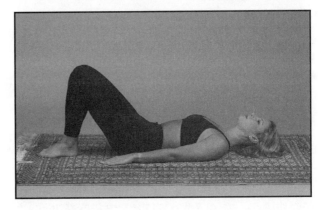

No matter how advanced you get, you can always benefit from pelvic tilts. They help to strengthen and readjust the spine if it's a little out of alignment.

➤ From relaxation pose, in which you lie on your back on the floor, inhale, turning the tailbone down and pushing the breath into the belly.

➤ Exhale, tucking the tailbone under and flattening the back onto the floor.

➤ Continue to tilt the pelvic girdle with the breath, inhaling and rolling the breath into those lower glands and organs, then exhaling, pulling inward and under, pushing the breath all the way out and rounding the back against the floor.

➤ Repeat through five full breaths.

Push Knee Series

➤ *Difficulty Level:* I

➤ *Powers:* The diaphragm muscle; also aligns the spine and strengthens the abdominal muscles.

➤ *Caution:* This pose is easy and comfortable, but performing it on a hard surface could cause some discomfort. Invest in a good yoga mat.

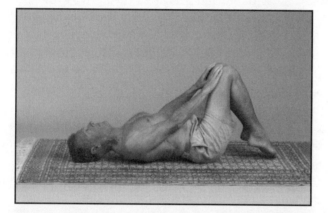

Push knee breath is like a fancy pelvic tilt. Inhale and push the knees away from the body.

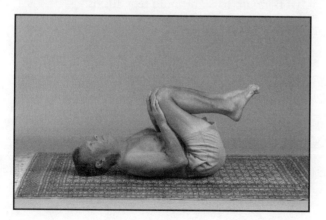

Pull the knees toward the body on the exhale in push knee breath. This motion with the legs helps to push air out of the body.

The Right Moves

Push knee breath is a nice massage for the abdominal area, great for relieving constipation and promoting elimination. The squeeze with the legs on the exhale literally massages the colon as you draw your knees in.

This great little movement is based on pelvic tilt, but with an addition that makes breathing even more productive. As we inhale, the body naturally arches, expands, and makes space for the breath, and with this movement, we help that expansion by pushing the knees away from the torso. As we exhale, the body naturally rounds and pushes the breath out. In push knee breath, we use the legs to help expel the breath.

➤ From pelvic tilt, place a hand on each knee with knees bent and toes pointed.

➤ Inhale and push the knees away from the body until the toes hit the ground about a foot beyond the hips. Arch the spine, keep the head on the ground, and straighten the arms as you push the knees away. Keep the movement controlled.

➤ Exhale and draw the knees tightly toward the chest, maintaining the same angle at the knee throughout the entire movement. Pull the tailbone slightly off the ground using only the lower abdominal muscles. This position is like worship to the supreme except we are on our backs, so it puts less stress on the body and is a greater abdominal strengthener.

➤ Variation: Push knee breath can become an even more powerful stomach exercise by placing the hands behind the head as if you were about to do a sit-up. Keep the elbows on the ground and press the toes to the ground as you inhale, then bring the knees to the chest as you exhale. Keeping the hands behind the head adds more of a challenge to the lower abdominal muscles.

➤ Repeat five times at first, working up to 30 or more repetitions.

Yoga Walks

➤ *Difficulty Level:* II

➤ *Powers:* The back, hips, and lower abdominal muscles.

➤ *Caution:* Stay strong in the abdominal muscles as you lift the legs to keep the pressure off your lower back.

Yoga walks is a great strengthener for the back, even though this wasn't my original intention when I developed this pose.

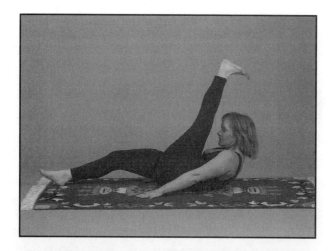

Yoga walks is based on the movement babies make when they lie on their backs and raise their legs into the air.

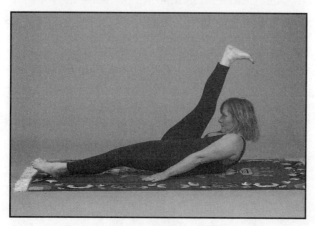

Bring the head up to meet the leg in yoga walks and you'll soon see the strengthening effects in the lower abdominal muscles.

I'm interested in the way babies move because their movements are purely natural. They move as necessary to get attention, build strength, and explore the world. If you've ever watched a baby lying on its back, you know that babies don't just lie flat and still like an exhausted adult. They bring their legs up in the air, into positions that would be daunting for the flexibility of most of us grown-ups. This position and movement massages the colon and the elimination center and strengthens the infant's abdominal muscles.

Babies can lie on the floor and wave their legs around all day. They make it look easy, but this position is far from easy for usually upright adults. Now let's see for ourselves what a challenge this movement can be.

Geo's Journey

I have my classes do yoga walks and after a few minutes of lying on our backs with our feet in the air, my students are exhausted! Knowing firsthand how tiring this movement can be may give you a whole new level of respect for babies.

➤ From push knee breath, extend the legs out, returning to a relaxed prone position.

➤ Inhale and reach way over your head with your arms, pointing the toes, stretching out the fingers, breathing from the tips of the toes to the tips of the fingers.

➤ Exhale and bring your hands by your sides, palms flat on the ground.

➤ Raise your head, setting the chin on the chest.

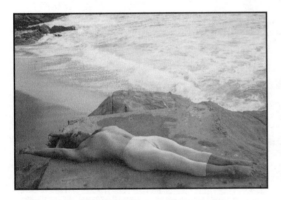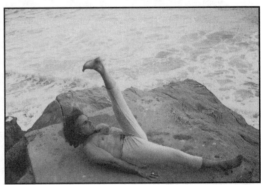

Geo performs yoga walks; inhale at left, exhale at right.

➤ Raise your right leg up, flexing the foot so the toes point back toward the head, pushing the breath out as you roll the right leg up. Leave the left leg on the ground.

➤ Inhale from this top position, stretching the leg back down across the floor, lowering the head to the floor, and reaching the arms back up over head.

➤ Exhale again and roll up with the left leg, setting the chin on the chest, hands forward, palms facing down.

➤ Begin with five repetitions and work up to 50, going back and forth, alternating legs. From there you can move up into 100 repetitions, and from there, you can alter the movement to raise both legs at the same time. But be sure you can do 100 repetitions first!

➤ Variation: As in push knee breath, you can also perform yoga walks with the hands behind the head for an added lower abdominal workout. After you've become very strong, try raising both legs at the same time, eventually coming all the way up on the shoulders, a great warm-up for shoulderstands.

The Wrong Moves

Don't rush to perform the advanced version of yoga walks, raising both legs at the same time. Unless your stomach muscles are strong enough, your lower back will compensate and you could sustain an injury. If you do try to raise both legs off the floor, concentrate on keeping the lower back pressed against the floor rather than allowing it to arch.

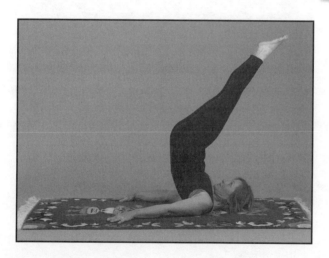

The advanced version of yoga walks brings both legs and the torso off the ground into a shoulderstand.

Arch with Knees Together

➤ *Difficulty Level:* II

➤ *Powers:* The thighs, hips, knees, lower back; the thyroid, parathyroid, and lymph system in the throat; also stimulates the base of the brain.

➤ *Caution:* Don't hold this pose so long that you feel a strain on your neck.

Begin the arch with knees together with a pelvic tilt, but keep the knees and feet pressed together.

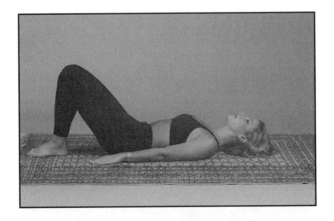

Continue the arch with knees together by exhaling and lifting the hips off the ground, keeping the knees and feet together.

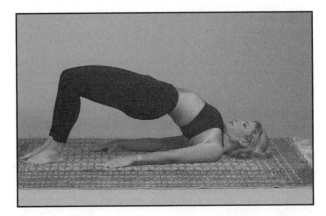

After the rounding of yoga walks, the body is ready for an arching pose.

➤ Bring the feet and legs together. Inhale as in pelvic tilt, turning the tailbone down but keeping the legs together.

➤ Exhale and lift the hips as high off the ground as possible, holding the knees together. Find the place where the hips can go no farther with the knees remaining together. Push down on the heels.

➤ Hold for one to five breaths, then lower back to the ground.

Eagle Crunchers

➤ *Difficulty Level:* III

➤ *Powers:* The abdominal muscles, which are squeezed by the crossing of the knees; also opens up the shoulders, elbows, hips, and knees. The crunch with the exhale makes for a very powerful stomach exercise that works very quickly.

➤ *Caution:* If you have bad knees, shoulders, or elbows, don't push your limbs into this position. Entwine them only as far as they will go comfortably.

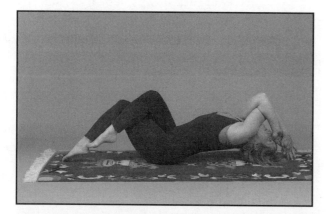

Eagle crunchers are sit-ups with a twist—literally! Entwine the arms and the legs for a great stretch.

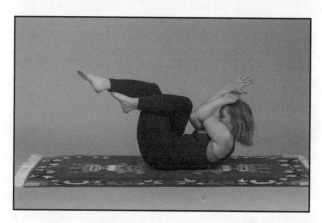

Bring the head and the knees toward each other on the exhalation in eagle crunchers.

Eagle crunchers is the traditional yoga eagle pose, but performed lying down on the floor. I prefer eagle crunchers to eagle pose because the twist in the limbs is gentler on the body in a prone position. This pose is a very powerful stomach strengthener and also activates the second chakra, stoking the digestive fire.

➤ After coming down from arching pose, bend the knees and place the right knee over the left knee. If your flexibility allows, hook the toes of the right foot under the left calf.

➤ Lay the left arm across the right arm, elbow over elbow. Reach around with the right hand, turn it, bend both elbows, and place the fingertips of the right hand on the inside heel of the left hand.

The Right Moves

When you practice the limb twists for eagle crunchers, you'll find that twisting in one direction is easier than twisting in the other direction. Your right knee might go easily over the left, but twisting the left knee around the right leg may feel awkward. To balance the body, try a few more repetitions of eagle crunchers on the side that feels less comfortable.

➤ Inhale and, keeping your arms and legs entwined, stretch your arms over your head, arch your back slightly, look back, and stretch your legs out, too, as in push knee breath.

➤ Exhale and roll into a ball, bringing your knees and elbows together, or at least toward each other.

➤ Continue with this movement, inhaling down, exhaling up. Start with 10 on one side, then reverse the position of your arms and legs, and do 10 on the other side. Then move to 20 on each side, then 25 on each side.

Arch with Knees Apart

➤ *Difficulty Level:* II

➤ *Powers:* The gluteal muscles and quadriceps; stretches, balances, and aligns the spine.

➤ *Caution:* Don't hold this pose so long that you feel uncomfortable pressure on your neck.

Arch with knees apart begins just like pelvic tilt.

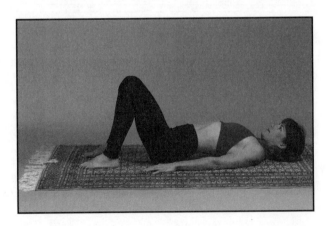

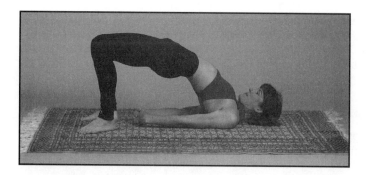

On the exhalation, lift the hips as high as you can, supporting the body with the feet, shoulders, and neck.

From here, we need a counterpose, and the perfect counterpose to eagle crunchers is hip raises with knees apart.

➤ From eagle crunchers, uncross your legs and arms so you are lying flat on the ground again.

➤ Raise your knees and keep your feet on the ground about hip-distance apart, hands by the sides, palms facing downward.

➤ Start with one repetition of a pelvic tilt. Inhale and turn the tailbone down, creating a slight arch in the back.

➤ Exhale, tuck the tailbone under, and flatten the back on the floor.

➤ Inhale again, then exhale and press the hips straight up, pushing down evenly on the heels, pushing up evenly on the hip.

These arching poses are excellent for the back, thighs, knees, and the back of the neck. This is a great lead-in and lead-out for shoulderstand work. They also make a great beginning to some of the other arches, wheels, and twists. So great, in fact, that we're going to repeat them at the beginning of the next chapter.

The Least You Need to Know

➤ The stomach and abdominal area are the body's center. Strength here imparts strength to the entire body.

➤ A strong stomach supports the lower back, lessening the chances of developing back pain.

➤ Great movements for stomach strengthening include pelvic tilt, push knee breath, yoga walks, and eagle crunchers.

➤ When working the stomach, be sure to include counterposes to stretch the stomach muscles. Arching poses work well for this purpose.

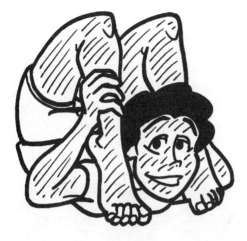

Chapter 20

Arches, Wheels, and Twists

In This Chapter

➤ You're never too advanced for a pelvic tilt

➤ Super-powered arches

➤ Mega-twists

I introduced you to tilts, twists, and arches in Chapter 7, "Tilts, Twists, and Arches." Now you are stronger, more flexible, and ready to advance a little farther with your arches.

Arches are wonderful poses to coordinate with your breathing, inhaling all the way down, exhaling all the way up, back and forth for two to five minutes or so. Five minutes of arch poses with the breath each day is a powerful, strengthening, and effective exercise for the knees, thighs, buns, lower back, thyroid and parathyroid (in the throat), and the back of the neck, where we carry lots of tension.

Once you are used to repeating this pose, the next step is to hold it. In each of the following arching poses (beyond pelvic tilt), begin holding the pose for about 20 seconds, hips up off the ground. Holding both the arch with knees together, arch with knees apart, and eventually, wheel pose, will increase your muscle strength and the flexibility of your spine.

Advanced Arch Series

Begin the advanced arch series with that good old standby, the pelvic tilt. This series can also flow right out of the tummy series of the previous chapter. Begin by unfolding from eagle pose to lie flat on the floor.

> ➤ Lie on your back and begin the pelvic tilt, turning the tailbone toward the floor and expanding the body with the inhale, pressing the back against the floor and tipping the tailbone up with the exhale. Move through this position for 5 to 10 breaths.

Pelvic tilt is a basic movement that can grow into many different routines, including the arch series of movements.

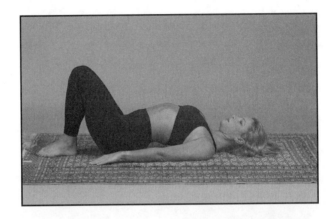

Press the back into the floor on the exhale in pelvic tilt.

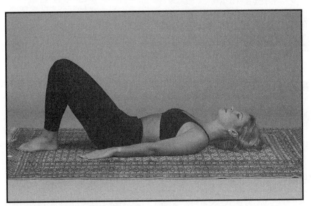

> ➤ Now move into arch pose, turning the tailbone toward the floor with the inhale, then lifting the hips off the floor with the exhale. Do 10 repetitions with legs together, then 10 repetitions with legs apart.

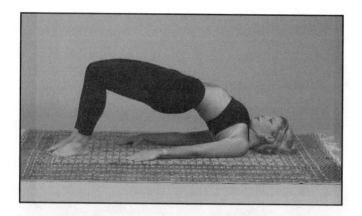

Arch pose, also called bridge pose, exaggerates the movement of the pelvic tilt for a greater stretch in the back, shoulders, and neck. Arch pose is shown here with feet, knees, and legs together.

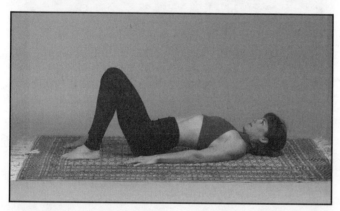

Inhale by arching the back slightly to prepare for arch pose with knees apart.

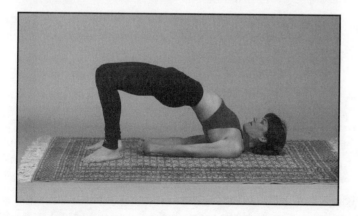

Arch pose is demonstrated here with feet, knees, and legs apart.

Wheel Pose

➤ *Difficulty Level:* IV

➤ *Powers:* An incredible stretch for the front of the body; strengthens the legs and arms, opens the hips, and flexes the spine.

➤ *Caution:* This pose takes a lot of arm strength. To prevent a fall, don't try to hold it longer than you are able. Move into and out of the pose with control.

The wheel pose brings the arch up even farther for a stretch along the entire front of the body.

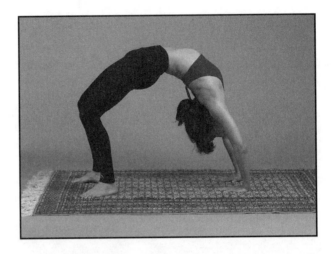

The Right Moves

To strengthen the inner thighs and inner gluteal muscles, work with the arch with knees together pose. To strengthen the outer gluteal muscles and the hips, work with the arch with knees apart pose.

Move straight out of arch with knees together pose into wheel pose, in which your knees will be apart and your feet separated.

➤ Come down from arch with knees together pose, and inhale again, turning the tailbone down slightly. Separate your feet and legs about hip distance.

➤ Bring the hands back next to the ears with the fingertips pointing under the shoulders.

➤ Exhale and push up onto the hands and feet, lifting the entire body off the floor—hips, chest, shoulders, and head.

➤ Let your head lie back and shift your body slightly to move your weight so it is evenly distributed over your hands and feet. In the beginning, do this pose with legs apart, and with plenty of distance between the hands and feet, so the arch isn't as extreme.

➤ Variations: When you get stronger and more comfortable in wheel pose, try it with feet together. This variation is a little more difficult and puts more stress on the back. You can also move your hands and feet closer together, to increase the stretch.

➤ Hold for one to five breaths, then come back down to the ground.

Elephant Pose

➤ *Difficulty Level:* V

➤ *Powers:* All the benefits of wheel pose, but with the added benefit of powering the focus and concentration to maintain the balance.

➤ *Caution:* You must feel very strong and confident in wheel pose to attempt elephant pose. If you aren't ready, you could tip over! It isn't easy to maintain a difficult balance when you are focusing while upside-down.

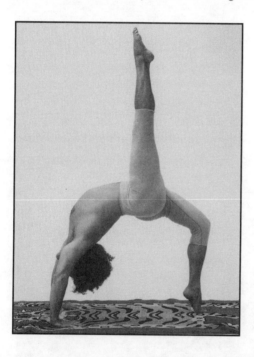

The elephant pose, sometimes called the one-legged wheel, is a challenging balance pose requiring great strength and flexibility.

Return to wheel pose to begin this challenging variation.

➤ Inhale and bring your hands back next to your ears, fingertips pointing under your shoulders, tailbone turned down.

➤ Exhale into wheel pose, and hold for 20 seconds, until you feel very stable and strong.

The Wrong Moves

When you do a lot of wheel poses, you may find your wrists getting very tired and sore. A lot of people have weak wrists, and in wheel pose, those small joints are supporting much of your body weight. Don't neglect your wrists. After coming out of wheel, shake out your wrists—rotate, flex, and bend until they feel comfortable again.

➤ Move your left foot toward the center, to maintain your balance.

➤ Slowly raise your right leg with knee bent, then extend the leg straight up overhead. Reach up with the toes and feel as if you are hanging from the sky by the tips of your toes. Eventually, you'll actually feel the body lighten as you focus on this hanging sensation.

➤ Hold for one to five breaths, then bend the knee, lower the leg to the floor, and come back down.

➤ Repeat on the other side.

Hug Yourself

➤ *Difficulty Level:* I

➤ *Powers:* Balances the body as a counterpose to arches and wheel poses.

➤ *Caution:* This easy, gentle pose is just what your body needs after a vigorous wheel pose. My only caution: Don't forget to do it!

Hug yourself counterbalances wheel pose by bending the spine in the opposite direction.

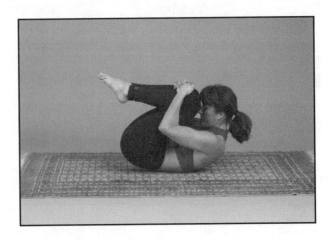

Hug yourself is a great pose to counterbalance many of the poses in this book. Whenever you arch your spine, hug yourself is the perfect balancing bend.

➤ After coming out of wheel pose or elephant pose, lie back down on the floor with knees up, arms at your sides.

➤ Exhale and draw your knees to your chest.

➤ Lift your head to meet your knees.

➤ Wrap your arms around your bent knees, interlocking your fingers.

➤ Hug yourself in this pose, rocking just a little as your spine finds its balance.

➤ If you can't get your knees all the way to your chest or if your head can't reach your knees, that's fine. Just be sure to wrap your arms around your knees so your spine can bend in the opposite direction that it was bending in the arches. This pose should feel very comfortable.

Advanced Twist Series

Now that we've worked the spine with arches and bends, we can work the spine side-to-side, with some more advanced twisting poses.

Geo's Journey

Twists have a very powerful effect on all the glandular systems of the body. Glands are organs that produce specialized chemicals to regulate blood chemistry and certain bodily secretions. The adrenal glands over the kidneys produce, among other things, epinephrine (adrenaline), helping the body to react appropriately in an emergency. The thymus gland in the chest produces immune-related hormones. The thyroid in the neck helps regulate metabolism. All these glands are twisted and activated in twisting poses.

Easy Back Twist

➤ *Difficulty Level:* II

➤ *Powers:* The lower back, neck, shoulders, and hips; also squeezes the colon, kidneys, adrenals, pancreas, lungs, and the organs of the lower abdomen.

➤ *Caution:* Move slowly into this position after arches and bends. Gently show your spine that you are now moving in a different direction.

Easy back twist gently stretches the entire back and loosens the hips and spine in preparation for more advanced twisting poses.

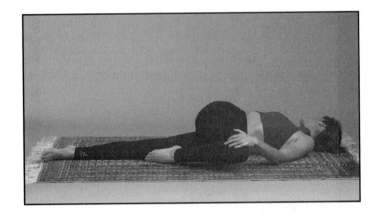

We worked on easy back twist in Chapter 7, but we'll repeat it here as a way to warm up the spine for more advanced twisting poses. Relax into this pose and let your spine get used to the twisting motion again. It takes about 20 seconds for the body to adjust to the pose. Give your spine at least 20 seconds on each side of this pose before moving on.

➤ After hug yourself, lie back down on your back with legs extended and arms at your sides. Inhale and feel your entire body expanding.

➤ Exhale and raise your right knee toward your chest, as if performing a one-legged hug yourself pose.

➤ Place your left hand on your right knee and bring your right knee across your body toward the floor to your left. If you can't bring your knee all the way to the floor, that's fine (although after all those hip- and spine-stretching arches, you may be surprised to see that your knee reaches the floor when it wouldn't before).

➤ Once your right knee is to the left, stretch your right arm straight out to the right, turning your head to look down your right arm. Make sure your right palm is turned down.

➤ As you roll over into the twist, you'll feel a nice stretch in the side of your hip and pressure across your ascending colon under your thigh. You'll also be twisting the kidneys, adrenals, lungs, and the organs of the lower abdomen.

➤ Hold this twist for one to three minutes. You should feel comfortable and relaxed, letting the weight of the body gradually deepen the twist. Concentrate on breathing into the open lung.

➤ Slowly turn your head so you are looking straight up, and with your left hand, lift your right knee back to center. Extend your leg back to the floor.

➤ Repeat the entire process with your left leg, twisting to the right side.

Geo's Journey

Remember that iliocecal valve, the place in the colon where the small and large intestine meet, which starts the colon's upward ascent on the right side of the body? Bent knee and straight leg twists put pressure on this part of the colon, and while this pressure stimulates the body's elimination system nicely, it also activates the second chakra. People "hold on" to more than waste matter in this area. Emotional baggage, things we are afraid to let go, can cause a physical holding back in the second chakra. Twists help to squeeze this area and get everything moving again, unblocking the dam when the twist is released.

Straight Leg Twist

➤ *Difficulty Level:* II

➤ *Powers:* The spine, the hips, the neck, the glandular systems of the body (especially the adrenals, thymus, and thyroid), and all the organs of the lower abdominal region.

➤ *Caution:* The weight of your leg becomes harder to control when the leg is extended. Don't let your leg fall over to the side or you could injure your lower back. Keep your movements controlled.

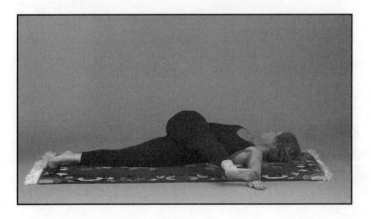

Straight leg twist is just like easy back twist, but with the leg extended, stretched up toward the hand, the foot placed on top of the hand.

Look over the extended arm in straight leg twist so that your extended arm forms a right angle to your body.

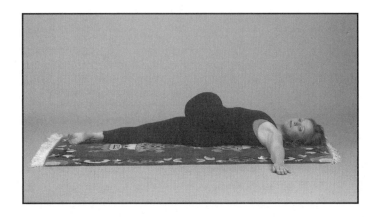

Straight leg twist is just like easy back twist, but, as the name suggests, with the leg extended.

The Right Moves

Twists are a lot of work, but they also provide a great opportunity for the body to rest. Don't rush out of twist poses. Hold them as long as you can, breathing and letting your body relax. Twists simultaneously accomplish two goals: a magnificent stretch and a well-deserved rest.

➤ After easy back twist, return to a prone position. Inhale and feel your entire body expanding.

➤ Extend both arms out to either side at right angles to your body, with palms down.

➤ Exhale and raise your right knee toward your chest, then extend your leg straight up.

➤ Inhale and lower your extended leg across the body to the left, keeping the motion controlled by pressing your hands against the floor and keeping both shoulders pressed to the floor. Scoot your hip back an inch or two to get a little arch in the back and a deeper stretch.

➤ Rest your extended leg at a right angle to your body at first. Then, when your flexibility allows, move the leg to about a 45-degree angle so your foot rests on the back of your left hand.

➤ Turn your head to look down your right arm.

➤ Hold for one to three minutes, breathing into the open side and feeling the body adjust and settle into the twist.

➤ Press your hands into the floor and raise your extended leg overhead, then bend the knee and lower the leg to the floor, extending it back into a prone position.

➤ Repeat on the other side.

Now you are ready to lie down on your belly and work the back of the body.

The Least You Need to Know

➤ Pelvic tilts prepare the body, no matter the fitness level, for more advanced arches.

➤ Arch with knees apart and arch with knees together strengthen the legs and gluteal muscles, as well as prepare the spine for the more extreme wheel pose.

➤ Hug yourself is a great counterpose for all arching poses.

➤ Easy back twist makes a good warm-up for more advanced twists, such as straight leg twist.

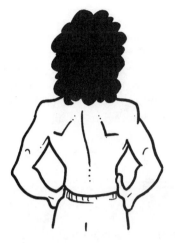

Back Power

We've just worked the belly and stretched the spine, so the natural progression will bring us around to those back muscles.

People today seem to have a lot of back pain. Whether this malady has to do with the fast pace of our society, too much sitting, lazy posture, weak stomach muscles, or a combination of all of these factors, the fact is that a lot of us really hurt!

Power Words

Osteoporosis is a thinning of the bones that often occurs in conjunction with aging, though it is not an inevitable part of aging. Osteoporosis leaves bones more vulnerable to fractures.

Back Up!

If you suffer from back pain, or even if you don't, your back can benefit from some targeted attention. A strong back results in better posture, more graceful movement, greater torso strength, a decreased chance of *osteoporosis* and other spine-related problems, and the energetic feeling that comes with a straight spine through which energy can flow freely.

Swimming Pose

➤ *Difficulty Level:* II

➤ *Powers:* A great warm-up and strengthener for the entire back, gluteal muscles, hamstrings, and deltoids.

➤ *Caution:* If you have lower back problems, begin with a very small movement. Even lifting your foot an inch or two off the ground is a good starting point.

Swimming pose is a great warm-up for the back, in preparation for more vigorous back-strengthening exercises.

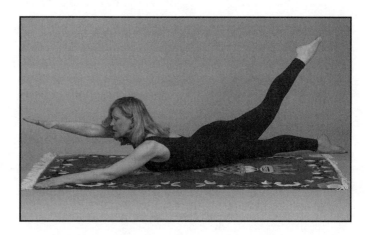

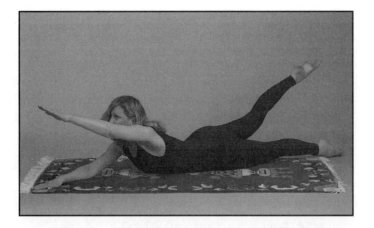

Swimming pose is a pose and a counterpose all in one, alternating the lift in the right arm and left leg with a lift in the left arm and right leg.

Before we begin working our backs too strenuously, we need to warm up the muscles. This is a great pose for anyone with lower back problems. It warms up the back and slowly begins to work muscles you may not have known you had.

➤ Roll over onto your stomach after finishing the twists in the previous chapter. Or, if you are starting here, lie down on your stomach.

➤ Stretch your arms over your head.

➤ Inhale and raise your right arm and left leg. Exhale down.

➤ Inhale and raise your left arm and right leg. Exhale down.

➤ Continue raising your opposing limbs with the breath for a minute or more, until you feel warm and your breath rate has increased slightly. If your back starts to feel strained, stop.

➤ Variation: People with really serious lower back trouble may find it difficult to lift the back foot off the ground at all, or to lift the head off the ground. Even bending the knee and raising the foot off the ground will begin the process of strengthening the lower back. Inhale and raise the right foot at the knee while raising the left arm in front of you. Exhale down. Inhale and raise the left foot at the knee while raising the right arm in front of you. Exhale down. This movement may seem small, but it will begin to make your lower back stronger.

Sphinx Pose

➤ *Difficulty Level:* II

➤ *Powers:* The gluteal muscles, legs, back, chest, and pectorals. Great stretch in the belly and the neck.

➤ *Caution:* Because this is a pose to get the back muscles prepared for more strenuous work, don't strain your back into an unnatural arch. Gently work it to gradually increase flexibility.

Sphinx pose stretches the back into an arch to increase strength and flexibility.

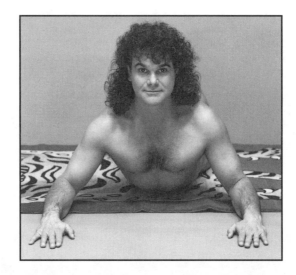

The arch in sphinx pose needn't be dramatic. If your lower back is tight, begin by simply lifting your upper body onto your elbows while keeping the lower body on the floor.

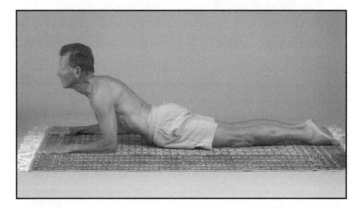

Sphinx pose is a basic back-stretching pose that moves the back into an arch without requiring too much strength. It is a great pose for slouchers because it helps your back to remember it can do more than just bend forward. It's also a great stretch in the stomach.

➤ Come back down from swimming pose with your arms to your sides, elbows bent, hands pointing forward, so that your arms form a U shape around your head.

➤ Bring your heels together, stretch out your legs, squeeze your thighs and buns.

➤ Inhale and raise your head and chest off the ground, keeping the elbows, forearms, and hands on the ground, pressing on them to help the stretch.

➤ Lift your chest and feel the stretch in the belly. You want to feel as if someone is sitting on your buns as you try to drag yourself forward.

➤ Hold for 20 to 30 seconds, working up to a minute.

➤ Exhale and come back down.

Locust Series

The Right Moves

When holding sphinx pose, try to capture a little of the feeling of the sphinx itself. Imagine you have been sitting in this position for 5,000 years, strong and powerful. Feel as if you are made of stone and nothing can compromise your ancient and invulnerable strength.

After the back is warmed up through swimming and sphinx poses, you are ready for locust series, a more challenging back strengthening series of exercises. Locust poses use the weight of the body to strengthen the back, doing what the body was designed to do.

Locust Head-Chest Raises

➤ *Difficulty Level:* II

➤ *Powers:* The upper and lower back, and the muscles of the chest and abdomen. Also tones the pancreas, liver, gallbladder, duodenal area, colon, and the entire area of the first three chakras.

➤ *Caution:* Your flexibility will only allow you to lift your body up to a certain point in locust pose. Find that point and work there, but don't try to force your body beyond it or you could injure your back.

This first locust pose is difficult for people who aren't used to working their back muscles, but it is the easiest of the locust poses and a good place to begin building strength in preparation for the more challenging variations. In this pose, you'll lift your head and chest off the floor.

➤ After sphinx pose, bring the legs and arms back down, then slide the hands back next to the hips, palms facing downward, fingers pointing behind you.

➤ Set your forehead on the floor and stretch your legs out with toes pointed, feet and heels together.

➤ Inhale, press down on your palms, raise your head up, and raise your shoulders and chest up off the ground.

Locust head-chest raises pose is the most basic locust pose for building strength in the back.

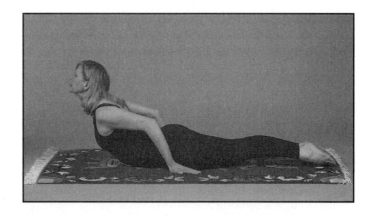

➤ Roll your shoulders back, leaving the top of your feet on the ground.

➤ Stretch your legs and the tops of your feet across the floor, rolling your heels together and squeezing your thighs and buns so you feel the front of the hips open as the back of the hips close.

➤ Roll your shoulder blades toward each other and feel your chest and heart opening.

➤ Exhale and bring your forehead to the mat.

➤ Repeat eight times.

You needn't lift your entire upper body off the ground in locust head-chest raises. Even if you can only raise your head off the ground, you will be building strength. Work within your body's limits.

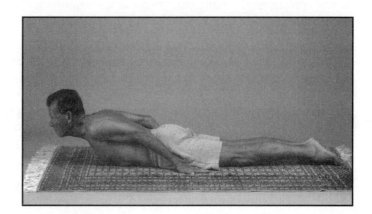

Locust Leg and Hip Raises

➤ *Difficulty Level:* III

➤ *Powers:* The lower back and gluteal muscles, stomach muscles, and pushes a lot of blood into the belly and all the lower glands and organs.

➤ *Caution:* Don't raise the body beyond the point your back will allow. Work your muscles to build strength, but don't cause yourself pain. You may only be able to lift your legs a few inches off the ground, and that's a fine place to start.

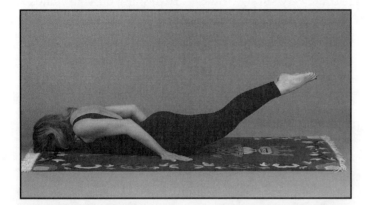

Locust leg raises work the lower back.

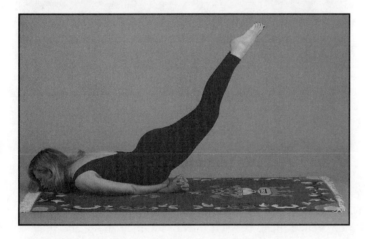

Locust hip raises take a lot of lower back strength.

The next step is to raise first the feet and eventually the hips off the ground.

➤ After locust head-chest raises, come back down and lie flat for a moment.

➤ Place your hands next to your hips again, but with a slightly greater bend in the elbow to get a little more pressure on the palms when you lift.

➤ Place your forehead on the mat. Some people like to do this with the chin on the mat. In either case, keep your forehead or chin pressed to the floor.

➤ Inhale and lift your legs off the ground.

➤ Exhale down.

➤ Variations: If at first you find it too difficult to lift your legs off the ground, begin by bending your knees and just lifting your feet off the ground. Soon you'll build enough strength to lift your legs, even if just a few inches off the ground. When you become very strong, you can try pushing on your hands and actually getting the hips all the way off the ground. This variation takes a lot of strength, so get very comfortable with the more basic locust poses first.

➤ Repeat eight times.

When raising the legs in locust leg raises, keep the knees slightly bent.

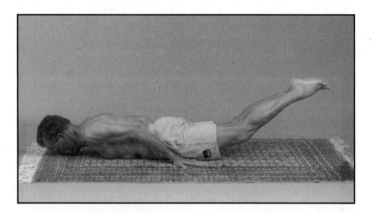

Geo's Journey

You've done locust poses before, whether you remember it or not! Every one of us did locust poses as babies. When babies lie on their bellies, they eventually get curious and want to see what is going on around them. They lift their heads, their chests, and their legs. Infants can do beautiful locust poses—and so can you.

Full Locust

➤ *Difficulty Level:* III

➤ *Powers:* The lower back and gluteal muscles, stomach muscles and chest; pushes a lot of blood into the belly and all the lower glands and organs.

➤ *Caution:* Work with head-chest raises and leg and hip raises until you have built a lot of back strength. Then, full locust will be relatively easy.

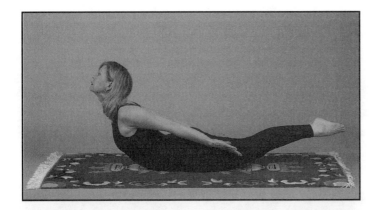

Full locust takes a lot of back strength, but regular practice can strengthen the back significantly.

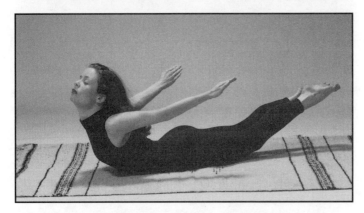

Full locust raises the arms, legs, and chest off the ground as if you were flying through the air.

This pose should make you feel a little like you are flying through the air.

➤ Return to a resting position on your belly, keeping your hands next to your hips.

➤ Inhale and raise your legs up, stretching the legs and squeezing the thighs and buns, as in locust leg raises.

➤ At the same time, raise your head and chest off the ground.

➤ Bring your hands up, palms facing downward and slightly outward so your shoulders roll open. Reach out through your fingertips. For an added shoulder stretch, turn your palms upward.

➤ Hold and breathe for 20 or 30 seconds, working up to about a minute.

➤ Exhale and come back down. Relax and feel how the pose is affecting your body.

Once you have gained a lot of back strength, you'll be able to raise your arms and legs high off the ground, leaving your belly as the only point of contact between you and the floor.

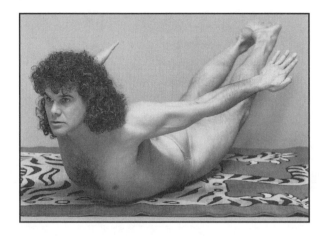

Bent Knee Locust

> ➤ *Difficulty Level:* III

> ➤ *Powers:* Just like locust pose, but with an added hamstring movement. This pose is very powerful in the lower back and gluteal muscles.

> ➤ *Caution:* Keep your feet pressed together to make the lift easier on your back muscles, which are probably fatigued by now.

Vary the locust by bending the knees for a slightly different muscle effort.

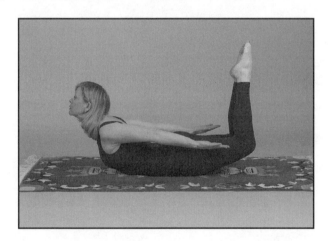

The next movement in locust pose is to bend the knees.

> ➤ From your stomach, bend your knees and bring your two big toes together.

> ➤ Set your hands by your sides, arms outstretched, palms facing down.

➤ Inhale and roll up, raising the head and hands off the ground.

➤ Using the muscles of the lower back and gluteal muscles, raise your knees off the ground an inch or two.

➤ Variation: Eventually, work toward keeping your knees, as well as your feet, pressed together in this pose.

➤ Hold for 20 to 30 seconds, working up to a minute.

The Right Moves

In both full locust and bent knee locust, keep your palms turned toward the floor. In some of the photos the model has her palms turned up. Once you are comfortable in this pose, rotating your palms upward gives your shoulders an extra stretch.

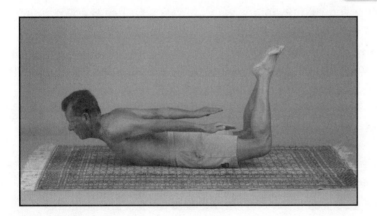

Bent knee locust can be adjusted for any fitness level. Begin by lifting your head and raising your knees just an inch or two off the ground.

Bow Pose

➤ *Difficulty Level:* III

➤ *Powers:* The structure of this pose drives a lot of blood into the belly, strengthening and nourishing all the glands and organs of the lower body; also a great strengthener for the back and opens the hips, thighs, knees, shoulders, chest, and heart. A great whole-body pose.

➤ *Caution:* Resist the temptation to rock back and forth when holding bow pose, for maximum effect in the belly and diaphragm.

In bow pose, the body forms a bow and the arms form the strings, so the arms should be held straight and taut through resistance with the feet.

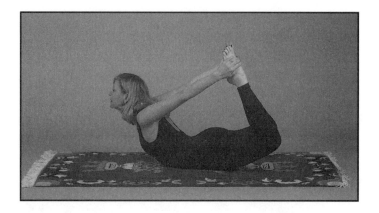

Move directly into bow pose from bent knee locust without coming down.

➤ After holding bent knee locust for 20 to 30 seconds, reach back and grab the feet. Later on, when you gain flexibility, you can walk your hands down your feet and grab your ankles.

➤ In bow pose, you want to make full use of your legs. As you hold your feet, push your feet away from your hips, pulling arms straight, opening the shoulders and lifting the hips off the ground.

➤ Keep your toes pointed toward the ceiling and arms straight. As you pull up higher and higher, your body will settle onto the belly and the diaphragm.

➤ Hold for 20 to 30 seconds, working up to a minute.

➤ Exhale and come down from bow pose, but keep hold of the feet, drawing the heels toward the buns for an extra quadriceps and knee stretch.

➤ Hold this stretch for 20 seconds, then slowly release the feet and come back down to the floor.

Bow pose opens the chest and heart while driving blood into the lower glands and organs.

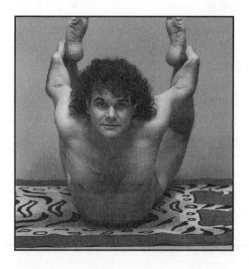

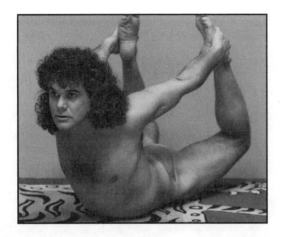

Keep the head up and the arms straight in bow pose, but resist the temptation to rock back and forth. Stay centered on the belly and pubic area.

Cobra

➤ *Difficulty Level:* III

➤ *Powers:* Strengthens the back and heart. Also powers the triceps, kidneys and adrenals; belly; strengthens thighs and buns; nice neck stretch affecting the thyroid and parathyroid, and releases pressure on the brain stem.

➤ *Caution:* Cobra is a great pose for the lower back, but don't strain it. You know you've gone too high if you feel pain or strain in the lower back.

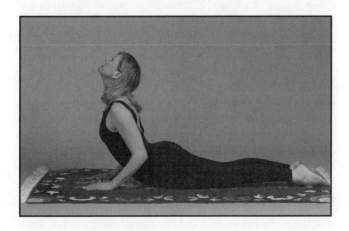

Cobra pose is like a more strenuous version of sphinx pose. The body is lifted higher and the muscles of the torso expend more effort to support the body.

Cobra pose is the final back strengthening pose before a well deserved counterpose. Similar to sphinx pose, cobra pose takes more effort and strength. The elbows come off the ground and the torso works to hold itself up.

➤ Place your hands next to the sides of your body, by the lower rib cage. Keep your elbows bent and in close to the body.

➤ Inhale and lift your upper body, keeping your elbows bent. Come up as high as you can, comfortably.

The Wrong Moves

When working on cobra pose, resist the temptation to let your shoulders come up around your ears. Try to keep your shoulders in their natural position, as if you were relaxing on the floor.

➤ At first, keep your feet apart. Later, when your back is stronger, you can press your feet, knees, and legs together in cobra pose.

➤ Keep your hips and pubic area on the ground as you roll the shoulders back and down into their natural sockets.

➤ Push down on your palms and pubic bone, stretching the stomach and lifting the chest and heart.

➤ Lay your head back and imagine you are a big, strong, powerful cobra, ready to strike.

➤ Exhale and lie back down.

➤ In the beginning, move in and out of this pose eight times. Eventually, hold the pose for 20 to 30 seconds, working up to a minute.

Cobra pose is an extremely powerful back strengthener when held for 20 to 30 seconds at a time.

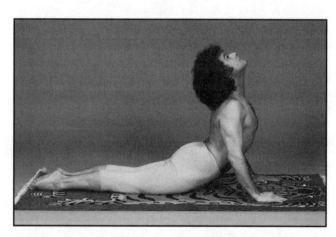

Yoga Mudra, American Style

➤ *Difficulty Level:* II

➤ *Powers:* Rests and balances the back; stimulates the organs of the lower abdomen; loosens the hips, thighs, and ankles.

➤ *Caution:* Keep your feet apart, making space for your body, until your knees are strong enough to support your weight.

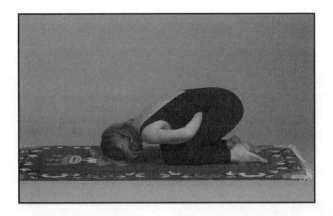

Yoga mudra, American style, serves as the perfect counterpose to back stretching poses by bending the back and pressing blood back out of the lower abdominal region.

Once again, every pose or pose series must have a counterpose, and by now, your back is more than ready to bend in the other direction.

The perfect pose to counter back strengthening poses like locust, bow, and cobra is yoga mudra, American style. This pose bends the back, relaxes the muscles, and has the added benefit of using the fists to compress the glands and organs of the lower abdomen, flushing out the blood that has collected there as a result of the exercises in this chapter, which lift the extremes of the body, encouraging blood flow to the center of the body.

Geo's Journey

Child's pose and yoga mudra pose have an additional benefit to your brain. As you rest your forehead on the floor, your head moves below the level of your heart. Suddenly the force of gravity compounds the force of your heart pumping blood to your brain. Your brain becomes flooded with blood, and all its accompanying oxygen and nutrients. What a boost for your brain! After child's pose and yoga mudra, you may notice you are thinking more clearly, or that your sensory perceptions are sharpened. That's because you've just charged your brain. This pose will also help you prepare for the inverted poses in the next chapter.

➤ After coming out of cobra, keep the hands by your sides and inhale, pushing your body back onto your bent knees, moving your hips back toward your heels as in Japanese sitting pose, but without sitting upright.

The Right Moves

Allow yourself to feel very comfortable and relaxed in yoga mudra, American style. Feel all your muscles relaxing and balancing. Let the tension drain away. You've had quite a workout, and your body needs and deserves a rest before you continue.

➤ Rest your forehead on the floor and feel the nice bend in your back. Keep your knees apart, making space for the weight of your body. Keep your hands resting at your sides. This is child's pose. Breathe here for at least 30 seconds, up to five minutes, letting your body relax.

➤ Now, raise your torso slightly, making room for your hands. Make your hands into fists and place them at the base of the lower abdomen so they are squeezed between your lower abdomen and upper thighs.

➤ Exhale, letting your fists help to expel the breath.

➤ Relax in this position for at least 30 seconds, up to 5 minutes ... or even 10 minutes!

Shoulderstands and inverted poses are the last poses in this book, so don't be in a hurry to get up out of your restful, rejuvenating yoga mudra pose. Rest up and get ready. The next chapter is tough, but you can do it!

The Least You Need to Know

➤ Many people suffer from back pain, but building back strength can eliminate the pain.

➤ Warm up the back with swimming pose and sphinx pose.

➤ The locust series strengthens the entire back and drives blood into the lower abdomen, flushing all the lower glands and organs with nutrients.

➤ Bow pose, sphinx pose, and cobra pose complete the back series.

➤ Yoga mudra, American style is a great counterpose to back-strengthening exercises like locust and bow pose because it bends the back in the opposite direction and helps to press the collected blood back out of the lower glands and organs.

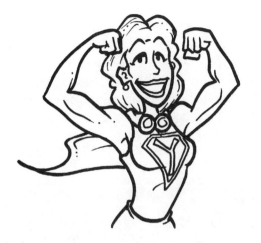

Super-Powered

This chapter and the next comprise the most challenging poses in this book. While most people should be able to do the first few poses (or variations of them), the poses in the second half of this chapter and in the following chapter take a lot of strength and balance. They are goals for the beginner, and challenges for the advanced. But once you can do them, they are great fun, incredibly strengthening, and give you a profound sense of achievement and confidence.

The poses in this chapter are inversions, which are very powerful. We spend most of our days upright and while our hearts have to supply blood to our brains, most of the body is below the heart, so it expends most of its energy pumping blood downward.

When you invert the body, however, suddenly the heart has to pump blood all the way *up* to the feet, making inversions strengthening for the heart. They also flood the head with blood through the force of gravity, giving the brain a great boost of oxygen and nutrients. Spend a little time inverted every day and your heart and brain will both benefit.

Add to that benefit the strength and balance required for some of the advanced inversions in the headstand series, and you've got yourself a Power Yoga routine truly worthy of the term "Power Yoga."

Yoga Rock 'n' Roll

➤ *Difficulty Level:* I

➤ *Powers:* Warms up and stretches the muscles of the lower and upper back and neck in preparation for shoulderstands.

➤ *Caution:* If you are very thin, you might need a pad or blanket to rock on, to take the pressure off your bones. If this bothers your back, stop.

The Right Moves

Yoga rock 'n' roll is like getting a massage. The floor and the weight of the body compress your back muscles. If your back is out of alignment, sometimes this movement will pop it right back in!

In shoulderstand, begin by warming up the body with a rocking motion. In this movement, the floor massages the back and neck, loosening the muscles in preparation for lifting the weight of the body.

➤ Lie on your back, then pull your knees up to your chest. Lift your head to your knees so your back is rounded like a rocking chair.

➤ Gently rock back and forth. As you roll forward, you'll feel the lower back stretch. As you roll back, you'll feel the neck and the upper body stretch.

➤ Continue for 30 seconds to one minute.

Shoulderstand Series

Shoulderstands are the most basic inverted poses. They stretch out the neck and loosen the shoulders as all the weight of the body is gradually centered over this area. Begin shoulderstands slowly, easing the body into the positions. Your neck probably isn't used to carrying all that weight. Your head only weighs about 15 pounds, but the rest of your body weighs a lot more.

Shoulderstand in Yoga Walks

➤ *Difficulty Level:* III

➤ *Powers:* The shoulders, neck, and abdominal muscles.

➤ *Caution:* Make sure your neck is warmed with yoga rock 'n' roll before swinging the weight of the body onto your neck and shoulders. People with detached retinas or very high blood pressure should avoid this pose. Also, shoulderstands and other reverse or inverted poses should generally be avoided during a woman's menstrual cycle.

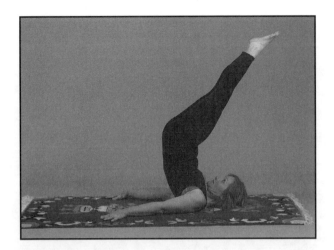

Shoulderstand in yoga walks is a good beginning inverted series pose because the body swings back and forth into a shoulderstand without holding the position.

In Chapter 19, "Tummy Series," I introduced you to yoga walks, and showed you the more advanced version, in which the body comes up onto the shoulders on each exhale. This is a good place to start the shoulderstand series.

➤ Relax the body after yoga rock 'n' roll. Keep your arms relaxed at your sides, palms down, legs extended.

➤ Inhale and reach over your head with your arms, pointing the toes, stretching out the fingers, breathing from the tips of the toes to the tips of the fingers.

➤ Exhale and bring your hands back to your sides, palms flat on the ground.

➤ At the same time, raise both legs and your hips off the floor, pushing the breath out as you roll up, supporting your body with your arms and hands by pressing them into the floor. As you get stronger, roll your back off the ground, too, so your shoulders, arms, and neck support your body on the upward motion.

➤ Inhale as you lower the body back down and raise the arms back overhead.

➤ Begin with five repetitions and work up to 50. From there you can move up to 100 repetitions.

Half Shoulderstand

➤ *Difficulty Level:* II

➤ *Powers:* The shoulders, neck, arms, abdominal, and gluteal muscles; this pose has a powerful effect on the sex glands and the back of the brain, and a secondary effect on the thyroid and parathyroid.

➤ *Caution:* Use the motion of your body to rock up into this pose rather than lifting straight up from a prone position, which could strain your back and neck.

Half shoulderstand puts less pressure on the shoulders and neck than full shoulderstand, and should be mastered first.

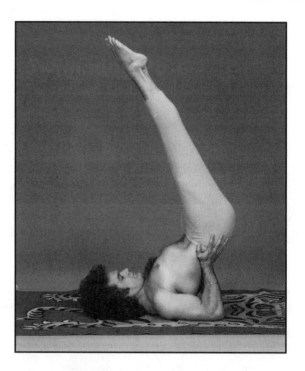

Geo's Journey

Half shoulderstand is one of the best inverted poses because it is easy enough for almost anyone to do, but it has all the benefits of the more difficult inversions. Reversing the body in half shoulderstand drops the blood pressure in your feet from 220 mg of mercury to about 20 mg in just 20 seconds, making this pose excellent for anyone suffering from varicose veins. Blood drops out of the legs and floods the hip area.

Now your shoulders and neck should be warm and limber. You are ready to begin holding the shoulderstand and reaping the full benefits of the inversion.

➤ On your final repetition of shoulderstand in yoga walks, as you rock up, bend your arms at the elbows and bring your hands up under your raised hips, supporting the hips with the hands.

➤ Point your toes toward the ceiling and center your weight over your hands and elbows. Feel the gentle stretch in the back of the neck. Your body should form a straight line from shoulder to hip, and then from hip to toe. Don't round the lower back.

➤ Hold the pose for 30 seconds to a minute, working up to five minutes.

➤ Variations: If you find it difficult to carry the weight of your hips, you can do this pose with your feet against a wall. Scoot up to a wall so your buns touch the base of the wall. Rest your extended legs against the wall as you relax on your back. Your body will form an L-shape. This is a great poseto hang out in for a while. Relax, breathe, meditate, and let the power of the inversion work for you!

The Wrong Moves

Half shoulderstand is a fairly easy pose, so your body should remain relaxed. If you feel tense and your neck is tight, ease the weight of your body forward over your hands and elbows. Your neck should be relaxed and should easily roll from side to side.

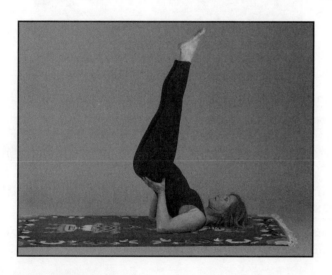

Half shoulderstand is an easy inversion giving you all the benefits of a full shoulderstand without the extra stretch in the neck.

Shoulderstand

➤ *Difficulty Level:* III

➤ *Powers:* Strong effect in the thyroid and parathyroid; nice stretch in the neck.

➤ *Caution:* This is shoulderstand pose, not "neck stand" or "neck-breaking" pose. Keep the weight primarily over the shoulders and don't strain the neck.

Shoulderstand brings the weight of the body over the shoulders, using the hands for steadiness only.

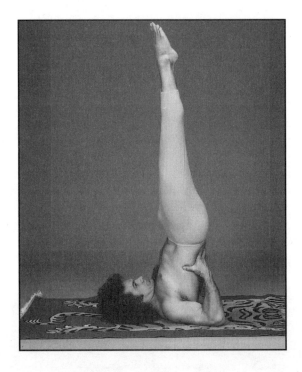

Like half shoulderstand, shoulderstand reverses the effects of gravity. In a short period of time, you get a lot of blood to the brain, which triggers the basal receptors on the side of the neck to lower your heart rate. This pose also gives a nice stretch to the medulla in the brainstem. Pressure tends to build up here because a lot of electrical energy travels through a narrow space. This pose helps to relieve that pressure.

You can come down from half shoulderstand, then back up into shoulderstand. Or, you can go right from half shoulderstand into shoulderstand.

➤ From half shoulderstand, push your hips and feet up over your head a little farther into shoulderstand. Feel the weight shift off your hands and elbows and onto your shoulders.

➤ Hold for 30 seconds to a minute, working up to five minutes in this position.

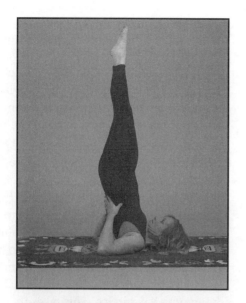

Don't worry if your body isn't absolutely straight. Your legs can come forward slightly to make the balance easier and to ease the strain on the neck.

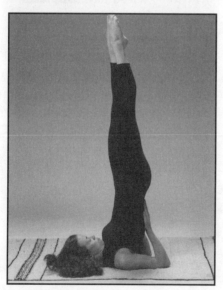

Point the toes in shoulder-stand for an extra stretch.

317

The Wrong Moves

This pose can be hard on the shoulders and neck, especially if you are new to the pose. Put a folded blanket under your shoulders to ease the pressure against the floor, keep the weight centered over the shoulders, not the neck, and don't worry if your legs aren't completely straight or exactly perpendicular to the floor. For most people, they won't be.

The Wrong Moves

When the neck is bearing weight, it should stay straight. You should be able to move your head a little in shoulderstand and plough poses and not be absolutely rigid. However, don't move your head around too much. Keep everything in line.

Plough Pose

➤ *Difficulty Level:* IV

➤ *Powers:* Powerful effect in the thyroid and parathyroid; good effect in the sex glands, the entire spine stretched and toned from the lower back right up through the top of the head; good stretch in the medulla and the brain stem; lots of blood to the brain; lowers heart rate.

➤ *Caution:* You don't want to keep reaching with your legs trying to touch the floor, stretching your neck beyond where it is ready to stretch. Find a place where you are comfortable and can hold this pose. It's a good idea, again, to have a blanket under the shoulders to lift them a little higher than they would normally be if you were lying on a flat surface. This takes the pressure off your neck.

Move into plough pose directly from shoulderstand.

➤ From shoulderstand, keeping your legs straight, slowly let your feet drop toward the floor, as far as they will go comfortably.

➤ Don't push your feet toward the ground. Let gravity pull them. If you can't reach the ground, don't worry about it.

➤ Hold for 30 seconds to a minute.

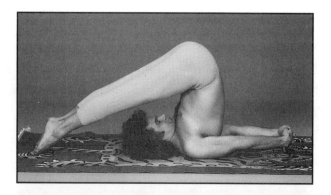

Plough pose imitates a plough sitting in a field and gives your neck, back, and shoulders a great stretch, too.

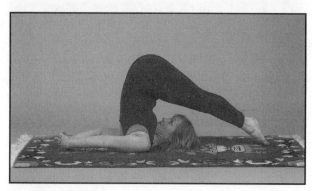

The goal in plough pose is to touch your toes to the ground. Don't worry if you can't get there yet. Flexibility like this takes some practice.

Ear Closing Pose

➤ *Difficulty Level:* IV

➤ *Powers:* Same as plough pose, but even more intense.

➤ *Caution:* This pose requires a lot of flexibility. Make sure you feel strong and comfortable in plough pose before adding an even greater stretch to the back and neck.

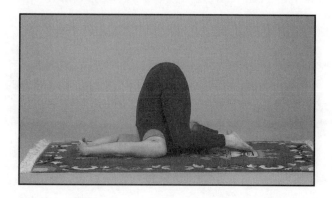

Ear closing pose is a more extreme variation of plough pose, in which the legs are bent and the entire lower leg from knee to toe rests on the ground.

319

The next step from plough pose is to bring the knees to the ground.

➤ From plough pose, slowly bend the knees and drop them by your ears.

➤ Let your entire shin, from knee to foot, rest on the ground. Keep your toes pointed behind you.

➤ Hold for 30 seconds to one minute.

➤ You can come down in two ways:

First, you can keep the knees bent and roll back down onto the back into yoga rock 'n' roll, stretching and massaging the back with gentle rocking. Keep your knees bent and your chin to your chest.

Or, you can straighten your legs back into plough pose, then roll your hips down slowly toward the ground, keeping your feet hanging over your head with just a slight bend in the knees. Put your hands at your sides to help control the lowering of the hips. Let your hips come down one vertebra at a time. Don't bend the knees too much or the weight will pull you down too quickly. Roll all the way back down and look behind you as you come down so that your upper back and neck arch slightly, until you are lying on your back once again.

Fish Pose

➤ *Difficulty Level:* III

➤ *Powers:* Opens the throat, neck, chest and belly; lifts the chest above the head and allows the heart to pump downward into the brain, lowering the heart rate; opens and charges the heart; strengthens the back and neck; great for people starting to get a double chin; brings a lot of blood into the face, revitalizing the complexion and hair. A wonderful all-around pose.

➤ *Caution:* Rest your head back gently so you don't force your body weight onto your head, injuring your neck. Use a pad or towel under your head if you find the position too uncomfortable, but really try to keep the weight off the head.

Fish pose balances shoulderstands by moving the spine and neck into an arch.

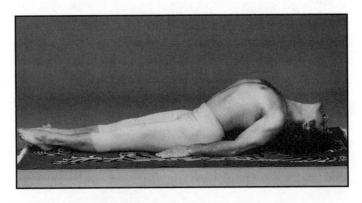

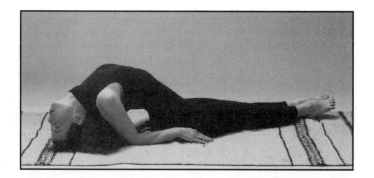

Fish pose with hands at the sides increases the stretch in the spine.

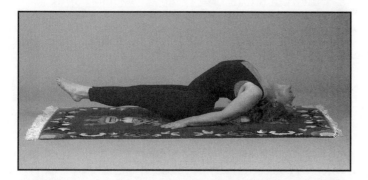

Fish pose with raised legs adds a stomach-strengthening component to fish pose.

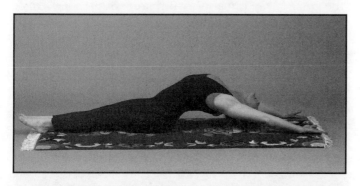

Fish pose with arms raised above the head adds energy and a shoulder stretch to the position.

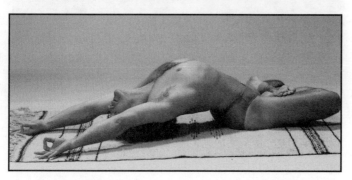

Fish pose in lotus position is an excellent full-body stretch, especially when the arms are brought overhead and the hands are held in Om mudra.

Power Words

A **mudra** is a hand position typically held during meditation or during certain yoga poses. The point of the mudra is to keep energy from escaping through the fingertips by closing the fingertips into a circuit, redirecting energy back into the body. **Om mudra** brings the tips of the thumb and first finger together into a circle.

The counterpose to all of the shoulderstand poses is fish pose. After bending your back and neck dramatically, both are ready for a nice arch.

I love fish pose, which was named after the Hindu god Vishnu. Supposedly, some yogis actually float down the Ganges River in this position, meditating. We all did this pose as babies, pushing our head back to start strengthening those muscles, lifting the chest and looking around at the world upside-down. High school wrestlers do this a lot, too, to strengthen their necks so they can lift their opponents and avoid getting pinned.

➤ Lie on your back with your hands at your side, after coming down from ear closing pose.

➤ Reach underneath your hips and lift yourself up onto your elbows with your legs on the ground. Lift the chest and lay the head back so the top of the head touches the floor.

➤ Variations: Try fish pose with the hands at the sides instead of under the hips, for an added stretch. Once you feel strong in fish pose, try raising your extended legs a few inches off the ground. You can also try fish pose with the legs crossed, or in lotus position, crossed with each foot lying on top of the opposite thigh.

Fish pose can be simple for beginners, or a highly advanced pose for those whose flexibility allows for variations.

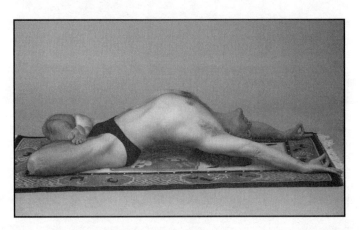

➤ Come down out of fish pose by slowly flattening the back against the floor and sliding the top of the head off the floor, to rest on the back of the head again. If necessary, move the arms back to the sides and extend the legs again.

Geo's Journey

Just as Mother always said, "Eat your fish; it's brain food." I say, "Do your fish pose; it's brain food!" Fish pose has a powerful effect on the brain, flooding your head with blood as you raise the heart above the head. The effect is so strong that when you come out of fish pose, you may feel a wave moving across your entire body. You are feeling the blood equalizing, moving back down out of your head.

Hand Balance Series

The next two poses are modified handstands. They look impressive and take a lot of strength and balance, but may not be quite as difficult as you think. Once you are strong enough, give them a try. They're a lot of fun!

Crow Pose

➤ *Difficulty Level:* IV

➤ *Powers:* Great for strengthening the wrists. Crow is almost an inversion, and encourages blood flow to the upper body, shoulders, and chest, as well as to the wrists and arms. The balance part of this exercise also hones focus and concentration.

➤ *Caution:* Don't try this pose until you've gained a lot of arm strength and have warmed up your wrists.

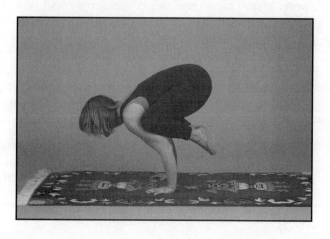

Crow pose is a difficult balance pose that women often believe they can't do. Barbara proves otherwise!

Crow pose is a difficult beginning handstand that takes arm strength. The key in this pose is to get the knees up high enough.

➤ After finishing fish pose, roll over on your stomach, then get up on your hands and knees.

➤ Place your palms on the floor under your shoulders, about shoulder-width apart.

➤ Slowly shift your weight over your hands so your elbows and chest are above your hands, your shoulders and head in front of your hands.

➤ Now, one knee at a time, bring your knees up to rest on the backs of your arms, high up by the shoulder joint. Try to get your hips up high enough that the weight of your body is centered over your hands.

➤ Keep your head up and focus on a spot on the floor in front of you.

➤ Hold for between one and five breaths—or as long as you can at first, which may be for less than one breath.

➤ Come back down onto hands and knees.

Peacock Pose

➤ *Difficulty Level:* V

➤ *Powers:* Strengthens the wrists, arms, and entire abdominal area; benefits the heart and lungs because of the physical effort involved; improves concentration.

➤ *Caution:* A very difficult pose. Master crow pose first. Women may find peacock pose particularly challenging, due to a lower center of gravity. For this reason, the lotus version of this pose may be easier for women.

Peacock pose is named for the snake-eating peacock, which can digest snake venom without harming itself. In this pose, the elbows push into both the ascending and descending colon on the right and left sides, forcing blood, especially with the lotus position variation, down into the colon.

➤ Spread the fingers on the floor, hands about shoulder-width apart, palms raised off the floor. At first, fingers can point to the sides, but eventually they should point back toward the feet. You can also do this pose on the fingertips with the palms off the ground.

➤ Bend the elbows and ease the body forward so the arms anchor the chest and the legs extend straight out behind the body.

➤ Keep the head straight and look directly down at the floor. If the head drops, you'll tip forward.

➤ The weight must be centered over the hands or the balance won't work. Each person must experiment with his or her own individual center of gravity to find the balance.

➤ Variations: Get into lotus position first, crossing the legs and placing each foot on top of the opposite thigh. Then, come up onto your knees and ease into peacock pose.

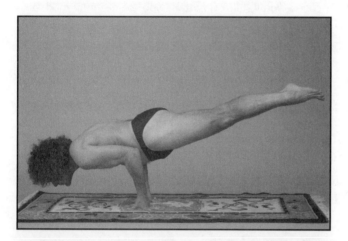

Peacock pose is a highly challenging balance pose that is easier for men than for women because men have a higher center of gravity.

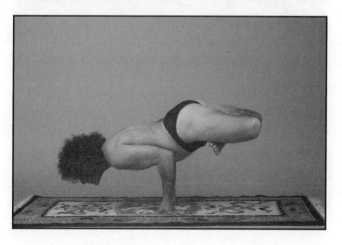

Peacock with lotus pose brings more of the weight toward the center of the body, so balancing is easier, although getting into the pose can be tough for those without adequate flexibility.

Geo's Journey

You may have heard stories about the incredible feats of yogis. One is that they can eat poison and survive. Maybe they do peacock pose because it drives blood into the belly, encouraging digestion and elimination. These days, you probably won't encounter real poison, but you may encounter fast-food hamburgers, deep-fat-fried food, processed food, and sugar, sugar, sugar. Your system will process that food better with a little help from peacock with lotus. Of course, you'll still feel better if you eat healthier food, peacock pose or no peacock pose!

The Least You Need to Know

➤ Always warm up the shoulders and neck before performing shoulderstands. Rocking on the spine with yoga rock 'n' roll is one good way to do this.

➤ Shoulderstands can be relatively easy and can function as a transition movement to go into and out of from yoga walks, or a half shoulderstand held for only a short period.

➤ Shoulderstands can also be advanced, such as in full shoulderstand, plough, and ear closing pose.

➤ Always balance shoulderstands with a good counterpose like fish pose.

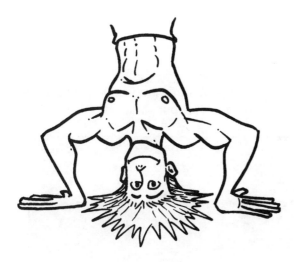

Chapter 23

Making Headway with Headstands

In This Chapter

➤ Headstands for strong necks

➤ Warming up with child's pose and camel pose

➤ Working into the headstand

➤ Uplifting headstand variations

➤ Coming down

The final series of balancing inversions is the headstand series. Headstands have all the benefits of inverted poses, but require an extra degree of neck strength. The neck and spine are supporting the weight of the body, so they must be strong, flexible, and well prepared. These poses aren't near the end of the book by coincidence!

In all the inverted poses, we see a reversal of the effects of gravity on the body. These poses are powerful for the heart because they teach it to pump uphill, against gravity. Headstands are great for your joints because they take the pressure off them and send all the blood to the brain.

Whenever you bring blood to the brain, you activate the basal receptor, that wonderful little thermostat on the right side of the neck that slows the heart rate. One of the ways to calm yourself when you are feeling anxious is to do an upside-down pose because after a few moments, the heart rate will actually slow down.

But first, let's warm up that spine.

Camel Pose

➤ *Difficulty Level:* II

➤ *Powers:* Opens the stomach and arches the spine in preparation for headstands.

➤ *Caution:* Lower yourself back slowly until you find your feet. If you miss your feet and fall back to the floor, you could injure your back.

Camel pose is a great counterpose for crunches and a good warm-up for headstand work.

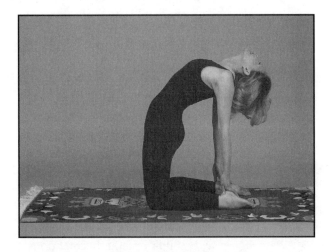

The Right Moves

If you do headstands as a final part of your workout, your body should be pretty warm. If you do them at the beginning of your workout, make sure you warm up your spine and neck sufficiently. Your neck will hold a lot of weight in these poses, so don't try them cold or you could sideline yourself for weeks.

Camel pose is a good counterpose for crunch-type stomach exercises, but I put it here because it also helps to prepare the spine for headstands, and is a counterpose for headstands.

➤ After finishing peacock, come back onto the hands and knees, then up onto knees with the top of the feet flat on the ground. Keep your knees about hip distance apart.

➤ Inhale and press the hips forward so they line up with the knees.

➤ At the same time, lay the head back and lift the chest to open the heart. Roll the shoulders back and reach your hands back toward the feet. Grasp your heels if you can. If not, just keep reaching.

➤ Hold for one to five breaths, then raise your right and then left hand off your feet to come back up onto your knees.

➤ Now exhale into child's pose, rolling forward, sitting between your legs and bringing your body to the floor, face down, arms extended.

➤ Repeat this movement, which is like a more advanced version of worship to the supreme, a few times until your spine feels limber and warm.

Geo's Journey

In the beginning, many people find it frightening to lay their head back because they aren't too sure about the strength of their neck muscles. In addition, laying the head back actually alters the brain chemistry slightly and you may experience the feeling that you are going to fall over on your head. This is a very vulnerable position, opening heart and neck, but when you let it go, your head will actually rest safely over the shoulder muscles. You'll soon get used to this pose and be able to let your head and neck hang back comfortably.

Half Headstand

➤ *Difficulty Level:* III

➤ *Powers:* Floods the head with blood; strengthens the arms, neck, and shoulders.

➤ *Caution:* Although a beginning headstand does not require as much balance, this pose can still be hard on the neck, so make sure your hands help to support the head in the right position, with the flat part of the head between the crown and forehead against the ground.

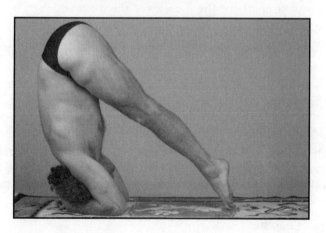

Half headstand is the first headstand pose, acclimating the body to the position without requiring a difficult balance.

The half headstand warms up the neck and spine and prepares the body for the more challenging headstand. In both the half headstand and headstand, the elbows should be just close enough to grasp each elbow with the opposite hand, forming a triangle with the head, to balance upon. If the triangle gets too wide, the weight is unequally balanced on the head.

The Right Moves

For headstands, position is everything. You want to be on the spot in front of the crown of the head, between the crown and the hairline. This is the spot called the fontanel on a baby's head—the soft spot, where the brain plates haven't yet fused. It remains flat in adults and provides the perfect spot for a stable headstand.

➤ From child's pose, clasp your hands and bring them against your head, forming a tight U-shape around your head.

➤ Push forward with your legs, raising your hips in the air and rolling onto the top of your head. Settle into the flat place on your head between the forehead and the crown.

➤ Walk forward with your feet until you bring the hips over your head, and hold that pose with the toes or the feet on the ground until you feel as if you are getting half of the weight of the body over the head. Use your feet more for balance than for weight bearing.

➤ Keep your hands firmly against your head for support.

➤ Breathe and hold for about 30 seconds to a minute.

Full Headstand

➤ *Difficulty Level:* IV

➤ *Powers:* All the powers of the inverted poses with an extra strengthening of the arms, neck, and spine; also strengthens the muscles of the torso and legs, which are used to keep the body balanced.

➤ *Caution:* If this pose hurts your head, try it on a mat or blanket. A pillow could be too thick to balance properly.

Headstands look impressive and are even something of a cliché when it comes to yoga. People tend to envision yogis either in full lotus poses (see Chapter 26, "Meditation for Your Life") or holding the headstand for hours on end.

I won't ask you to hold the headstand for hours. In fact, even five minutes in a headstand is a long time. At first, you need only stay up for a breath or two. Even half a breath is a good beginning. If you've followed the Power Yoga program throughout this book, I suspect you'll find the full headstand isn't as difficult as you might have imagined.

Move into full headstand from half headstand.

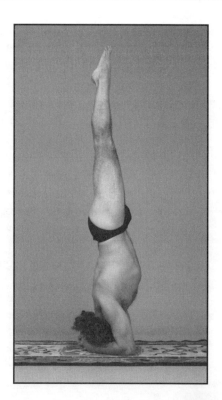

Full headstand takes a strong neck and good balance, but may not be as difficult as you think.

Geo's Journey

Headstand is not a pose to stay in for 10 or 15 minutes, like people seem to think they're supposed to do. Especially in the beginning, you should be working in headstand, not just hanging out and letting the pressure build up in the brain. Five minutes is a long headstand. I've seen people do it for 30 minutes, and I've done it myself, but that takes a lot of practice. You can get the same benefits holding the pose for a minute or two.

➤ From half headstand, bend your knees and bring them in to your chest, then raise your legs straight up. If you are very strong and confident in the headstand, you can raise them straight up from half headstand without bending them first, but this is more challenging.

➤ Make sure you are centered over the strong spot on your head, in front of the crown.

331

➤ Continue to use your arms to stabilize the head and the muscles of the torso to stabilize the body. Imagine you are hanging from the sky by the tips of your toes, so that balance is unnecessary. Let your body lighten as you visualize the sensation of hanging.

➤ Feel the weight evenly distributed between the elbows, across the forearms, and on the head, not just on the neck. As you reach up with the toes, feel the knees open, the ankles open, the spine opening and stretching. You don't want to feel compression here. If you feel compression, you aren't lifting enough and you may not be strong enough for this pose yet. Continue to visualize hanging from the toes. You'd be surprised how much this helps adjust your position!

The Wrong Moves

If you get too far back onto the crown or high spot on the head, you'll create too much of a bend in the neck. If you get too far for-ward, toward the front or top of the forehead, you'll create too much of an arch in the neck. In any pose that puts pressure on the neck, keeping the neck very straight and neither too arched, nor too bent, is extremely important.

➤ Variation: If you find the balance of headstand difficult, try it against a wall for a while. You can work with the position of your body with-out falling. Then, when you feel confident enough, you can move away from the wall. In the beginning, you'll feel even more secure try-ing this pose in the corner, about eight inches out. This is a very safe way to hold this pose. Bend your knees rather than leaning into the wall so your neck stays straight and doesn't arch too much.

➤ Hold for 30 seconds up to five minutes, then come down either by bending your knees and bringing your legs into your chest, then extend-ing them down into half headstand, or by low-ering your legs straight down into half head-stand.

➤ Roll back into child's pose and hold for five breaths.

➤ Lift your torso back up into camel pose and hold for five breaths.

➤ Roll back into child's pose, back into half headstand, then back into full headstand in preparation for feathered peacock.

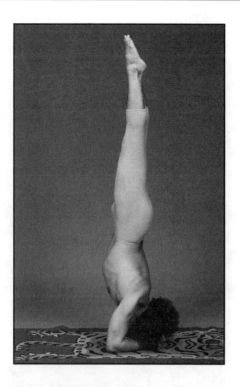

If your head is uncomfortable on the floor, try headstand on a mat or blanket.

Feathered Peacock

➤ *Difficulty Level:* V

➤ *Powers:* A literally uplifting pose that opens the belly, strengthens the back and arms, and is excellent for focus and concentration.

➤ *Caution:* It takes a lot of strength, balance, and focus to lift from headstand into feathered peacock. You should feel very confident in headstand before attempting this pose.

Use visualization to help you move from headstand into feathered peacock.

➤ From headstand, unclasp your hands and bring them down to the floor, side by side, fingers separated and pointing forward, thumbs together. Find an equidistant triangular stance with elbows shoulder-width apart to hold the body.

The Wrong Moves

Your back will arch slightly in this pose, but be careful not to let it arch so much that you feel pressure in your spine. Just as in headstand, you should feel the back opening, not compressing. If you feel compression, pressure, or pain in the spine, you aren't doing the pose properly. Keep visualizing the feet being lifted. If you still feel pressure, come back down and wait until you are stronger to try this pose again.

➤ Remember how you were hanging from the sky by your toes? Reach up with the legs and imagine being pulled up from above. Draw your weight back onto your elbows and lift your head.

➤ Hold for a few breaths and work up to a minute. One minute is a goal you can work toward.

Feathered peacock is a beautiful and challenging balance inversion that lifts out of headstand.

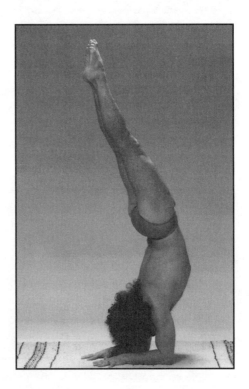

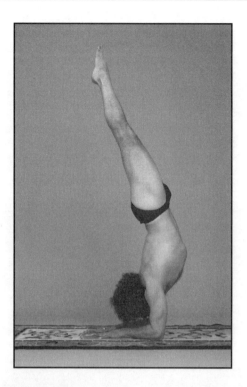

Feathered peacock is as mentally challenging as it is physically challenging. The mind must focus to maintain the lift and balance.

Scorpion Pose

➤ *Difficulty Level:* V

➤ *Powers:* All the powers of the inversion, plus opens the chest, heart, and belly, and puts a nice, deep stretch in the spine.

➤ *Caution:* You may have to shift, adjust and experiment in this pose to find the right balance, which is different than the balance required for feathered peacock.

Scorpion flows out of feathered peacock, dropping the feet over the head to evoke the shape of a scorpion.

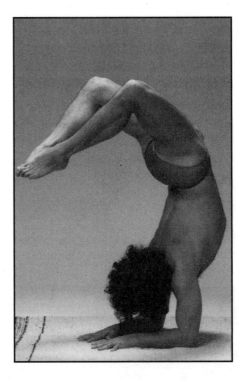

The scorpion pose has a similar effect as the feathered peacock except with scorpion pose, you drop the feet further over the head by bending the knees. Some lucky people have the flexibility to put their feet right on top of their heads. I like to reach out with my feet instead of moving them toward my head, creating a greater stretch in the stomach.

Remember, you should feel no pressure in the lower back, but instead a lifting and opening feeling.

➤ From feathered peacock, slowly bend your knees, keeping your toes together, and drop your feet back over your head.

➤ As you drop the feet back, maintain your balance by shifting your arms back, bringing your upper arm perpendicular to the floor. Center your weight over your straightened upper arm and shoulders so it falls mostly on the elbows, but is also supported by the forearms and over the hands.

➤ Hold for a few breaths and work up to a minute.

Geo's Journey

Believe it or not, scorpion pose really isn't that difficult to do once you find your balance. The head and the feet help to balance each other, and the lifting of the head helps to keep you from going over onto the feet. This pose actually serves as a good counterpose for headstand, and flows nicely into dolphin pose.

Dolphin Pose

➤ *Difficulty Level:* V

➤ *Powers:* Strengthens the back and the triceps; stretches the belly, feet and legs; sends blood to the brain and upper body.

➤ *Caution:* This balance is different from both feathered peacock and scorpion. Again, you'll have to shift and experiment to find it. Work carefully and be sure not to twist your neck or fall onto your chin.

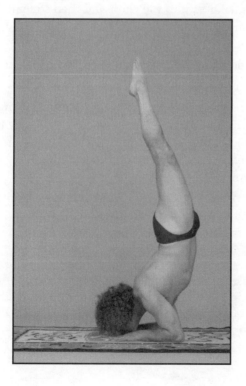

Dolphin pose flows from scorpion, bringing the forehead near the floor.

Dolphin pose flows from scorpion pose. The position looks like the pose some dolphins are trained to hold when they come up on the side of the pool and lift their tails into the air. A more helpful image, however, might be to imagine your feet as the head of the dolphin as it lifts out of the water to jump. Feel this same lifting feeling to help open the spine and lessen the pressure on the neck, as if you were sailing upward, feet first.

➤ From scorpion, slowly straighten the knees again and bring the legs up overhead, as in feathered peacock.

➤ At the same time, bend the elbows to create a deeper angle, shifting the upper body forward as the legs move backward.

➤ Gently drop your head and move your face forward onto the center of your hands where your thumbs touch. Your chin and forehead should be about an inch from the floor.

➤ Hold for a few breaths and work up to one minute.

➤ Now, return to headstand. Slowly roll your head until the strong flat part of your head touches the floor again.

➤ At the same time, shift your weight with the help of your legs to straighten your body above you. Hold for a few breaths.

➤ Now, drop the legs back into half headstand again, either by lowering your straight legs or by bringing the knees into the chest and then straightening the legs back to the half headstand position, feet touching the floor. Hold for a few breaths.

➤ Roll back down into child's pose and hold for a few breaths, up to a minute.

➤ Lift the body back into camel pose. Hold for a few breaths.

➤ Return to child's pose and remain here for up to five minutes, allowing your body to adjust and equalize after being inverted for so long. You may feel the blood slowly returning to your extremities, warming them. Let your muscles and your mind relax after the intense focusing workout. Breathe naturally and allow your breath to return to normal.

➤ As you lie in child's pose, begin to focus on the rise and fall of your breathing. Don't try to control it. Just be aware of it, in preparation for winding down our Power Yoga workout with some breathing exercises.

There you have it—the "workout" part of your Power Yoga workout, in full. But don't go jumping up and rushing off just yet. Warming down is at least as important as warming up, to reap the full physical and mental benefits of your workout. The next and last section of this book will take you through the final phases of the Power Yoga routine, the winding down.

The Least You Need to Know

➤ Headstands are powerful inversions that strengthen the neck and arms, send blood to the brain, and relieve the pressure on the joints and extremities of the upper body.

➤ Headstands help retrain the heart to pump blood *up* to the body.

➤ Warm up for headstands with child's pose and camel pose.

➤ Beginners can learn the headstand by first working in half headstand, and then trying headstand against a wall or in a corner.

➤ Once headstand is easy, try more advanced variations on the headstand that bring the body up onto the arms, including feathered peacock, scorpion, and dolphin.

➤ Warm down from headstands by returning to child's pose and camel pose.

Part 6

Winding Down

Time to come down, and you deserve it! We'll start with some breathwork, to build the breathing muscles and make the best use of the body's breathing mechanisms. Most people don't take full advantage of their lung capacity, and so aren't enjoying the full power and vitality of a body filled with life-force energy. I'll teach you how to breathe correctly, and give you some techniques for energizing or calming you, depending on what you need at any given moment.

Then, we'll come down to the floor and relax with some basic, easy, calming poses, to help the body re-establish its equilibrium.

Last of all, we'll talk about meditation. The original purpose of yoga exercises was to keep the body under control so it wouldn't interfere with meditation. Just five minutes of meditation each day can change your life. Try any or all of my favorite techniques described in the last chapter of this book.

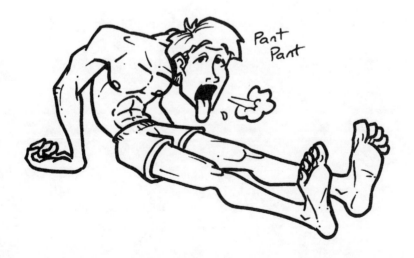

Pant
Pant

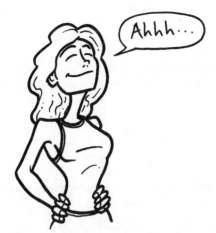

Chapter 24

Ahhh...

Breath of Life

In This Chapter

➤ How the breath works

➤ Know your lungs

➤ Infuse your body with life-force energy

➤ Breathing techniques

➤ Locks and retentions for concentrated energy

➤ Breath work and Power Yoga

I wouldn't consider any Power Yoga routine complete without a portion of the workout devoted to breathing. Breath is life, and learning to control the breath can bring you to amazing places, increasing your vitality, your energy, your health, even your attitude. So, while I've got you down on the ground after that vigorous Power Yoga workout, let's talk about breathing.

The Mechanics of Breathing

All day long, every time we inhale, our body arches and expands and makes space for the breath. Every time we exhale, the body collapses, compresses, and forces the breath out, and goes into a little forward bend. When it comes to breathing, our bodies are like big balloons.

Power Words

The **diaphragm** is the breathing muscle. It sits at the base of the rib cage between the right and the left side, protected by an armor-like skeleton.

Actually, we do have two balloon-like organs in our bodies: the lungs. The lungs fill up a large portion of your chest cavity, and they expand and contract with the breath, just like a balloon. With each inhalation, the large breathing muscle at the base of the chest cavity called the *diaphragm* pulls down, creating a vacuum that helps to draw air into the lungs.

The three lower ribs are the breathing ribs. They're designed to expand outward. The lungs are pear-shaped, so our bodies are made to expand at the bottom of the lungs first, as we inhale. As we exhale, the lower ribs roll back in and help the diaphragm push the air out of the bottom of the lungs.

These days, unfortunately, people have forgotten how to breathe. They have not forgotten how to breathe completely, of course, but how to breathe correctly. The lungs are pear-shaped, as I mentioned earlier, with the largest portions at the bottom. The average adult rarely utilizes the breathing muscles below the heart. Most people tend to carry and hold stress in the diaphragm and belly, which constricts the breathing and allows very little movement in the lower reaches of the lungs. This means that we're all breathing out of the smallest part of our lungs! That's certainly not efficient, nor healthy.

When I tell my students to take a deep breath, they'll often breathe in way up high in the chest for about three seconds, fill the upper part of the lungs, then exhale, puffing what little amount of air they could get in those three seconds back out. They think they're taking a deep breath. Any opera singer, or any singer who has had training, as well as people advanced in a yoga practice, know that breath is life and the bigger and deeper the breath, the more power we have for living.

Geo's Journey

We can go without food for months. I've seen people fast for 220 days taking in only lemon and water. We can go without water, depending on conditions, for a couple of weeks (only for a few days in very hot, dry conditions). But we can only live without air for a matter of minutes. Without the breath, we're gone, history, dead. Most of the energy, the life force, the nourishment our body needs to function comes not through the food we eat, but through the air we breathe. Each inhalation draws in new life and energy, each exhalation gets rid of what we don't need any longer.

Also notice that as the breath gets shallower, the *intercostal* muscles and lower ribs lose strength and flexibility because they aren't being used. If we don't use the intercostals, if we don't push the breath way down low into the lungs, the ribs won't expand and the intercostals can become dormant and stiff.

One of the first places in which new students experience soreness when starting a Power Yoga routine is in the intercostals, the muscles that expand and contract the ribs. Side stretches and triangle poses stretch the intercostals and muscles along the side of the body. So many people are locked up on the side of their bodies, continuously breathing more and more shallowly, getting less energy and less oxygen to the brain. Although people live longer due to modern science and medicine, many people exist in a daze. They just aren't getting enough oxygen to the outer reaches of the brain and body.

Power Words

The **intercostals** are the muscles between the ribs that help expand and contract the ribs when we breathe. The lungs expand and contract in two ways: by the downward and upward movement of the diaphragm, which lengthens and shortens the chest cavity; and by the elevation and depression of the ribs, which increase and decrease the diameter of the chest cavity.

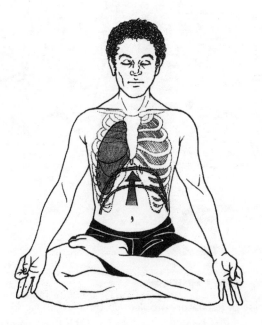

The lungs, ribs, intercostal muscles, and diaphragm muscle all work together on the inhale and exhale.

Breathing and the Body

If your lungs are like balloons, they aren't like empty balloons. They are filled with branched, broccoli-like structures called bronchioles ending in air sacs called alveoli. The alveoli have very thin tissue walls and are surrounded by capillaries. When blood enters the lungs through the capillaries from the heart, it has a high concentration of carbon dioxide. The air in the alveoli has a high concentration of oxygen. The body likes to equalize things, so carbon dioxide moves into the lungs and is exhaled, while oxygen moves into the blood and is carried back to the heart. It's an efficient system.

The heart and the lungs work together to remove carbon dioxide from the body and bring oxygen into the blood. Although you have little control over your heart, you have a lot of control over your breathing, so breath work is a great start for cleansing, clearing, and strengthening your body and your life-force.

The heart and lungs work together on each inhalation and exhalation. The diaphragm muscle helps move air into and out of the lungs. The alveoli facilitate the oxygenation of the blood and the removal of carbon dioxide.

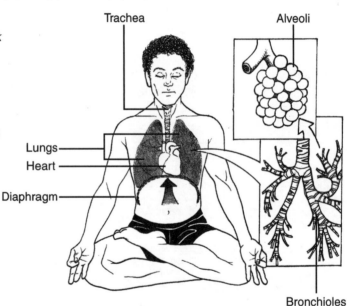

Trachea

Alveoli

Lungs

Heart

Diaphragm

Bronchioles

Geo's Journey

I suspect two causes for the increase of respiratory problems in the modern world: shallow breathing and pollution. But the reality of living in a polluted world is that complete breathing, especially complete exhalations, become imperative. We need to push that stuff out of the bottom of the lungs, to get rid of the pollution that, due to gravity and shallow breathing, will otherwise settle deep into our lungs and stay there.

One type of breath work is deep breathing, a way to re-train the body to get more out of each breath. It is the process of consciously manipulating this muscle activity to exaggerate the contractions of the internal intercostals and the diaphragm on the inhale, and to contract the external intercostal muscles and abdominal muscles, forcing the diaphragm back and up, and forcing air out of the lungs on the exhale. Deep breathing draws more air into the lungs and pushes more air out than normal breathing, so the effects of breathing are exaggerated, as well. More carbon dioxide is purged from the body and more oxygen is taken in.

Breathing brings in air, but it also brings in prana, the force of living I talked about back in Chapter 5, "A Word About Energy." If we can deepen, lengthen, expand the breath, take in more air and prana, then we're going to have more energy.

How do we do it? I don't just tell my students, "Breathe more deeply." That doesn't help. They might do it for 10 breaths then go right back to their old, shallow breathing habits. The tension of life and work encourage shallow breathing and constriction of the chest.

Better to re-train the body with new habits. The strong, dynamic movements of Power Yoga help stretch and open the body as we inhale, arch, and create space, then push out every bit of used breath with the exhale with such movements as forward bends.

> **The Right Moves**
>
> In yoga, the exhale is more important than the inhale. If we don't completely exhale, it's impossible to completely inhale because there is no space. The lungs are still filled with residual breath.

Your Spiritual Filtration System

When you maintain a diligent practice in breath work, in a very short time you'll find that all your bodily processes strengthen, and you'll also notice a not-so-subtle power developing inside you.

Breathing exercises teach your body to move and release the negative energies deep inside. Simply becoming more aware of your breathing helps the body move the way it was meant to move when breathing, without constriction and obstruction. Internal organs get compressed the way they are meant to be compressed.

Your body inherently knows the movements that are natural for it, and breath work helps your body to remember these movements, stirring up and rejuvenating the entire body. The whole body becomes activated and excited. Endorphins start pumping from the brain, and the body is infused with a wonderful sense of pleasure.

I interpret this sense of pleasure as a sign of great, glowing health. Unfortunately, many people don't experience this level of good health even though it isn't difficult to attain. It begins subtly, on the very first day you practice yoga. This glowing health can be yours. You can release this energy because it is innate to your body. If we breathe too shallowly over a long period of time, a lot of the residual life-force that's deep inside of us becomes dormant as well and, for some, is lost forever.

However, with a Power Yoga program, we start to stimulate and awaken all those different areas. It's amazing to watch the body come back to life.

Breathing and the Mind

The other important aspect of breathing is the way it affects the mind. If we go outside and walk up a big hill, we'll find that our breathing soon quickens, and if the hill is too steep for us, breathing and heart rate becomes very irregular and we have to stop.

The tension of climbing the hill causes irregular breathing, just as the tension and stress of everyday society causes irregular breathing, and may actually encourage people to breathe shallowly. Tension and stress may cause breathing to shorten, which in turn further stresses the mind and increases tension and stress. Fear causes a similar reaction.

If we slow the breathing down—if, for example, we go out and sit on a cliff and look out over the ocean—we'll notice that breathing becomes longer, quieter, and slower. Calm, tranquil environments have the opposite effect on breathing as fearful or stressful environments. Even what you think about can change your breathing.

The good news is, just as the mind affects breathing, breathing can affect the mind. Relieving stress isn't easy, and people try all sorts of methods. They go to psychologists on psychiatrists, they read books, they try to think themselves out of their stress. All these avenues can work, but they'll work better if you also change your breathing. Changing breathing is a clever way to sneak up on stress. A smooth, deepening breathing exercise will immediately have a calming affect on the mind. Slow, calm, and steady the mind by slowing, calming, and steadying the breathing.

I like to think that each of us is a special spirit that is reflecting into the world now as a unique rhythm. Our rhythm becomes affected by all the other rhythms around us, and the goal in yoga is for each of us to be ourselves, to move at the speed of our own rhythms. True power eventually manifests as we become more and more ourselves and are less and less affected by the rhythms of everyone else.

When we live in our own smooth, natural rhythm, we actually tend to affect the world around us in a more profound way. If we can slow down and lengthen the rhythm of our breathing, we're going to get closer to our natural rhythm. Everything in our bodies will work in a more natural way.

We are designed to be healthy. Every part of the body is meant to work and if it's not working, we have to look at what we are doing and how we are living. If something doesn't work for you, change it. If your breathing isn't enhancing your life, change it.

Geo's Journey

We're all searching for this thing called "enlightenment." An enlightened human being is a happy human being. A person who is happy, delighted to be right here in this world today, experiencing everything as a unique individual, is enlightened.

For centuries, yogis have worked to take advantage of the effect of breathing on the mind by creating breathing exercises. Some are simple counting exercises: for example, inhaling to a count of six, holding for a count of three, then exhaling for a count of six. An exercise this simple is a step toward learning to control your breathing.

Breath Watch

Before we get into the details of breathing exercises, I'd like you to simply try being aware of your breathing and the ways in which your body naturally moves with the intake and expelling of the breath. Power Yoga is built around the principle that the body moves in a certain way with the breathing.

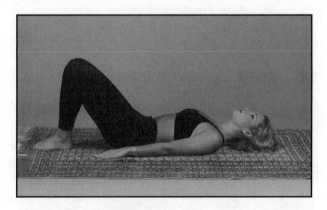

Relax on the floor with knees bent and pay attention to the way the breath moves the body with each inhalation and exhalation.

➤ Lie on your back with your knees bent, feet about hip distance apart, hands at your sides, palms down, shoulders back, focusing attention on the area of your diaphragm, just below the rib cage.

➤ Bring your attention to the natural fall and rise of the breath. See and feel how the body expands as you inhale. See and feel how the body naturally falls, compresses, and relaxes as you exhale.

➤ Don't try to control your breathing. Just watch the rise and fall, the natural flow and motion.

349

The Right Moves

Babies and animals know instinctively how to breathe correctly. Watch a baby inhale. His belly moves out and down with the inhale, the whole body expanding. As he exhales, his whole body collapses. So it is with any animal—next time your dog or cat is sleeping, watch it breathe.

When we ask people to breathe deeply, they try too hard to breathe. Trying too hard makes breathing incredibly difficult. We can't try to breathe. We were meant to breathe unconsciously, with our bodies taking care of this function for us. Just lie on your back and pay attention to the movement.

Now, move your awareness deeper into your body.

➤ Imagine breathing down into the base of the spine. When you breathe low, you press the breath down into the lower lungs, putting pressure on all the lower glands and organs, including the colon, stomach, intestinal tract, and liver. You also expand the breath.

➤ Once you've begun breathing more deeply, notice how your whole spine is involved in breathing. The spine or tailbone will naturally turn down with the inhale, activating the muscles of the lower back.

➤ As you exhale, notice the back collapsing and the sacrum tucking under as the stomach drops. The diaphragm will actually push up and under the rib cage to force the air out of the lungs, and as that happens, the back tends to round and the lower back tends to move toward the floor.

Pelvic Tilt

Remember the good old pelvic tilt? I use it in every class, and it is an important beginning pose for breath work because it is basic, essential, and one of the simplest ways to focus on the breath.

Inhale in pelvic tilt, expanding the front of the body and arching the back slightly.

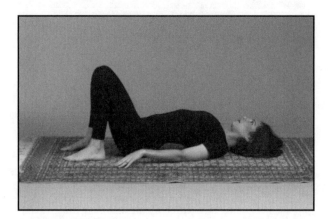

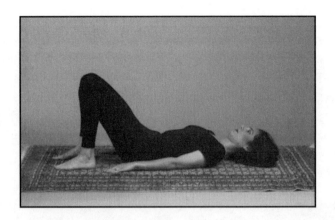

Exhale in pelvic tilt, collapsing the body and pressing the spine against the floor.

➤ Continue to breathe as you have been, but gradually, as you focus, begin to turn the tailbone down deliberately as you inhale, making more space for the air.

➤ Consciously turn the tailbone under, flattening against the floor as you exhale. Feel your back muscles working.

➤ Move back and forth with the breath in this movement for at least a minute, preferably longer, until you really have a feel for the way the breath moves the body.

Deep Complete Breath

This next exercise helps you to focus on a method of deep, complete breathing while lying down, letting the body move naturally, but making a conscious effort to work on pushing the breath out.

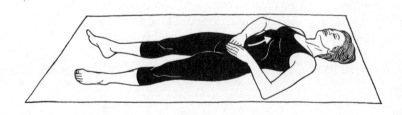

On the exhale, feel the diaphragm muscle push the breath up and out of the lower lungs. The deep, rhythmic breathing massages your body's glands and internal organs as you relax, while speeding fully oxygenated blood to each part of you. This will give you an energy boost when you've completed this exercise.

351

➤ Continue to breathe, but now focus all your attention on the exhalation. Don't worry about the inhalation. You need to push out all the old air to make space for the new. Do this by drawing the muscles of the stomach way up and under the rib cage as you exhale, literally pushing out every ounce of air.

➤ Stop for just a moment between the exhale and the inhale, and between the inhale and the exhale.

➤ Gradually lengthen each exhale, letting the breath out more and more gradually, with control.

➤ Continue for one to five minutes.

You can use deep complete breath while lying on the ground, but you can also try it in any yoga pose to see how deeply you can breathe while working the body in different ways. Put yourself into different poses, stressful poses, then consciously slow the breath, lengthening as if nothing at all were happening.

Ultimately, you'll be able to take deep complete breath into your life. Instead of getting panicky when things get out of control, you'll be better able to focus.

Some years ago, I had a boating accident. A rope wrapped around my hand and tore off the ends of two of my fingers. It was a holiday and I had to wait for eight hours for a hand surgeon to show up and take skin off my wrist and make me some new fingers. Without the doctor there, they didn't want to give me anything for the pain, and being a hardheaded yogi, I didn't really want anything. But I can tell you that with all the nerve endings at the ends of the fingers, it was pretty painful.

I had to focus on my breathing to cope with the pain. I slowed my breath down, kept it smooth, regular, and deep. Soon I slipped into a light trance. I remember a guy walking by my little cubicle and saying to the nurse, "Give me whatever you gave that guy!"

When the doctor finally showed up, I was just as calm and composed as can be. I went through the operation and was told my fingers would take six months to heal. It took me seven weeks to get back to normal, and I attribute this largely to my work with breathing, my understanding of the body, and the perfection of the body and its ability to heal and take care of itself.

Ujiya Breath

In yoga, we call a deep, controlled breathing ujiya breath. Literally, the term means "chest breathing," which is interesting because most people breathe in the chest, while we want to breathe more deeply than that. The key to ujiya breath is actually the control of the breath as it comes in and out using the back of the throat.

To find the right spot, suck in some air through your mouth and feel where it hits the back of your throat. This is the spot you can use to control the inflow and outflow of breath. We don't have much conscious control over the movement of the lungs, or even of the diaphragm, but this spot in the throat we can consciously control.

➤ Compress the back of the throat, then inhale to create a hissing sound. Inhale slowly, controlling the air as it enters your lungs through this narrowed space in the throat.

➤ Exhale, keeping the throat compressed and continuing the hissing sound. Controlling the breath from this space in the throat is like letting the air out of a balloon by holding your fingers around the neck of the balloon and letting the air squeak out. You control the rate at which breath enters and escapes.

➤ Inhale again, drawing the breath through your compressed throat, and focus on that spot. Feel your breath entering your lungs. When your lungs are full, hold the air in for about a second.

➤ Exhale very slowly, hissing the breath out. After your lungs are empty, stop for a few seconds before inhaling again. Stopping the breath between the inhale and the exhale, and controlling its flow with the throat are important steps to gaining control over the flow of the breath.

➤ Breathe with ujiya breath for one to five minutes. This breathing exercise is very calming. Eventually, work this breathing method into your yoga postures.

Locks and Retentions

Some other yoga methods to be used in conjunction with breath work are locks and retentions. *Locks*, also called *bandhas* in yoga, are exercises that close off parts of the body, much the way you closed off your throat in ujiya breath to hold the breath in or out between the inhalations and exhalations. Locks are held in conjunction with the exhalation of the breath. They compress, isolate, and concentrate energy inward, into the chakras and the glands and organs. Imagine stopping up a stream. As the water continues to gather in one place, the stream gets deeper.

Locks are very powerful exercises for energizing and activating the body. Three main locks are common to yoga: the throat lock, the stomach lock, and the anal lock. The most important of the *bandhas* is stomach lock.

Retentions are the opposite of locks. Retentions are held in conjunction with the inhalation of the

Power Words

Locks, or **bandhas,** to use the Sanskrit term, are powerful exercises that concentrate energy in the chakras, glands, and organs by creating a vacuum at certain points in the body in conjunction with the exhalation of the breath. The three primary locks of yoga are the throat lock, stomach lock, and anal lock. **Retentions** are the opposite of locks. These are held in conjunction with the inhalation of the breath, and press energy outward, through the chakras, glands, and organs, to flush and clear them.

breath, and they press energy outward. Imagine unblocking the dam in that stream we created with the lock and forcefully flushing the water down the stream bed. Retentions are more advanced and should be done with caution because they can raise blood pressure.

Stomach Lock

The stomach is an important area, and one where people tend to hold a lot of tension. The first three chakras are all down in this lower abdominal area, and the third chakra, located over the navel, is the place where we bring in energy and feel the physical sensations of emotion—the butterflies before a big event, for example.

Stomach lock concentrates the body's energy by blocking its flow to the stomach.

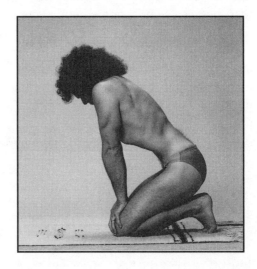

Emotionally sensitive people tend to protect this area, rolling forward when breathing to shield the third chakra from the influx of strong emotion. Because we're afraid of its power, we hold the third chakra in. When you start moving the belly and pushing the breath down as you inhale, this area begins to open up. The stomach lock, which involves sucking the stomach and diaphragm way up and under, has a powerful opening effect in that sensitive center and pushes the breath completely out.

People also have a tendency to hold in their stomachs for other reasons. Many people are self-conscious that their bellies are too big, even hanging over their belts! This kind of holding blocks the third chakra, too, but stomach lock will help to flood the third chakra with energy. Rather than stifling this important energy center, it floods the chakra with energy, opening and activating it. It will feel great!

The stomach lock creates a very powerful vacuum in the body that is especially wonderful for the heart, great for all the lower glands and organs, and fabulous for the lungs. The stomach lift puts pressure on the nerves on the inside of the spine, one of the very few ways we can get to these nerves.

Stomach lock may well be one of the best of all stomach exercises. All the glands and organs in the abdominal area—pancreas, liver, gall bladder—are affected. The diaphragm is strengthened immensely, so this is great for anyone with asthma or any other kind of lung problems.

The Wrong Moves

Stomach lock develops the stomach muscles, aids in elimination, and helps relieve constipation, but because it puts such compression on the stomach, it (and all yoga) should always be done on an empty stomach, at least two hours after a small meal, longer after a large meal.

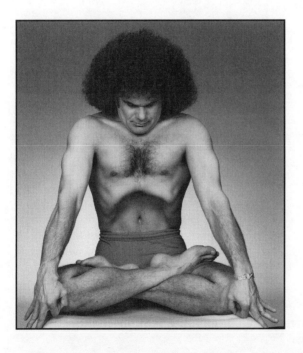

Stomach lock is a strong, powerful pose that compresses the energy in the chest and heart. This photo also shows the chin lock, which further concentrates energy in the chest.

➤ Sit up after deep complete breath and cross your legs. If you have the flexibility, put each foot on top of the opposite thigh in lotus position.

➤ Exhale fully, then stop the breath before inhaling.

➤ Suck your stomach way up under your rib cage. In order to do this, you have to get the breath all the way out. You can't suck in the stomach when you still have residual breath hanging out in the bottom of your lungs because the stomach and diaphragm won't fit under there if air is in the way. Pulling the stomach in can actually help you to exhale completely, expelling the last molecules of air.

➤ Hold this lock for a few seconds, then release.

➤ Inhale, letting the belly roll out and down, arching the spine slightly.

➤ Variation: Nauli is actually an extension of the stomach lock. After the lock is in place and the stomach and diaphragm are pulled far up under the ribs, Nauli isolates the rectus abdominus muscles, the muscles that run vertically from the top of the ribs down to the lower abdomen, along the center of your torso. Push these muscles outward using the concentrated energy of the stomach lock.

Nauli is an extension of stomach lock that pushes out the rectus abdominus muscles, isolating them from the stomach and diaphragm, which are pushed up under the rib cage.

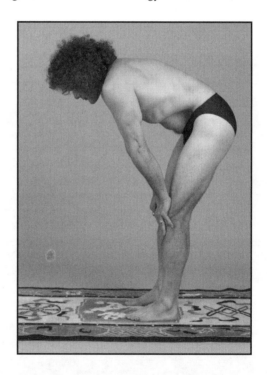

If you do nothing but pelvic tilts, deep breathing, and stomach lifts, you'll be practicing very powerful yoga.

Geo's Journey

You may have to work at stomach lift for a while to get the hang of it. Most people aren't used to exhaling fully, so first you have to learn what that feels like. When you think you've exhaled everything, give your lungs a little push with the belly and see if you can't "poof" some more breath out of your lungs. Then, get used to the feeling of sucking the stomach and diaphragm up under the rib cage. This motion actually massages the nerves of the spine and is one of the few ways to get to this area. After you've got it and repeated this lock for a while, you'll be amazed at the way your spine will open up and move more freely.

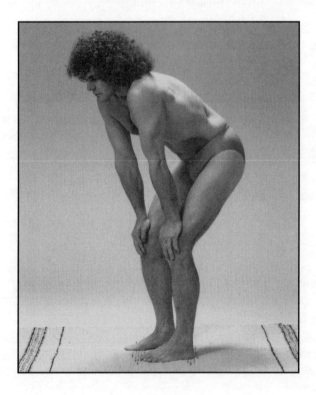

Stomach lock can also be performed from a standing position, with the hands on the knees for support.

Stomach Retentions

Retentions are the opposite of locks. Retentions push energy through the body, raise the blood pressure, and bring blood into the brain. They strengthen the heart and the brain, but are for the more advanced yogi.

The stomach retention is most powerful in the first chakra, located at the base of the spine. Yogis say the first three chakras are where we relate to the world. The sacrum is the center of our physical body, grounding us to the earth. Everything is affected by the hips, sacrum, and the first chakra. The sex glands lie in this area, and probably influence us in more ways than we understand. This area can also become blocked by our tendency to hold in our basic human nature. Stomach retention helps to push energy through this first chakra.

Start slowly with retentions, using little movements. You've got your whole life to do them, so don't try to do too much too fast.

The Wrong Moves

If you have high blood pressure, heart problems, a history of stroke, or a detached retina, skip the retentions.

➤ Release stomach lock and inhale fully. As you inhale, turn the sacrum sharply down, allowing the belly to roll down and out.

➤ After you've inhaled fully, hold the breath in as you keep the stomach pressed out.

➤ Feel the front of the body and the belly release while the muscles of the back activate.

➤ It takes muscle to turn the tailbone down. We start to activate and strengthen the lower back muscles in a very gentle, easy way with this retention.

➤ Hold the breath for a few seconds, then exhale slowly.

Breath of Fire

Now that we've calmed the body through deep breathing and activated the body's energy through locks and retentions, we can begin to energize ourselves again through breathing. Runners get high off this very breath, and you can use it whenever you need a boost of energy.

Yoga calls this breathing exercise breath of fire. It is a powerful exercise for the heart and the brain. It stimulates the heart, increasing blood pressure, blood flow, and heart rate. It also increases blood flow to the brain, releases *endorphins,* and stimulates the glands and organs of the head.

Breath of fire, also sometimes called charging breath, forces the exhale, while basically ignoring the inhale. Imagine the breathing sounds a runner makes when running down the street.

Breath of fire is one of the easiest and most powerful exercises there is. I have a friend with Parkinson's disease who has used this breathing technique to stay alive for several more years than he would have without it. It's a powerful breath, strengthening the abdominal muscles and all the muscles associated with breathing.

This technique pulls in the diaphragm to strengthen the abdominal muscles, pushing breath out with force, almost as if you had been hit in the stomach.

Power Words

Endorphins are a feel-good chemical released by the brain that relieves pain and induces a feeling of euphoria after physical exertion. Endorphins are chemically similar to morphine, but are a completely natural response by the brain to the body's needs. For example, they make physical exertion pleasurable, something that helps us to survive because we need to move and work to live.

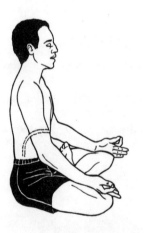
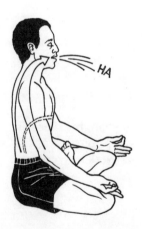

HA

Breath of fire is a deeply empowering breathing exercise. Do it for 10 to 15 minutes every day.

➤ Exhale quickly by pushing the breath out forcefully with the stomach muscles. You can make a breathy (not vocalized) "HA" sound as you force the breath out.

➤ Let go of the stomach muscles, and the air will naturally flow back in. Make no effort to inhale.

➤ Exhale again, forcefully pushing out the breath, then let go and allow the air to flow back in. Push breath out, release. Push breath out, release.

The Right Moves

Exhaling through the nose warms and builds heat in the body. Exhaling through the mouth releases heat from the body to create a cooling effect.

Repeat for a few minutes. The breathing is actually fairly fast, about one "HA" per second. This technique is an amazing pick-me-up. If you practice breath of fire for 10 to 15 minutes each day, you'll be in better shape than ever before.

Eventually, the goal is to incorporate breath work into your Power Yoga routine. You can directly affect your mind in two opposite ways during your Power Yoga routine by using breath work. Slow, calm, and relax the body by keeping the breathing slow, smooth, and regular; or activate the body by breathing with a quicker, more energized rhythm.

Breath work can be performed while sitting, lying down, or in any yoga posture, or with any yoga movement. Lengthening the breath will affect the performance of a Power Yoga movement or series in one way; quickening the breath will affect your performance in another. You can move in and out of postures with slow breaths, but take quick breaths while holding postures, or vice versa.

Begin experimenting with breath work in the following poses:

➤ Cobra

➤ Back stretching pose

➤ Alternate leg stretches

➤ Spear thrower and swordsman

➤ All the arching poses

The body is always moving and changing. Focusing on different breathing techniques takes mind control, which develops breath control, which develops everything in the body and being. Let breathwork work for you.

The Least You Need to Know

➤ The body naturally moves with the breath, expanding and arching with the inhalation, collapsing and bending with the exhalation.

➤ The diaphragm is the main breathing muscle that helps to pull air into the lungs and push air out of the lungs. Its effect can be exaggerated through deep breathing techniques.

➤ Breathing techniques help to regulate, control, and concentrate life-force energy in the body.

➤ Pelvic tilt, deep complete breath, and breathe of fire are breathing exercises to help master breath control.

➤ Locks and retentions help to manipulate and concentrate energy in the chakras.

➤ Breath work, in conjunction with a Power Yoga routine, will add immense power and energy to the body.

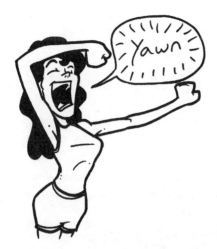

Chapter 25

Warm-Downs

In This Chapter

➤ You're busy; can you skip the warm-down?

➤ Maximum benefit for a minimum effort

➤ Working down to the floor

➤ A relaxation routine your body will love

You've worked hard, and you deserve a nice, relaxing warm-down. Your body requires a warm-down, too. You've bent, arched, stretched, and twisted your body, and now you need to regain your equilibrium.

Warm-downs help your body to adjust to what it has learned, equalize blood flow, regulate the breath rate and heart rate, and ease your mental processes back into the daily flow of life.

Warm-downs do more than just allow the body a gradual transition back into every-day life. They also ease the transition from a focus on the physical to a focus on the mental. In fact, the original purpose of yoga exercises was to keep the body healthy, strong, and under control so it won't interfere with meditation (the subject of the next and last chapter of this book).

After the last chapter's breathing exercises, you aren't coming straight out of vigor-ous physical poses, but breath work, which is hard work, too. Now it's time to slow things down. Relaxation is the key here. In a broader scheme, relaxation is the "counterpose" to a workout, so to keep everything in balance, don't skip this final portion of your Power Yoga routine.

Yoga Mudra, American Style

➤ *Difficulty Level:* II

➤ *Powers:* Relaxes and stretches the spine and neck; slows the heart rate; helps to align the spine; massages the colon and the glands and organs of the lower abdomen.

➤ *Caution:* This pose should be very relaxing. If you feel any strain, shift your position. Put a pillow between your feet to reduce the strain on your knees.

Yoga mudra, American style is an easy relaxation pose to hold for as long as you have time.

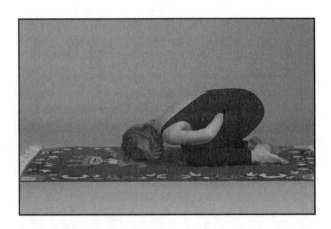

The Wrong Moves

If your fists are uncomfortable against your abdomen in yoga mudra, American style, don't feel bound to keep them there. Lay your hands at your sides or over your head. You won't get the same colon massage, but comfort is the primary concern in this pose. You should be able to stay in this pose for two to five minutes.

The best way to begin to warm down is with a nice, easy yoga mudra, American style. Unlike the standard yoga mudra (see the next section), you sit on or between your feet rather than with your legs crossed. This position makes the forward bend easier.

➤ You've probably either just finished your workout, ending with Chapter 23, "Making Headway with Headstands," in child's pose, or just completed breath work. In either case, you are probably down on the floor.

➤ From child's pose, raise your body and press your fists into your lower abdomen so they are sandwiched between your abdomen and the base of your thighs.

➤ Lean forward over your fists until your forehead rests on the floor.

➤ Hold for two to five minutes. Relax completely and breathe normally.

Yoga Mudra

➤ *Difficulty Level:* II–IV, depending on your sitting position

➤ *Powers:* Opens the spine; massages the lower glands and organs; relaxes the mind.

➤ *Caution:* Don't try this in the lotus pose unless you are comfortable in this position. Also, don't force your head to the ground or you could injure your lower back.

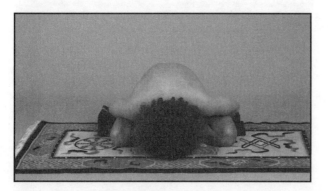

Yoga mudra is a very relaxed position that you should be able to hold comfortably for several minutes or longer.

The only difference between yoga mudra and its American counterpart is that in classic yoga mudra, you sit with the legs crossed and the arms at your sides.

➤ From yoga mudra, American style, raise your body and sit back onto the floor. Bring your legs out in front of you, then gently and slowly cross your legs into *perfect pose, half lotus,* or *lotus pose,* depending on which your flexibility allows. These poses are very stable sitting poses that encourage the body to sit back on the sitting bones rather than slumping forward. Don't worry if you can't get into lotus pose, which is too difficult for most people. Perfect pose is very comfortable.

The Power Words

Certain body positions are ideal for sitting comfortably on the floor. **Perfect pose** is a basic cross-legged pose that brings the heels in to the body. **Half lotus** takes more flexibility, bringing one foot on to the opposite thigh. **Lotus pose** is too difficult and uncomfortable for most people, but if you are flexible enough, it is a very secure, stable pose in which each foot lies on top of the opposite thigh.

365

Perfect pose is a basic cross-legged pose with the heels brought all the way in so they press against the body.

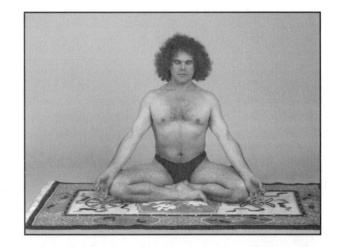

Half lotus is a cross-legged position in which one foot is brought onto the other thigh. Be sure to counter the pose by doing it both ways.

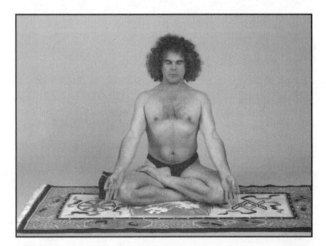

Lotus pose requires flexibility in the hips, but once mastered, it is a very stable and comfortable position.

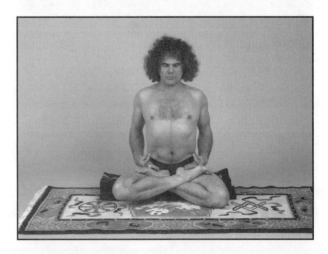

366

➤ Let your arms extend behind you on the floor and slowly lower your forehead back to the ground.

➤ Relax into the pose and breathe, letting all your muscles and joints release.

➤ Variations: How you place your legs and where you put your arms in yoga mudra is really a matter of choice. You can cross your legs but lean over your fists; you can sit on your legs but keep your arms to your side; you can sit between your legs and do the shoulder stretch described in the next exercise. Tailor yoga mudra to your personal preference and maximum comfort.

➤ Hold for five breaths, up to five minutes.

Geo's Journey

Lotus pose is a difficult pose that takes a lot of work to get the body to be able to hold comfortably. It is a beautiful, symmetrical pose, meant to evoke the beauty and symmetry of the lotus flower. If you can get to the point where you are comfortable in lotus pose, you'll find it a useful and very stable pose for relaxation and meditation, helping the body to stay easily upright and in the correct position.

Yoga Mudra with Shoulder Stretch

➤ *Difficulty Level:* II

➤ *Powers:* Powerful stretch in the upper shoulders, back, triceps, arms; drives blood into the brain from the extended arms; the heels massage the colon and pancreas; this is a good pose for people with diabetes.

➤ *Caution:* If you can't straighten your arms or raise them up in this pose, that's okay. Don't strain your shoulders. Instead, begin with the elbows bent and the arms lowered. Straighten and raise the arms just enough to feel a stretch.

*Inhale in yoga mudra
with shoulder stretch by
lifting the head up with
arms extended behind
you, fingers interlocked.*

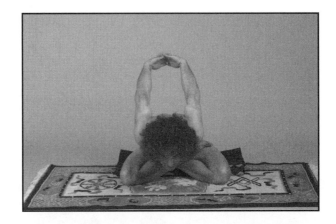

*Exhale in yoga mudra
with shoulder stretch by
lowering the forehead
to the floor with arms
extended behind you,
fingers interlocked.*

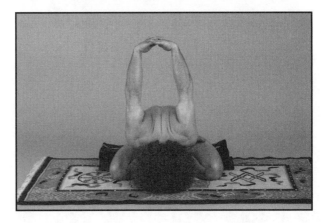

People tend to carry a lot of tension in their shoulders. Adding a nice, gentle shoulder stretch to yoga mudra helps that tension to flow out of the body.

➤ From yoga mudra, bring the hands together and interlock the fingers. Raise the arms, with elbows straight or almost straight, up behind your back.

➤ Inhale and raise your head to look in front of you, keeping the arms raised behind you. Your lower back will arch slightly as you raise the weight of your head.

➤ Exhale and lower your head back to the floor, keeping the arms high.

➤ Repeat for five full breaths, then release the hands and lower them back to your sides, returning to yoga mudra.

Relaxation Pose

➤ *Difficulty Level:* I

➤ *Powers:* Relaxes the entire body and mind, bringing both back into equilibrium after a vigorous workout or a stressful day.

➤ *Caution:* If you know you have somewhere to be after your workout, you might want to set your alarm. You wouldn't be the first person to fall asleep in this pose!

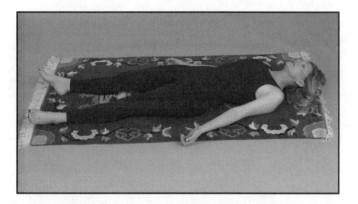

Relaxation pose is just like it sounds. The entire body relaxes into the floor.

Relaxation pose, called shavasana (literally, "corpse pose") in yoga, is an important pose for any workout. Without it, your body cannot benefit fully from the great physical exertion you've just made. Relaxation pose gives the body a chance to adjust to the work it has done, strengthening muscle tissue, relaxing the joints, and calming the mind.

Relaxation pose is easy on the heart because the heart doesn't have to work against gravity to pump blood to any part of the body. It is easy on the lungs because breathing slows. It allows the muscles to rest and best of all, it calms, slows, and eases the mind after the focused exertion necessary for a Power Yoga routine.

The Right Moves

Some people who have previously suffered from insomnia have found relief with relaxation pose. Although the goal isn't to fall asleep, relaxation pose can help nudge an overtired body and mind toward dreamland.

The following instructions are guidelines to help you get the most out of relaxation pose, but you'll defeat the purpose if, as you lie on the floor, you have to keep picking up this book. If you listen to my CD, *Geo's Power Yoga*, you'll find this pose described as follows. You can listen to the CD while you lie on the floor in the pose. (See Appendix C, "Study with Geo," for ordering instructions.)

Or, you can read the following section onto a cassette tape that you can play back for yourself while you do this pose. Even when you are familiar with the process, it's nice to have a voice directing you through the relaxation process. If you do make a tape of this section, read slowly with a soothing tone, and pause for five to 10 seconds between each bullet, so you'll have sufficient time to respond to—and relax to—the instructions.

➤ From yoga mudra, roll over onto your back. Separate your legs a comfortable distance. Bring your hands away from your body, palms facing up. Straighten the back of your neck. Relax your lower jaw.

➤ Now focus just below your rib cage on your diaphragm, your breathing center. See your body naturally expand from here as you inhale, taking in new life. Feel your body gently release, relax, and let go as you exhale, giving back to life.

➤ Relax and watch the rhythm of your breathing, the gentle rise and easy fall. See the body naturally expand, feel the body gently release and let go. Meditate on the breath, on the rhythm of your breath, the rise and the fall of your breath, like waves in the ocean of life. Follow the waves.

➤ Don't control your breathing. Just be aware of it. Watch it, almost as if you were watching someone else breathing. Rise, fall. Expand, release. Pay attention to the rhythm your breath falls into, your natural rhythm.

➤ Stay here, watching the breath, feeling the rhythmic waves of breath, feeling your own personal rhythm, for five minutes or more. Ten minutes is exquisite. (If you are taping these instructions, let five to 10 minutes of tape run at this point. Fill the space with relaxing music if you like.)

➤ As you watch your breathing, remember for a moment that you are special, blessed with your own wonderful spirit, like a snowflake with your own beautiful patterns of body and mind, blessed with life, to live in your own way.

➤ As you watch your breathing, remember that you are blessed.

➤ Now move your attention from your breathing down the body and into your feet. Be conscious of your toes and arches, the way your heels touch the ground. Internally, speak to the feet. Tell your feet to relax. Relax and let go.

➤ Focus just a bit higher on your calves now. Let your feet hang comfortably open and feel your calves relax. Relax.

➤ Move into your knees and the area behind your knees. Relax your knees. Tell your knees to relax and feel a warm wave move down your thighs and through your knees. Relax.

➤ Focus on your thighs, the biggest, strongest group of muscles in your body. They represent your strength. Now speak to your thighs and tell your thighs to relax and let go.

➤ Move into your hips, the center of your physical body. Let your legs hang comfortably open and tell your hips and legs to relax. From the waist down, feel as if you are just fading away. Let go. Relax.

➤ Focus on your stomach. Soften and relax your stomach from deep inside. Relax and let go.

➤ Move into your chest now and relax the outer shell of skin, the muscles, the bones. Let your armor drop away.

➤ Drop down into your lungs. Stop the breath a minute, then take little "barely breaths," barely inhales, then barely exhales, just what you need to stay alive. Let your lungs relax and be as still as they can possibly be. Barely breathe. Relax into stillness.

➤ Drop down deep into your heart, into the center of your being. From deep inside, tell your heart to relax and let go. Relax and let go of any hurt, any pain, any fear. With all that out of the way from deep inside, let go of any love you've held back. Feel your heart open and just let go. Relax.

➤ Move down your arms and into your hands and fingers, your palms, your thumbs. Tell your hands to let go. Let your forearms relax. Let your upper arms, biceps, and triceps relax. Relax your shoulders, feel them move softly away from each other.

➤ In your mind's eye, picture your spine. Now gently relax from the base of the spine to the base of the brain. Let your spine melt like butter, melting into the floor. Relax.

➤ As you move toward the top of the spine, relax your neck, the front of your neck, the back of your neck.

➤ Relax your lower jaw again. Just let it hang. Soften your lips.

➤ Relax your face now. Feel your skin go perfectly smooth. Relax all the muscles in and around your eyes. Soften your eyes.

➤ Relax your forehead, the top of your head, the back of your head.

➤ Now drop down into the center of your brain. Tell your brain to relax. Feel it drop into the back of your head. Relax and let go. Totally, completely. Just relax.

➤ For just a few moments now, think about someone you love, anyone at all, young or old, real or imaginary, alive or not. See them just the way you love them and see yourself with them doing the things you love to do. For just a little while, be with someone you love.

➤ May the light in your heart guide you always. From the unreal into the real, from darkness into light, from fear into love, guide you always into love.

➤ Slowly, gently, easily now, start to come back. Begin to feel the rise and fall of your breath again.

➤ When you feel you are ready, bring your feet together, stretch your arms over your head, stretch up from the waist, and feel good about your upper body.

➤ Stretch down from the waist and feel good about your lower body.

➤ Stretch out the right side, reaching the right arm out.

➤ Stretch out the left side, reaching the left arm out.

➤ Feel good about yourself all over, head to toe, inside and outside.

➤ Finally, bring your awareness back to the present moment. Open your eyes and gently roll up.

I hope you're feeling absolutely fabulous by now. You should be relaxed, calm but energized, content but joyful.

At this point, you may choose to continue on with your day. Or, you may choose to meditate. Meditation works at the end of a workout, although some people prefer it first thing in the morning, last thing at night, with the sunrise or sunset, or in the middle of a hectic day. Whatever works for you, great.

In the meantime, congratulations on finishing a spectacular workout from start to finish. You are already more powerful.

The Least You Need to Know

➤ Warming the body down after a workout is an important part of the workout and shouldn't be neglected.

➤ Warm-downs allow the body to regain its equilibrium and derive the maximum benefit from physical exertion.

➤ Begin the warm-down with forward bends, then sit on the floor for yoga mudra and yoga mudra with shoulder stretch.

➤ End with relaxation pose, to fully relax and calm the body and mind.

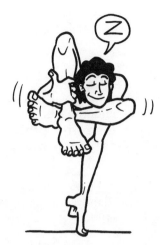
Meditation for Your Life

In This Chapter

➤ Meditation, the culmination

➤ How, when, and where to meditate

➤ Which form of meditation suits you?

➤ Move, breathe, relax, meditate, and know thyself

I have to start with a little story about meditation. I have this wonderful friend, Vince, who is a great yoga teacher. He's been teaching yoga for years. Some time ago, he went to India to study with a yogi to learn meditation. He'd read all the books on meditation and knew all about the different forms and systems.

When he got to India, he sat in front of the great yogi he had come to see and at one point, he raised his hand to ask a question. He said to the yogi, "What form of meditation do you find to be the best?" The yogi looked at him quizzically and said, "Form? Form? You sit, you meditate." He had no understanding of this concept at all.

We, in the Western world, tend to be overly rational about everything. We have to have rational explanations and categories for everything, but meditation is really a flow into that other side of the mind—not the rational mind, but the subconscious.

The more you meditate, the more you will begin to understand that non-rational side of the brain. You open the door to the subconscious mind and its rhythms, and peek inside. But most of us aren't yet as advanced as that great yogi in India. We do categorize. We do rationalize. So we do have to start working with meditation in a way we understand. "You meditate" isn't all that helpful for a beginner, especially someone from this culture, so let's think about meditation first in terms everyone understands.

You Already Meditate

We all go into meditative states at different times in our lives. Just like yoga, meditation is a natural part of being human. It probably comes out of our animal brain, from back when we were able to hibernate. During hard times with harsh weather and little food, being able to shut the body down for a while was a survival mechanism. Somewhere deep inside, we still have that ability.

And we use this ability all the time! Have you ever unconsciously shifted your gaze into a softer focus and let your mind float away for a minute or so until you snapped yourself back to reality? We all have. You see kids doing it all the time.

Do you get involved in your work, your play, your hobbies, or your art so that time passes so quickly, you can't believe a day is gone? You've been in a meditative state.

Tuning out the outside world isn't an outmoded skill. Our modern world almost demands it. We are so bombarded with stimuli that without it, we would go into overload. We wouldn't get anything done, and we certainly wouldn't get any satisfaction out of our activities. We need to recharge.

Geo's Journey

There are still yogis who can slow their heart rates down so much that you can't even tell they have a heartbeat. They can let their breath become so shallow you can barely detect it. This is a form of hibernation. Impressive, perhaps, but is such a skill really necessary, or just a novelty? Actually, tuning out the external world is a great survival skill to have in the present day. If we don't give our minds a rest from constant activity and intense stress and stimulation, they won't perform as well as they could, and may even break down.

But like everything else in the world today, we have to be reasonable in our approach. If you tell yourself you are going to meditate an hour a day, I'm guessing you probably won't do it, at least not for more than a couple of days. Who has the time? Or the patience? Besides, for a beginning meditator, an hour of meditation is pretty tough. But if you tell yourself you will meditate five to 15 minutes a day, you have a much more realistic goal, and one that would have an absolutely wonderful effect on your life.

The world is full of rhythms, and we are affected by all the rhythms in the world, from electronic devices to heavy machinery, cars, computers, voices, and the rhythms of the people around us. We're so over-stimulated by everything going on in this technologically sophisticated, often over-crowded information age that it becomes very difficult for anyone to actually sit still and relax, let alone meditate.

Just because it's difficult doesn't mean our bodies don't need it—quite the contrary. All the stimuli we are exposed to means we need meditation even more. It's important for us to pull away and spend private time alone.

The average person will go into meditation quite naturally under certain conditions. Some people go into a meditative state when they listen to music, some when they are driving down the highway, some when they run or jog.

Any form of rhythm starts to open up the subconscious mind, allowing us to move into the non-rational part of our brains. But because we start from the rational mind, we have to start with a rational approach to meditation.

So let's look at meditation very rationally. Meditation is described in the *Yoga Sutras* as absorption. When we become absorbed in anything, we're in a meditative state. I know a guy who works on transmissions, and he loves his work. He gets involved in all the fine little gears and mechanical details. He is very precise, and can work on a transmission all day long. For him, the time just flies because he's completely immersed in a meditative state when he's working. And of course, he does a phenomenal job. If you ever have a transmission problem, this is the guy to fix it.

Becoming absorbed in anything—music, making love, the rhythm of the road when driving—puts you into a meditative state. But it is nice to be able to control when this meditative state happens, to be able to sit down and say, "Okay, now I'm going to get into a meditative state for a period of time."

The Right Moves

If you are a runner or a jogger, you are probably familiar with the meditative state you enter as you run. The rhythm of running, of the feet against the ground, is very conducive to invoking a meditative state. Walking will have the same effect, and walking meditation is a centuries-old form of meditation practiced in many different cultures and religions.

Power Words

The *Yoga Sutras* is a text by the Indian sage, Patanjali, written somewhere between 200 B.C. and A.D. 400, consisting of a collection of aphorisms that define the nature of yoga.

Each person has certain procedures that will help induce that meditative state, but once in a meditative state, all is one. In the beginning, there is the meditator, the process of meditation, and the object of meditation. In the end, everything becomes absorbed into the object of meditation, and everything becomes the object of meditation.

For example, if you are meditating on light, the sun, or a candle, then at first, there is you; there is the process of meditating on the sun, light, or candle; and there is the sun, light, or candle itself. Eventually, when you are fully immersed in the meditative state, the only thing that exists is the light. You and the process become completely absorbed into the one entity. All is one.

The Nuts and Bolts

First let's talk about you, the meditator. The meditator must be in a comfortable sitting position. Sitting up straight and comfortable can result in the best meditation sessions. Many people are stiff in the hips and tight in the hamstrings, and find it very difficult to sit in a cross-legged position and be comfortable. The tightness pushes you back on your tailbone, but a better position is to sit forward on the sitting bones, cocking the tailbone back a little to sit forward right where the thigh bone hits the hip bones.

In order to accomplish this, some people sit in the lotus position, which rolls the hips back and puts you right onto those sitting bones. However, for the average person, lotus position isn't an option. It is a pose the average person has to work on for a long time before it becomes comfortable. If your seat isn't comfortable, if you are in any pain, you can't meditate. You can't meditate if you are scared or worried about things. You have to get all that out of the way first.

Getting all that mental baggage out of the way is actually the original purpose of yoga poses, which were developed because the yogis knew they couldn't meditate if they were sick or in pain. Yoga poses relieve the stress on the joints and muscles, creating a healthier, stronger body that can sit comfortably in meditation, not be drawn away from the meditation by any pain or discomfort.

The Right Moves

If you just can't get comfortable on the floor, you can certainly meditate in a chair, but be sure to sit up straight in your chair, not slumped against the back. Feel your body being lifted at the crown, so sitting feels effortless and your body feels light and open.

You'll also want to wear comfortable, loose clothing; meditate outside or in a well ventilated room; and meditate on an empty stomach, so your body isn't distracted by the work of digestion.

Because meditation works best on an empty stomach, before breakfast in the morning is a great time to meditate. Many people find it easiest to meditate early in the morning when the head is clear and fresh from sleep. In the evening, you often have too much on your mind to meditate easily, although meditation before you go to bed is good for clearing your head.

I find it easiest to get up early in the morning and meditate first, before I do anything else. I go into my little meditation room where I have my *altar,* and I meditate. Then I get up, take a shower, and do my yoga. I think early morning meditation is easier because you are still close to your dream state, so meditation is an easy transition.

But not everyone can meditate in the morning; each person has to find the place in his or her schedule where meditation will fit. If you have to close your office down for five minutes in the middle of the afternoon and sit comfortably in your office chair to meditate, then that's great. Meditation will recharge you and make your life better, no matter what you are doing or how you are living.

Sitting up straight is absolutely vital. Whether you are in a chair or on the floor, keep that arch in the lower back and the chest and heart up and open.

You also want to close off the outside world in meditation, both literally and symbolically. Meditate in a room where you won't be disturbed and where you will be comfortable and relatively free from physical distractions. You'll also find it helpful to cross the ankles and bring the first finger and thumb together, to close off the energy flow, keeping it inside you, and keeping outside energy outside you. You are, in a sense, temporarily sealing off your internal environment. Bringing the hands together in prayer fashion will also close you off. All the saints and yogis of old closed off the world in some similar way.

Cross your legs and arms to protect your chakras from outside influences, because meditation is a journey inward, not an exploration outward. Protect your body so you don't have to feel vulnerable and can move inward with greater confidence.

Power Words

An **altar** is a special place that inspires you spiritually. It is generally raised off the ground and decorated in a way that is meaningful to you: candles, pictures, or statues of saints, objects collected from spiritual journeys, anything that connects you to the spiritual.

Forms of Meditation

Even though a great yogi may be puzzled by the idea that meditation could come in different forms, on an initial level, it does. The goal may be the same, and the meditative state, once entered, may be the same no matter how you get there.

But how do you get there? You have many options, and because meditation isn't the focus of this book, I can't begin to get into them all. For a more complete handling of this subject, check out *The Complete Idiot's Guide to Meditation* (Alpha Books, 1999).

While I can't explain all of these methods in detail, I can tell you about some of my favorite forms of meditation, many of which are great for beginners.

The Right Moves

The meditative state experienced while running or jogging is similar to walking meditation, but the physical exertion required for running is more of a focus than the sensory perception of the world around you.

Walking Meditation

Catholic priests have a morning walking meditation every day. They walk, say their prayers, think about the coming day, and contemplate the spiritual mysteries. Walking is an excellent form of meditation because it puts the body into a rhythm and naturally helps the body slide into that meditative state. If you do nothing else, take a 15-minute walk every morning. Walk smoothly, pay attention to your breathing, and listen to your heartbeat and the sounds of the environment around you. Keep your eyes wide open and your senses tuned to everything. Be awake and acquaint yourself with the day.

Sunrise and Sunset Meditations

This is a fabulous light meditation that I love. I'll get up early in the morning before the sun comes up and climb up to the top of a hill. I'll sit there with my eyes closed, and get into a nice, straight position. When the sun comes up, I'll feel the rays hit my third eye, that sixth chakra.

You can try this, too. Go outside before sunrise and sit comfortably. Softly close your eyes (you don't want to damage your eyes by looking directly at the sun) and focus on the area between your eyebrows, the third eye or sixth chakra, and wait to feel the sun. It's a beautiful meditation. The warm sun comes up and the early morning sunlight fills your being. You get so sensitive that you can almost hear the rays of light. It's an intense meditation and one of my favorites.

Sunset meditation is lovely, too, and a great way to tune in to the natural world around you. Animals and birds do sunset meditation, or at least, they seem to. They all sit quietly at sunset and an exquisite calm fills the air. Sit outside and focus on the natural world around you. Take in everything your senses can perceive. It's a nice way to end your day if you can, to calm yourself for the move into evening.

If you start each day with a sunrise meditation and end each day with a sunset meditation, your days will be beautiful indeed.

Power Words

A **mantra** is a word or short sequence of words chanted during meditation used as a focus for the attention. Some mantras are also thought to vibrate in such a way that they activate the body's energy.

Mantra Meditation

One of the more traditional forms of meditation taught everywhere in the world and also one of the easiest forms of meditation is *mantra* meditation. Transcendental Meditation, or TM, a form of meditation very popular in the West, is a mantra meditation.

Churches and saints have been using mantra meditation, or the repetition of prayers, for centuries. Mantra meditation makes use of short, subtle, quick sounds that move us internally.

Geo's Journey

In India, you'll see a lot of people wearing beads around their necks that they call a mala. If you go to any of the Christian Eastern Orthodox or Catholic churches, you'll notice the priests and nuns all wear beads as well, called rosaries. In Greece and through-out the Arabic peninsula, you'll see wrist beads called worry beads. These are used to bring your focus back to your meditation. If you tried to say a Catholic rosary, with all the different prayers in that rosary, your mind would inevitably drift and you'd lose your place. The tactile sense of the beads between your thumb and your first two fingers brings you back, reminds you where you are, and keeps your attention during meditation. You can also use a "worry stone" for a tactile focus. This can be any flat, smooth stone you find that you rub between your thumb and first two fingers.

Mantra meditation is a repetition of a sound or prayer over and over for as long as you want to meditate. I remember doing a meditation once in India where I sat for days in a cave in front of a statue and meditated. Finally, I realized that my mantras had a rhythm to them. Whatever the mantra was, it always seemed to develop a rhythm that was my rhythm, and the sound of that particular rhythm would start to open up my subconscious mind and move me into a meditative state.

Mantra meditation is something anybody can do. You can use simple little mantras like "I live in love. I live in love. I live in love. I live in love." Repeat it rhythmically to yourself and focus your attention on the words, the sound, the meaning.

Or you can use a more traditional yogic mantra like "Om mani padme hum," which can be translated as "You and I are one."

This mantra speaks to the universe. It represents the microcosmos, you, talking with the macrocosmos, the universe. You are one with the universe, a particle in the universe, a cell in the body of God. This is a lovely concept and a lovely mantra.

Geo's Journey

I named the highest part of myself Takoma. When I do mantra meditation, I want to bring out the highest part of myself, so my personal mantra meditation is "I am Takoma, I am Takoma, I am Takoma," which says that I am the highest part of myself. It's a good idea to give the highest part of yourself a name. Talk to this side of you and be with that side of yourself as often as you can, so that side becomes a larger portion of you.

Another great little mantra is also part of a familiar saying: "I am healthy, wealthy, and wise." (Feel free to leave out any of the adverbs or substitute others.) You can probably think of many other mantras that might suit you. Whatever is short and meaningful to you will work. Experiment with different words, sounds, and phrases until you find a mantra you feel is truly "yours." Then, work with it, chanting it until you fall into a rhythm that sounds to you like your rhythm. The mantra is already working its magic!

Sound Meditation

Sound meditation is different than mantra meditation. You start this meditation by sitting up nice and straight, as usual. Close your eyes and focus on only what you hear. Listen to everything around you. Hear the electricity in the walls, the refrigerator going on and off, the birds or wind outside, people in the next room, people in the next house. Don't pretend anything isn't there. Just focus on all the sounds around you.

Listen for about five minutes, then draw your focus in, right between your ears, and listen right there. From there, hear the way all the sounds come together in your ears.

We learn to differentiate sounds. All the sounds come together and affect the sound center at the back of the brain. Over the years, we learn to distinguish that one sound is this, another is that. We discriminate, we shut out certain sounds, let in certain sounds, get used to sounds.

But if we focus right between the ears, we start to hear where all the sounds start to come together, including the sounds within: the internal sounds of the blood rushing through the brain and the arteries, the heart pumping, the brain waves. All the sounds inside of us, all the sounds outside of us come together in a wave, in what we call the AUM (it rhymes with "home") or Om in yoga.

The Om is the sound of all things. When you first hear the Om, it is both surprising and familiar. I mentioned earlier in this book that I remember first hearing the Om when I was seven years old in Portland, Maine. It was early in the morning, and it was like a pulse, almost a wah-wah-wah kind of sound.

I was just lying there, not quite ready to get up. I started listening and pretty soon, I noticed that all the sounds came to me in one sound, that all the sounds had the same basis behind them, the same wave behind them. All sound comes to us as a sound wave, and that's what the Om is, that larger wave of sound that contains all the smaller sounds.

Sit and listen to the Om. Hear it inside you as you hear all the outside sounds come to you. This is a very quieting form of meditation that I've been doing since I was seven, and I love it to this day.

Sound meditation can take different forms and result from all kinds of hidden opportunities. I remember years ago, when I was meditating one morning, there was a baby next door crying like crazy, and at first I let myself get a little irritated. I thought, "How can I meditate? This baby is making so much noise, I wish they'd just quiet her down!"

But then I just let go of the frustration. I started listening to the baby, and I noticed how she started off with very high-pitched sounds, very disturbed and upset. These high-pitched sounds affected me in the upper chakras.

As the baby continued to cry for the next 20 minutes, gradually the tones got deeper and lower, from the high "eees" to the lower "ahhs," which I found affected me more in the middle of my body. Then the sound deepened into the "mm-mm-mms" that affected me down in the lower chakras.

The Wrong Moves

Listening is difficult. Many people don't listen these days. We've gotten out of the habit. We are all so anxious to push our own thoughts out there that we don't take the time to listen. But let's not waste such a wonderful opportunity for personal growth. Let's take time to just sit back and listen, letting go of the feeling that we need to make noise.

I suddenly realized that the baby was doing sound meditation. She was upset, and what she was doing naturally was balancing her chakras by listening and creating all the different tones, all the way down. Finally, when she got down into the "Mm mm mm mm," she fell asleep, and that was the end of the crying.

Breathing Meditation

Another great thing to meditate on—and one of the easiest—is the breathing. We focus on the breathing in relaxation exercises, such as the one in the last chapter.

We focus on the breathing in our yoga poses, paying attention to and moving in concert with the natural flow and motion of the breath.

The breath also provides an anchoring focus for meditation. Breathing meditation is very quieting, and something you can do at any time. You've always got your breath.

Feel your body naturally expand as you inhale, release and let go as you exhale. Meditate on the rise and fall of your breath. Feel your body take in new life as you inhale, feel your body release, relax, and let go, giving gently back to life as you exhale. Keep bringing your attention back to the breathing.

Even though you practiced following the breath in the last chapter while lying down, I don't like to do breathing meditation while lying down in my classes. People tend to fall asleep, and if you fall asleep, you aren't meditating. You are sleeping. So try it sitting up, straight and comfortable, on the floor or in a chair.

I also like to use a process called barely breathing. Barely breathing is almost like dropping into a hibernating state. When you start to barely breathe, taking in just what you need with little inhales and little exhales, you'll see it takes you very subtly into that hibernation state the impressive yogis have mastered. Eventually you can learn to slow your heartbeat, your breath rate, and your metabolism until you are using almost no energy at all.

Heart Meditation

This next meditation is a meditation I use a lot now. It came to me some years ago when I was meditating on a flower one day in the mountains above Los Angeles. I was focusing on the flower, looking into it, and softening my eyes.

Pretty soon I noticed movement, and I looked a little deeper and I realized that the flower wasn't moving—I was. I recognized how my heart, set slightly to the left, was pulsating downward and driving the blood downward. This caused me to pulse toward the right, creating a little circular motion.

No matter how still I tried to be, I still moved subtly with the beat of the heart and the flow of the breath. So I started meditating on the heart, which led me to a whole new form of meditation. I realized that if I was meditating on the heart, I could meditate on all the chakras.

To try this meditation method, start by bringing your thumb and fingers together. Notice the heartbeat in your fingers. Keep your awareness there, until you find the pulse.

From there, move your awareness into the middle of your chest. Close your eyes, relax your body, and go into a very small circular motion, feeling the heart pulse. Sit and focus on the beating of the heart, right in the middle of the chest, feeling your body pulsate and throb with the rhythm of the heart.

Now, move through the chakras, spending about one minute in each chakra, working up to about five minutes:

➤ Move your focus and attention down into the first chakra, down at the base of the spine. Feel the heartbeat at the base of the spine, pulsing red.

➤ As soon as you establish the heartbeat here, move to the second chakra, right into the belly button area. Feel the heartbeat deep in the belly, the blood throbbing and the heart pulsing in the belly, an orange pulsing rhythm.

➤ From there, move into the solar plexus. Relax the chest and belly, and feel the heartbeat in the solar plexus. See the beautiful chakra here, a pulsating yellow rhythm.

➤ Then come back into the heart and see the heart again, but now as a very green rhythm, the fourth chakra.

➤ Now move into the throat and start to feel the energy in the throat, the blood moving through the throat, a light sky blue pulse.

➤ After focusing on the throat for awhile, move into the third eye and feel the heart beating between the eyebrows. Focus on that for about a minute and feel it pulsate here between the eyebrows, a deep blue pulse.

➤ Now move your attention right to the top of the head, the crown chakra, your connection to the divine. Focus there and feel as if your body is pulsating upward through that area. See it as violet pulses, a violet rhythm pulsating through the top of the head. Hold on to that for about a minute.

➤ Now drop back down into the third eye, feeling the heart beat here. Drop back down to the throat, feeling the heart beating in the throat. Then drop back down to the heart and focus here, staying here as long as you comfortably can. Meditate on your heart. Let the body relax and pulse, meditating on the center of your spiritual being, the seat of your spirit.

The Right Moves

I've heard stories of yogis going into meditative states for a whole day or week or two weeks. They are barely breathing. They aren't ever totally still, of course, and neither will you be, but you can reach a point where the heartbeat and breath can barely be measured. It is a subtle, delicate, but attainable state.

As you get stronger with this meditation, you can spend more time on the heart when you return to it for the third time. Start to visualize the heart as holding a wonderful little god or goddess sitting on a throne in the middle of your heart. The god or goddess is the divine aspect of you sitting right there in the middle of your heart, all-powerful, all-knowing, all-loving. This is the secret part of you.

Each of us has a special spirit that is here looking after us, taking care of us, loving us more than anything else in the world. You can think of this spirit as your higher self, your guardian angel, or the part of God within you. You can touch that spirit, be with that spirit, talk to that spirit, name that spirit, and know that spirit. Be still and know the spirit that resides within you and is always with you, loving you, with no other reason to be here right now than to take care of you.

Internal Focus Meditation

We don't always have a beautiful sunrise or sunset to focus on, but we can always internalize our focus by looking through our third eye. You can actually stimulate the third eye by softening the focus of the eyes, bringing them down slightly, and staring at the tip if your nose. When you stare at the tip of your nose, it centers everything in your being. The stare isn't difficult. It's a soft stare, looking with both eyes toward the center, barely focusing. You can see everything around you, but you hold your focus right at the tip of your nose. I think you'll be surprised at how it affects you.

Power Words

Samadhi and **nirvana** are both Sanskrit words that, to simplify, refer to a state that is the ultimate goal of yoga and meditation. It is a state of ultimate bliss in which the self becomes one with the object of contemplation and, by extension, with all of creation.

Eventually you can incorporate this internal focus into your Power Yoga routine. Once you have the routine down and it is very familiar, like a smooth, graceful, powerful dance, focus your attention through the entire dance to the area of your third eye. Turn your eyes up gently and soften the focus, and start moving through the Power Yoga routine, all the while keeping the focus at the third eye, imagining an inverted triangle or pyramid right between the eyebrows.

The effect is absolutely amazing—by the end of the yoga session, you will be euphoric. It's very intense. Once you know the dance well, whatever your routine might be, as long or as short as it may be, try it while focusing on the third eye in this way. You'll see everything else around you, peripherally, but your center of focus will be at the third eye. Drawing your attention to your middle seems to open the door, allowing you to feel the pulse on either side of your body and opening your awareness to that euphoric mind, the epiphany state, the *samadhi* or *nirvana* state we all search for, in which we attain ultimate bliss.

The Process Ends ... and Begins

Like Power Yoga, meditation is a process. We started with very basic movements in yoga. We learned, gradually, to move the focus inside and to increase consciousness, focus awareness in different places, to see whether this hand is coming up, that hand or leg is stretching, if the shoulders are rolling back and the chest rolling open, or if the body is closing or bending. The more we focus, the more conscious and aware we become.

As the body gets stronger and healthier, the consciousness and awareness also get stronger and healthier. We move that ultimately into our relaxation exercises and then into meditation, for the big payoff: a fully integrated, actualized, aware self. The ability to focus clearly carries us into that next realm, the subconscious mind, that euphoric yogic state, which is the yogi's goal.

It's a fascinating process to watch, but an even more fascinating process to experience. I'm happy to have experienced it with you, and I hope you will continue on your journey of growth, because the process doesn't end here. It is just the beginning of a lifelong quest for self-knowledge.

Keep building strength and flexibility, opening your chakras, heightening your awareness, spiraling into yourself and your own being, learning who you are, and living. It's a wonderful time to be here, awake and alive, in this body-mind that can do so much if you will only give it the opportunity ... and the power.

The Least You Need to Know

➤ Meditation is the final goal of yoga. Yoga poses were originally developed to keep the body from becoming a distraction during meditation.

➤ Meditation is easiest first thing in the morning, but is also beneficial at the end of the day.

➤ The meditative state is one of complete absorption into the object of meditation until meditator, process, and object of meditation are one.

➤ A variety of meditation techniques exist, including walking meditation, sunrise/sunset meditation, mantra meditation, sound meditation, breath meditation, heart meditation, and internal focus meditation. Each individual can experiment to find the form or forms that work best.

➤ The yoga process leads to greater self-knowledge, but it is a journey that never ends.

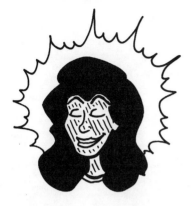

Alternate Power Plays

Alternate Power Plays

This book is organized so that you can move through the chapters in order, taking as much, or as little, of the routine as you like for your personal use. Once you've mastered the poses in this book and the sequence in which they are presented, however, you may want to try something different. The following variations also make great Power Yoga routines.

Repeat this entire sequence for as long as you can.

Level I Standing Series

Pose	Chapter Reference
Marine pose	6
Windmills (twist the body from side to side, letting the arms swing)	(no chapter reference)
Reed	11
Grasses blowing in the wind (move the arms over head and the torso from side to side, like blowing grass)	(no chapter reference)
Butterfly	6
Linebacker	6
Bear pose	16

continues

Level I Standing Series   (continued)

Pose	Chapter Reference
Spear thrower	12
Swordsman	12
Extended warrior	12
T-balance	12
Triangle pose	14
Extended triangle	14
Angle pose	14
Extended angle pose	14
Bent knee forward bend	12

Level I Ground Series

Pose	Chapter Reference
Pelvic tilt	7
Bridge pose (feet apart)	7
Push knee breath	19
Yoga walks	19
Bridge pose (feet together)	7
Hug yourself	7
Easy back twist (roll over onto all fours)	7
Bear pose	16
Cat pose	8
Prowling tiger	8
Japanese sitting pose	8
Child's pose	8
Downward stretching dog	16
Worship to the supreme	8
Swimming pose	21
Sphinx pose	21
Yoga mudra, American style	21
Relaxation pose	25

Level I Back Series

Pose	Chapter Reference
Marine pose	6
Windmill	(no chapter reference)
Butterfly	6
Spear thrower	12
Swordsman	12
Tree balance	13
Reed pose	11
Cat pose	8
Prowling tiger	8
Pelvic tilts	19
Push knee breath	19
Hug yourself	7
Power arch (knees apart)	19
Simple bent knee twist	21
Child's pose	8
Relaxation pose	25

Level II Stomach Series

Pose	Chapter Reference
Pelvic tilt	7
Yoga walks	19
Bridge pose (legs together)	20
Eagle crunchers	19
Wheel pose	20
Hug yourself	7
Easy back twist	7
Cobra pose	21
Camel pose	23
Worship to the supreme	8
Child's pose	8
Relaxation pose	25

Level II Ground Work

Pose	Chapter Reference
Monkey pose	15
Single leg forward bend	15
Pigeon pose	15
Pigeon hip stretch	15
Pigeon quad stretch	15
Yoga split	15
Boat pose	18
Sun pose	18
Back stretching pose	18
Alternate leg stretch	18
Side stretching pose	18
Gate latch pose	18
Yoga rock 'n' roll	22
Half shoulderstand	22
Fish pose	22
Eagle crunchers	19
Bridge pose	20
Wheel pose	20
Hug yourself	7
Easy back twist	7
Locust series	21
Cobra pose	21
American yoga mudra	21
Perfect pose (for meditation)	25
Relaxation pose	25

Level II Standing Series

Pose	Chapter Reference
Marine pose	6
Windmills	(no chapter reference)
Grasses blowing in the wind	(no chapter reference)
Butterfly	6
Linebacker	6

Pose	Chapter Reference
Bear pose	16
Standing prayer pose	11
Reed pose	11
Standing forward bend	16
Dead lift	16
Standing forward bend	16
Flat back pose	18
Reed pose	6
Standing prayer pose	11
Spear thrower	12
Swordsman	12
Extended warrior	12
T-balance	12
Half moon pose	13
Twisted half moon	13
Standing split stretch	13
Tree pose	13
Triangle	14
Extended triangle	14
Twisted triangle	14
Angle pose	14
Bent knee forward bend	19

Level III Burpee Series

Pose	Chapter Reference
Standing prayer pose	11
Reed	11
Standing forward bend	11
Dead lift	11
Standing forward bend	11
Flat back pose	11
Squat	11
Burpee	16
Board	16

continues

Level III Burpee Series   (continued)

Pose	Chapter Reference
Push-up	16
Downward stretching dog	16
Alligator	16
Upward stretching dog	16
Downward stretching dog	16
Squat	11
Standing forward bend	11
Dead lift	11
Standing forward bend	11
Flat back pose	11
Reed pose	11
Standing prayer pose	11

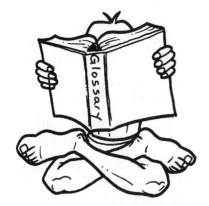

Power Talk: Glossary

abduction   To move a body part away from the midline. For example, imagine a line through the center of your body. Lifting your arms out to the side away from this line, as you would for the spear thrower movement, would be abduction.

Achilles tendon   This tendon attaches the gastrocnemius, or calf muscle, to the heel bone.

adduction   To move a body part toward the midline. Returning your arms to your sides as you move out of the spear thrower movement would be adduction.

adrenal glands   Located above the kidneys, these glands produce hormones such as adrenaline in the body in response to stress.

adrenaline   Also called epinephrine, this hormone is produced by the adrenal glands in response to stress. It revs up the body, preparing it for action.

altar   A special place that inspires you spiritually. It is generally raised off the ground and decorated in any way that is meaningful to you: candles, pictures, or statues of saints, objects collected from spiritual journeys, anything that connects you to the spiritual.

anaerobic respiration   The process that takes over when the lungs and circulatory system are no longer able to supply muscles with enough ready oxygen and nutrients during strenuous activities. In anaerobic respiration, the body breaks down glucose to synthesize the chemical needed to power muscle contractions (called adenosine triphosphate, or ATP). During the complicated process involved in producing ATP anaerobically, lactic acid is produced and accumulates in muscle tissue, causing the burning sensation people call "sore muscles."

anatomy   The study of the structure of bodies, including humans, other animals, and plants.

ascending colon   The part of the colon that travels upward, against gravity, along the right side of the body.

aura   The electromagnetic field surrounding the body. Although some claim that everyone can see auras with practice, some people seem to see them more easily than others. Certain photographic techniques can reveal auras on film.

bandhas   The Sanskrit word for "locks," or exercises used in conjunction with breathing to concentrate and intensify prana or energy within the body.

biceps   The large muscle in your upper arm that you think of when you imagine people "showing some muscle." This muscle flexes and supinates (turns upward) the forearm.

cecum   A pouch in the colon connected to the iliocecal valve.

chakras   Energy centers associated with certain glandular and organ systems. Chakras aren't physical structures, but energy vortices that exist along the midline of the body, from the base of the spine to the crown of the head.

chi   The Chinese term for life-force energy that flows through the body and also exists outside the body in everything around us.

coccyx   Another word for the tailbone, or the last vertebra in the spine.

colon   Also called the large intestine, this organ moves waste material out of the body after the small intestine has digested and absorbed the usable parts of the food we eat.

deltoid   The large, rounded muscle that covers the top of the shoulder. This muscle is largely responsible for the movements of the shoulders and arms.

descending colon   The part of the colon that travels down the left side of the body.

diaphragm   A large, flat, plate-shaped muscle that divides the chest from the abdominal cavity and is instrumental in breathing.

endorphins   The feel-good chemical released by the brain that relieves pain and induces a feeling of euphoria after physical exertion. Endorphins are chemically similar to morphine, but are a completely natural response by the brain to the body's needs. For example, they make physical exertion pleasurable, something that helps us survive because we need to move and work to live.

epinephrine   *See* adrenaline.

etheric body   The part of the body extending beyond the physical body, consisting of energy.

extension   Increasing an angle at a joint. For example, coming out of the chair pose increases the angle of the knee from bent to straight.

flexion Decreasing an angle at a joint, such as the angle between your thigh and lower leg, by drawing the lower leg up toward the thigh. Moving into the spear thrower position decreases the angle at the knee as you lunge forward.

gastrocnemius The muscle of the calf. This muscles helps flex the knee and the foot.

gluteus maximus The "buns" muscle, and the largest muscle in the body. It abducts, rotates, and extends the thigh.

gluteus medius The muscle that runs along the side of the hip and abducts and rotates the thigh.

hamstrings The biceps femoris, semitendinosus, and semimembranosus, three muscles that flex the knee and extend the hip.

iliocecal valve The place where the small and large intestines connect. This valve moves waste matter into the cecum.

intercostals The muscles between the ribs that aid in breathing.

lactic acid A product of anaerobic respiration that causes the feeling of sore muscles.

large intestine The colon.

latissimus dorsi Muscles that wrap around the torso from front to back, moving the arm backward and downward and rotating the arm inward.

locks Exercises used with the exhalation of breath to concentrate and intensify life-force energy in the body. Locks involve setting the body in certain positions—most notably at the chin, the stomach, and the rectum—to keep energy inside and redirect its flow.

mantra A word or short sequence of words chanted during meditation used as a focus for the attention. Some mantras are also thought to vibrate in such a way that they activate the body's energy.

medulla oblongata The enlarged extension of the spinal cord that connects to the brain. This nerve-rich area is responsible for regulating the heart muscle, constriction of the arteries, and the rate of breathing.

metabolism The process, occurring in all living things, in which food is broken down in the body and converted to energy.

mudra A position, often used to refer to a hand position typically held during meditation or during certain yoga poses. The point of the hand mudras is to keep energy from escaping through the fingertips by closing the fingertips into a circuit, redirecting energy back into the body.

nirvana   A Sanskrit word that, to simplify, refers to the enlightened state that is the ultimate goal of yoga and meditation. It is a state of bliss in which the self recognizes that all is one and one is all.

niyamas   Traditional yoga observances: Be pure, be content, be disciplined, be studious, and be devoted.

obliques, internal and external   The muscles along the sides of the torso that flex the upper torso and spinal column.

Om   A Sanskrit word that yoga practitioners have used for centuries to describe the resonating sound of the universe. Saying "Om" on the exhalation while you're doing Power Yoga can help you focus on your breathing and get in tune with the universe.

Om mudra   A yoga hand position in which the tips of the thumb and first finger come together into a circle.

osteoporosis   A thinning of the bones which often occurs in conjunction with aging, though it is not an inevitable part of aging. Osteoporosis leaves bones more vulnerable to fractures.

parathyroid glands   Located on each lobe of the thyroid gland and also behind it, these glands produce a hormone that regulates the level of calcium in the blood so the bones can absorb it.

pectoralis major   The primary chest muscle, extending from the center of the rib cage to the underarm. This muscle is also influential in moving the arm, primarily in forward and downward motions.

physiology   The study of the processes and mechanisms of life in humans, other animals, and plants.

Power Yoga   A moving, flowing form of yoga that is almost dance-like in its grace. In Power Yoga, traditional (and nontraditional) yoga poses are tied together to affect many different aspects of the body with an entire routine. Traditional Hatha Yoga tends more to work specific areas and hold poses to strengthen certain areas. Power Yoga strings these together to bring out the natural, innate power of movement in the human body.

prana   The Sanskrit word for life-force energy that flows through the body and exists outside the body in everything around us.

pronation   To move a body part downward, toward the floor. For example, turning your torso toward the floor in the bent knee forward bend.

protraction   To move a body part forward, such as opening the chest in exalted warrior.

psychosomatic   Refers to a physical disorder that either originated from or is worsened by the emotions.

quadriceps   The four muscles of the thigh, and the largest muscle group in the body. These muscles extend the knee joint.

rectus abdominis   Stomach muscles that run vertically from the pubic bone to the ribs. These muscles help to flex your torso and tense your abdomen. They are also used in certain yoga breathing exercises (see Chapter 24, "Breath of Life").

retentions   The opposite of locks, retentions are used with the inhalation of the breath to push certain areas of the body such as the stomach outward, pressing energy through the body.

retraction   To move a body part backward, such as caving in the chest with cat pose.

rhomboids   Muscles helping to power the upper back. These muscles help to move the shoulder blades toward the spine.

rotation   Revolving a body part on an axis, such as rotating your head to look to the right or left. Some rotation is called external or internal, depending on whether it moves the body part away from or toward a midline. For example, a midline is a line between your feet. Turning your feet outward is external rotation; turning your feet inward, toward the midline, is internal rotation. Rotating your head at the neck to look up in angle pose is an example of rotation.

sacrum   The lower part of the backbone, between the hipbones, horizontally, and between the upper spine and the tailbone, vertically.

Samadhi   A state of ultimate bliss in which the self becomes one with the object of its contemplation and, by extension, one with the universe.

sattvic   The term used to describe foods (and other things) that are pure, healthful, and bestowing energy. The word *sattva* is a Hindu word that refers to the purest aspect of the self, and sattvic foods are those that promote life energy, clarity of mind, strength, and inner contentment. Traditionally, these foods are fresh, clean, hearty, nutritious, organic, unprocessed, in natural form, and free of sharp, strong, bitter, pungent, or spicy tastes.

sigmoid colon   An S-shaped part of the colon that empties into the rectal area, where waste is stored until it is expelled through the anal canal.

small intestine   The part of the intestine that digests and absorbs the usable parts of the food we eat.

solar plexus   A network of nerves in the abdomen, behind the stomach, corresponding with the third chakra.

splenius capitis   One of the larger neck muscles responsible for rotating the head and drawing it back.

sternocleidomastoid   The neck muscle that runs along the front of your neck from your ear to your chest. It helps you to flex your neck and rotate your head.

supination   To move a body part upward, toward the sky. For example, turning your torso upward, as in revolving triangle.

T'ai Chi   A martial arts system commonly used today in the East and West as a method of moving meditation and exercise.

thymus gland   A gland near the heart linked with the effectiveness of the immune system, particularly in children.

thyroid gland   A gland in the throat that produces hormones that stimulate the body's metabolic rate, or the rate at which nutrients are consumed and energy is produced in the body.

transverse abdominis   The abdominal muscle that runs horizontally, tensing the abdomen from the pubic area up through the lower ribs.

transverse colon   The part of the colon that travels horizontally, connecting the ascending and descending colon.

trapezius   A large muscle that attaches to the spine and stretches all the way over the shoulder to the collarbone. This large muscle helps to move the shoulder blades and the head.

triceps   The smaller muscle on the back of the arm that balances the biceps. The triceps muscle helps to extend the forearm.

vertebrae   The bones of the spine.

vinyasa   The Sanskrit term for a series of yoga poses used in a practice, and also for a series of poses performed in a row with flowing movements. The root *vi* means "in a special way," and the root *nyasa* means "to place."

vision quest   A personal spiritual journey that can take many forms. Typically, the questor goes into nature alone for a few days, fasts, and meditates until he or she experiences a spiritual revelation.

yamas   Traditional yoga abstentions—not harming others, not lying, not stealing, not lusting, and not being greedy.

yoga   From the Sanskrit word *yuj*, meaning "to yoke." Yoga is just that—a yoking of the different sides and forces of the self, through various techniques. Most yoga practiced today in the West, including Power Yoga, is based on a type of yoga called Hatha Yoga. The root *ha* means "solar" and the root *tha* means "lunar." Hatha Yoga, then, is the balancing or yoking together of the solar and lunar aspects of the self. All forms of movement yoga are based on Hatha Yoga.

Yoga Sutras   A text by the Indian sage, Patanjali, written somewhere between 200 B.C. and A.D. 400, consisting of a collection of aphorisms that define the nature of yoga.

Study with Geo

Geo offers retreats, seminars, and classes. You can also purchase his workout CD. To get in touch with Geo Takoma for CDs or information, call 949-494-3656 or write to Life's Natural Design, 825 La Vista Drive, Laguna Beach, CA 92651.

If you would like to take some serious personal time and master the art of physical and spiritual self-discipline, consider a vacation at the Ashram in Calabasas, California, a retreat where you can take Power Yoga classes from Geo and get your physical, mental, and spiritual sides in shape. But get ready for some serious discipline. No resting in mud baths at this retreat! For more information, contact the Ashram at 818-222-6900.

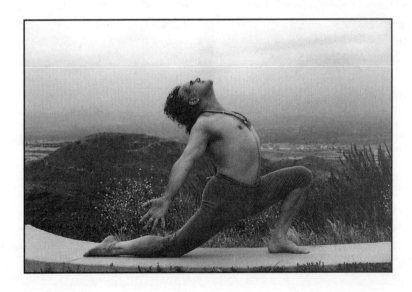

Index